Practical Trends in Anesthesia and Intensive Care 2017

Davide Chiumello
Editor

Practical Trends
in Anesthesia and
Intensive Care 2017

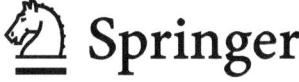 Springer

Editor
Davide Chiumello
Department of "Scienze della Salute"
University of Milan
Milan
Italy

ISBN 978-3-319-61324-6   ISBN 978-3-319-61325-3   (eBook)
http://doi.org/10.1007/978-3-319-61325-3

Library of Congress Control Number: 2017959198

Printed on acid-free paper

This Springer imprint is published by Springer Nature
The registered company is Springer International Publishing AG
The registered company address is: Gewerbestrasse 11, 6330 Cham, Switzerland

Preface

The book is a useful guide to the management of the most-debated hot topics of practical interest in anesthesia and intensive care. It reviews the state of the art of issues related to both intensive care medicine and anesthesia, such as assisted ventilation, ultrasound assessment of renal function, sedation during non-invasive ventilation, subarachnoid hemorrhage, coagulation disorders in septic shock, difficult airways management and hemodynamic monitoring during anesthesia.

Written by leading experts and including updated references, it provides a comprehensive, easy-to-understand update on anesthesia and intensive care. The book clearly explains complex topics offering practicing clinicians insights into the latest recommendations and evidence in the field while, at the same time, making it a valuable resource for students new to the study of anesthesia and intensive care.

Milan, Italy   Davide Chiumello, MD

Contents

Maxillofacial Trauma and Airway Management

Silvia Coppola, Sara Froio, and Davide Chiumello

1.1 Introduction

Maxillofacial trauma represents a challenge for the anesthesiologist in the emergency airway management. This kind of injuries can often compromise the patient's airways and become potentially life threatening.

Maxillofacial injuries may occur as an isolated damage or as a part of traumatic injuries [1].

The American College of Surgeons in Advanced Trauma Life Support (ATLS®) system represents the "gold standard" for the polytrauma patient management.

Within the ATLS® protocols, the first priority is always represented by the maintenance and the protection of the respiratory tract together with the cervical spine protection.

In-hospital mortality and morbidity of trauma patients often result from pitfall related to airway management.

In a large study population (2594 patients), Gruen et al. found the errors in the airway management are the most common factors related to mortality (2594 patients were analyzed) [2].

Current literature points out the complexity of this clinical scenario characterized by potentially life-threatening injuries [3–5].

Together with the assessment of maxillofacial trauma patients applying ATLS® protocols, it is necessary to understand specific features of this scenario: priority can conflict or suddenly change and hidden pitfalls can arise [3, 6, 7].

S. Coppola • S. Froio
ASST Santi Paolo e Carlo, Milan, Italy

D. Chiumello (✉)
ASST Santi Paolo e Carlo, Milan, Italy

Dipartimento di Scienze della Salute, Università degli Studi di Milano, Milan, Italy
e-mail: davide.chiumello@unimi.it; chiumello@libero.it

© Springer International Publishing AG 2018
D. Chiumello (ed.), *Practical Trends in Anesthesia and Intensive Care 2017*,
http://doi.org/10.1007/978-3-319-61325-3_1

This chapter aims to provide an overview of the maxillofacial airway management for anesthesiologists and intensive care physicians on the basis of recent literature.

1.2 A Complex Scenario

Beside the anticipated difficult airway, other factors can complicate this clinical setting. C-spine injury, unexpected vomiting, facial bleeding, and facial fractures pose additional problems both for the decision-making and for the practical approach. Identifying major difficulties and pitfalls may help the clinician to choose the best strategy for the airway management.

1.2.1 Cervical Spine Injuries

Cervical spine injuries are reported in 1–10% of patients presenting with facial fractures [7]. Cervical injuries should always be suspected in patients with lower- and midface trauma until it can be clinically or radiologically excluded. However, frequently clinical exclusion is not possible in a patient with altered Glasgow Coma Scale (GCS) and alcohol or drug intoxication [4]. In these cases a computed tomography (CT) scan evaluation is needed [8].

In general, based on the reported maxillofacial trauma, it is possible to hypothesize the most frequent associated C-spine injuries [9]:

- Midface injuries are associated with C5-7 trauma.
- Lower-face injuries are commonly associated with C1-4 trauma.

Complete C-spine diagnosis can take hours, and in the meanwhile the patient's C-spine has to be protected by a semirigid collar and spinal immobilization in the supine position, avoiding neck movements. If endotracheal intubation is needed, in-line stabilization has to be maintained during the procedure. Unfortunately, manual in-line stabilization has demonstrated to reduce the laryngoscopic view. It has been suggested the use of videolaryngoscopy rather than the direct laryngoscopy to minimize neck movements [10].

1.2.2 Unexpected Vomiting

The maxillofacial trauma patient should always be considered to have a "full stomach": he often bleeds from the facial injuries and fractures and swallows blood, with a high risk of vomiting. Furthermore, the patient may have recently eaten or taken alcohol or drugs. At the same time, opioids for pain relief and brain injury can trigger nausea and vomiting [1, 4]. However we don't suggest the insertion of a nasogastric tube to decompress the stomach in maxillofacial patients who are confused and not cooperative, because the maneuver itself could represent a trigger for vomiting [11].

Vomiting that occurs in the presence of facial injuries represents a threat to airway protection, especially when C-spine lesions coexist. Vomiting may occur suddenly so that it is mandatory to identify patients, which are at highest risk of pulmonary aspiration and require intubation to secure the airway. Conversely, patients with minor facial injuries and preserved state of consciousness could not vomit, and the indication to protect the airway is not impelling.

Moving from these considerations, it is important to remember that the decision to intubate the patient may be influenced by the need for an intra- or extra-hospital transport. The goal is to minimize risks and maximize safety for patients during transport.

However, anesthesia and intubation are at high risk of pulmonary aspiration; in fact, the assessment of risks and benefits of an early intubation requires the judgment of an expert help [11].

- In case of early episodes of vomiting in the emergency department, when the patient is still on a spinal board, the inclination of the board will be useful to lower the head together with a high flow suction of the airway. Trendelenburg position allows the vomit following into the oropharynx, thus reducing the aspiration risk.
- If repeated episodes of vomiting occur in patients with moderate brain injury, drug intoxication and/or full stomach together with maxillofacial trauma, and a high risk of lung aspiration, airway protection should be ensured.
- After an accurate airway evaluation, the anesthetist decides whether to proceed with tracheal intubation with spontaneous breathing patient or with a rapid sequence induction. Preoxygenation will always be provided and in-line spine stabilization maintained during these maneuvers.
- Sellick's maneuver (cricoid pressure) is suggested during rapid sequence induction; however it is contraindicated in a patient who is vomiting because of the esophageal rupture risk. Furthermore this maneuver can worse the laryngeal view, making endotracheal tube placement more difficult [12, 13]. Definitely, cricoid pressure is part of an overall approach of rapid-sequence induction to minimize the risk of aspiration, but it can be reduced when the laryngeal view is impeded.

1.2.3 Bleeding

Blood loss from maxillofacial bleeding is rarely life threatening and at the same time only in few cases induces hemodynamic instability or hypotension. Nevertheless, it can represent a pitfall in airway management. Then, clinicians should always consider that:

(a) Small bleedings, in supine awake patients who swallows, can trigger vomiting.
(b) Profuse bleeding (from extensive tissue disruption or from distinct vessels) may contribute to acute airway obstruction.

Prompt hemostasis and tracheal intubation, when feasible, should be considered according to ATLS® guidelines [6].

Hemostasis can be achieved externally or internally by:

- Direct pressure
- Sutures
- Packing in the oral cavities
- Balloon tamponade
- Reduction of facial fractures

When conservative treatment fails, arterial embolization or surgical approach of the bleeding vessels may be considered [14]. After hemostasis is achieved, maxillofacial injuries do not require immediate repair [15].

1.2.4   Facial Fractures and Timing of Surgery

Surgical maxillofacial treatment can often be deferred until life-threatening injuries have been managed, except for upper airway obstruction and profuse hemorrhage [16].

Most patients with maxillofacial trauma present a stable airway, but there are specific situations associated with this kind of trauma that require emergency airway. Conditions at higher risk for airway obstruction are presented in Table 1.1 [17].

Moreover, C-spine injury, severe neurological impairment, soft tissue neck injury and smoke aspiration are considered conditions at high risk for airway obstruction and require endotracheal intubation in the emergency room [18, 19].

Apart from mentioned specific clinical conditions that need early and emergent airway control, optimal time for repairing maxillofacial fractures is still debated.

Conditions that need immediate treatment:

- Control of profuse hemorrhage
- Stabilization of bleeding fractures

Conditions needing urgent treatments within few hours:

- Reduction of open fractures.
- Surgical repair of contaminated wounds.
- All injuries that could lead to severe infections or lasting functional impairment should be treated within 24 h [20–22].

Table 1.1 Conditions at higher risk for airway obstruction

Injuries	Nature of airway obstruction
1. Posteroinferior displacement of a fractured maxilla	Nasopharyngeal obstruction
2. Bilateral fractures of the anterior mandible	Loss of tongue support in supine patient
3. Fractured teeth or bone fragments	Obstruction or the airway anywhere
4. Profuse oronasal hemorrhage	Airway bleeding
5. Soft tissue swelling and edema	Upper airway obstruction
6. Fractures of the larynx and hyoid	Swelling of the glottis

Conditions in which surgical treatment can be safely deferred (within days):

- Patients with associated clinical life-threatening injuries require urgent tracheostomy for the risk of increasing facial edema.

In this setting the maxillofacial surgeon should be early involved in the trauma team's decision-making process [3].

1.3 Airway Management

Maxillofacial trauma often presents a problem of difficult mask ventilation and a predicted difficult intubation, because of:

- Suspected C-spine injury
- High risk of vomiting and aspiration of gastric content
- Oronasal bleeding
- Soft tissue disruption
- Rapidly evolving clinical picture

The fourth National Audit Project of the Royal College of Anesthetists (NAP4—Major complication of airway management) recommends that senior staff should be available in the emergency department, because the complication rate of intubation in this clinical scenario can exceed 20% [23–25].

The anesthetist will choose the best approach, balancing the risks and benefits in relation to the patient's characteristics, airway, signs of impending obstruction, and staff experience (Fig. 1.1):

- Monitoring in awake, spontaneously breathing patient
- Early tracheal intubation [11]

When the airway is patent and no emergency intubation is needed, anesthetists can assess the airway to identify patients who may have difficult anatomy.

Airway difficulty can depend on several factors [26]:

- Poor patient's cooperation
- Difficult mask ventilation
- Difficult supraglottic device placement
- Predicted difficult laryngoscopy
- Difficult endotracheal intubation
- Difficult surgical airway access

When the anesthetist decides on early intubation approach with a predicted difficulty, different options exist. It is important to consider consultation with surgeon and a review of recent imaging studies before proceeding with the airway management [27]:

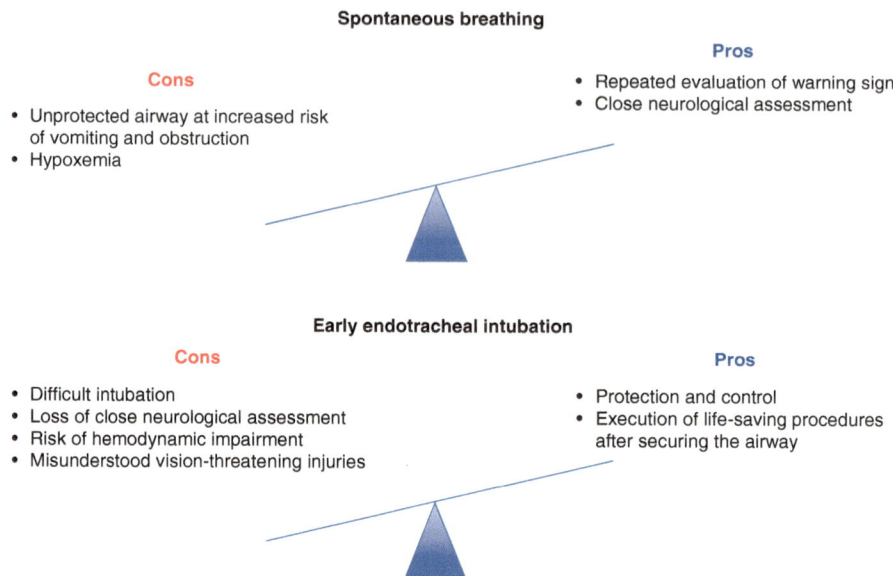

Fig. 1.1 Risks and benefits of the spontaneous breathing approach compared to early tracheal intubation

- Endotracheal intubation in awake spontaneous breathing patient versus intubation after general anesthesia induction
- Noninvasive versus surgical techniques

When difficult intubation is anticipated, guidelines strongly recommend [27, 28]:

1. Adequate patient's position, equipment for primary intubation including capnography in the emergency department and other alternative devices, adequate size of supraglottic device, and additional skilled help and "exit strategy" in case of failed intubation after three attempts
2. Preoxygenation with 100% of inspired oxygen for 3 min of tidal volume breathing

Intubation failure should be declared after three attempts, according to the Difficult Airway Society and the Canadian recommendations on management of the unanticipated difficulty airway.

In this clinical setting when general anesthesia is induced and patients are adequately oxygenated, exit strategies include:

1. Wake the patient
2. Supraglottic device positioning
3. Additional equipment and expert help for further controlled tracheal intubation attempt
4. Surgical access

If oxygenation fails after failed intubation, it is strongly recommended to make one attempt at placing a supraglottic device. Then, if oxygenation is still not adequate with this device, immediate cricothyrotomy should be done.

When tracheal intubation is achieved, periodical reassessment of the stability of the tube should be performed. In fact, patient transport (radiological department, operating room, evolving edema) can result in tube displacement.

1.3.1 Noninvasive Techniques

1.3.1.1 Orotracheal Intubation: Direct Laryngoscopy

Direct laryngoscopy with orotracheal intubation is not the method of choice in maxillofacial surgery because the presence of an oral tube can interfere with surgical maneuvers.

Lee et al. considered direct laryngoscopy as the fastest technique in the emergent airway management of patient with facial fractures in the operating room setting; however it is mandatory to approach this technique with the appropriate expertise [28]. In fact, direct laryngoscopy is indicated in case of emergency airway in a "can't intubate can't oxygenate scenario" with nasal pyramid fractures and skull base fractures or when maxillo-mandibular fixation is not required [16].

On the other end, direct laryngoscopy is contraindicated in case of trauma that can limit mouth opening after general anesthesia induction, of laryngeal trauma, or when maxilla-mandibular fixation is required [15].

1.3.1.2 Nasotracheal Intubation

Nasotracheal intubation often represents the option of choice for elective airway management of patients scheduled for maxillofacial surgery. This technique offers the surgeon better visibility and the possibility of maxilla-mandibular fixation, and it is in patients with reduction of mouth opening. Nasotracheal intubation can be also done in awake patients (fiber-optic intubation under local anesthesia and spontaneously breathing patients) or after general anesthesia induction (direct laryngoscopy) or by a "blind" approach [15].

In the end, it is important to remember that it is contraindicated in case of basal skull fractures with nasal fractures for the risk of intracranial placement during blind insertion. No cases of intracranial placement of tube are reported when fiber-optic intubation is performed [29].

1.3.1.3 Restricted Visual Intubation Techniques

Anatomic abnormalities and the presence of foreign materials decrease the success rate of tracheal intubation to 80% especially when severe oronasal hemorrhage coexists [14].

In case of tracheal intubation with a restricted view (direct laryngoscopy Cormack-Lehane 2b–3) despite continuous suctioning of the oral cavity, the tracheal tube introducer should be considered (recommendation for the airway management—Canadian Airway Focus Group).

Gum elastic bougies and lighted stylet have been proposed as support devices to facilitate tracheal intubation. The gum elastic bougie is considered more effective when the best view is Cormack-Lehane 3 [30, 31]. However, when a rigid device is inserted, great care must be taken to not apply excessive force [23].

The lighted stylet technique is based on the principle of the transillumination of anterior neck soft tissue to guide endotracheal tube. This device can be used during direct laryngoscopy or combined with the intubation through a laryngeal mask (*aintree* catheter). Lighted stylet is considered an option for difficult intubations in maxillofacial trauma [32–34].

As pointed out before, this technique should be only performed by an expert anesthetist; obviously when neck or laryngeal abnormalities preclude transillumination, the lighted stylet is not appropriate [35].

1.3.1.4 Visual Intubation Techniques

Difficult airway algorithms describe visual intubation techniques for the management of anticipated difficult airway [27, 36].

Rigid fiber-optic laryngoscopes can facilitate intubation in patients with suspected or known unstable C-spine injuries: they do not require head or neck movements to obtain a clear view (Wuscopes, Bullard laryngoscopes) [37, 38]. The American Society of Anesthesiologists (ASA) and the Italian Society of Anesthesia and Intensive Care Unit (SIAARTI) include videolaryngoscopes among the alternative intubation devices when a failed intubation is declared and oxygenation is adequate [27, 36, 39].

A recent systematic review underlined that the use of videolaryngoscopy is strongly recommended in patients at higher risk of difficult laryngoscopy, but it is cautiously recommended in patients with known difficult direct laryngoscopy [40]. In trauma setting videolaryngoscope provides a better laryngeal view maintaining cervical in-line stabilization [41], but it is well known that a clear visibility is essential for a correct use of these devices (fogging, secretions, blood, and vomit in maxillofacial trauma can impair the vision).

In patient with anticipated difficult intubation and difficult mask ventilation, fiber-optic intubation under local anesthesia in spontaneously breathing patients is the first choice [27, 36]. Unfortunately, it is challenging and sometimes not practical in maxillofacial trauma because of oral bleeding, vomit, or secretions that can occlude supraglottic structures. Nevertheless, although time-consuming, fiber-optic intubation has been used by skilled clinicians in patients with penetrating neck trauma, oronasal bleeding, and unstable fractures [15].

1.3.2   Alternatives to Tracheal Intubation

Supraglottic devices (SGD) have a limited role in this kind of trauma patients because they have to be placed blindly and do not provide an airway protection, with the risk of displacement and aspiration of gastric content [23]. However, SGD are recommended as "exit strategy" when intubation is failed after induction of anesthesia in adequately oxygenated patient or when oxygenation fails after failed intubation attempt [36].

Of note, SGD allow the passage of a tracheal tube with a blind technique or under fiber-optic guidance. Fiber-optic assisted intubation via a place classic laryngeal mask should be considered only when dedicated laryngeal masks are not available [31].

Similarly, the Combitube can be inserted quickly and may also protect against the aspiration of gastric content or blood. It is important to keep in mind that its insertion may cause complications in the upper esophageal tract, particularly when disruption of the anatomy and tissue damage are present [42].

1.3.3   Surgical Techniques

A surgical airway is mandatory in emergency [43]. Cricothyrotomy is recommended over tracheostomy by the Canadian and Italian guidelines and ATLS® because it is less time-consuming, easier, and causes fewer complications. The cricothyroid membrane is less vascular and more palpable. Canadian guidelines recommend that cricothyrotomy should be done with a percutaneous needle-guided wide bore cannula or surgical technique, because the percutaneous insertion of an intravenous type cannula is associated with the highest complications and failure rates and does not allow the placement of a cuffed tracheal tube to ventilate, although it is advocated by ATLS® to buy time while preparing for a definitive airway [36].

Tracheostomy can be considered in a patient with a previously secured airway when the severity of maxillofacial trauma or the associated multi-organ injuries require prolonged mechanical ventilation. In some cases, after expert evaluation of the patient's clinical conditions and local anatomic abnormalities, tracheostomy under local anesthesia could be performed. Progressive soft tissue swelling can often require an elective tracheostomy at the end of other surgical procedures. To avoid tracheostomy, which is associated with higher morbidity, maxillofacial surgeons have described submental and retromolar intubation in selected patients with maxillofacial trauma [15]. In fact, several maxillo-surgical procedures preclude the conventional oral intubation route. The submental surgical route described by Hernandez-Altemir, performed after orotracheal intubation, might offer an effective option for the surgeon and the anesthetist to obtain an unobstructed surgical field and ensure the maintenance of a secure airway [44].

1.4   Vision-Threatening Injuries

Maxillofacial trauma can also result in various degrees of orbital floor fractures, so that a compartmental syndrome can develop. A reduction in perfusion pressure and ischemia of the optic nerve can occur within 2 h [21, 45]. Moving from these considerations, an urgent ophthalmic assessment is needed in all patients with periorbital lesions (Fig. 1.2).

Fig. 1.2 Vision-threatening injuries

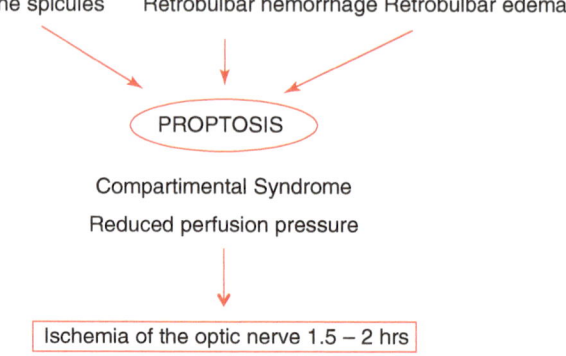

Recognition and appropriate treatment of vision lesions should be performed at the end of the "A, B, C, D, E" evaluation and should not delay life-saving interventions. The management of vision-threatening injuries consists in globe protection: high-dose steroids and surgical decompression (under local or general anesthesia). Before surgical treatment, a computed tomography scan will be helpful to clarify and identify anatomical structures. However, proptosis per se is rarely an indication for urgent surgery [21, 45, 46].

Conclusions

In conclusion, maxillofacial trauma may be challenging for the decision-making process and clinical management. Knowledge of the priorities and of specific potential complications together with the cooperation among different professional figures in a multidisciplinary team is crucial for the successful management of patient with maxillofacial trauma.

References

1. Perry M, Dancey A, Mireskandari K, Oakley P, Davies S, Cameron M. Emergency care in facial trauma–a maxillofacial and ophthalmic perspective. Injury. 2005;36:875–96.
2. Gruen RL, Jurkovich GJ, McIntyre LK, Foy HM, Maier RV. Patterns of errors contributing to trauma mortality: lessons learned from 2,594 deaths. Ann Surg. 2006;244:371–80.
3. Perry M. Advanced Trauma Life Support (ATLS) and facial trauma: can one size fit all? Part 1: dilemmas in the management of the multiply injured patient with coexisting facial injuries. Int J Oral Maxillofac Surg. 2008;37:209–14.
4. Perry M, Morris C. Advanced trauma life support (ATLS) and facial trauma: can one size fit all? Part 2: ATLS, maxillofacial injuries and airway management dilemmas. Int J Oral Maxillofac Surg. 2008;37:309–20.
5. Coppola S, Froio S, Merli G, Chiumello D. Maxillofacial trauma in the emergency department: pearls and pitfalls in airway management. Minerva Anestesiol. 2015;81:1346–58.
6. American College of Surgeons. Advanced trauma life support program for doctors. 9th ed. Chicago: ATLS; 2012.
7. Beirne JC, Butler PE, Brady FA. Cervical spine injuries in patients with facial fractures: a 1-year prospective study. Int J Oral Maxillofac Surg. 1995;24:26–9.

8. Dupanovic M, Fox H, Kovac A. Management of the airway in multitrauma. Curr Opin Anaesthesiol. 2010;23:276–82.
9. Lynham AJ, Hirst JP, Cosson JA, Chapman PJ, McEniery P. Emergency department management of maxillofacial trauma. Emerg Med Australas. 2004;16:7–12.
10. Robitaille A, Williams SR, Tremblay MH, Guilbert F, Thériault M, Drolet P. Cervical spine motion during tracheal intubation with manual in-line stabilization: direct laryngoscopy versus glidescope videolaryngoscopy. Anesth Analg. 2008;106(3):935–41.
11. Krausz AA, El Naaj IA, Barak M. Maxillofacial trauma patient: coping with the difficult airway. World J Emerg Surg. 2009;4:21.
12. Haslam N, Parker L, Duggan JE. Effect of cricoid pressure on the view at laryngoscopy. Anaesthesia. 2005;60:41–7.
13. Rice MJ, Mancuso AA, Gibbs C, Morey TE, Gravenstein N, Deitte LA. Cricoid pressure results in compression of the postcricoid hypopharynx: the esophageal position is irrelevant. Anesth Analg. 2009;109:1546–52.
14. Cogbill TH, Cothren CC, Ahearn MK, Cullinane DC, Kaups KL, Scalea TM, Maggio L, Brasel KJ, Harrison PB, Patel NY, Moore EE, Jurkovich GJ, Ross SE. Management of maxillofacial injuries with severe oronasal hemorrhage: a multicenter perspective. J Trauma. 2008;65:994–9.
15. Robertson CG, Doucet JC. Helping anesthesiologists understand facial fractures. Oral Maxillofac Surg Clin North Am. 2013;25:561–72.
16. Kellman RM, Losquadro WD. Comprehensive airway management of patients with maxillofacial trauma. Craniomaxillofac Trauma Reconstr. 2008;1:39–47.
17. Ghabach MB, Abou Rouphael MA, Roumoulian CE, Helou MR. Airway management in a patient with Le Fort III fracture. Saudi J Anaesth. 2014;8:128–30.
18. Dunham CM, Barraco RD, Clark DE, Daley BJ, Davis FE, Gibbs MA, Knuth T, Letarte PB, Luchette FA, Omert L, Weireter LJ, Wiles CE, EAST Practice Management Guidelines Work Group. Guidelines for emergency tracheal intubation immediately after traumatic injury. J Trauma. 2003;55:162–79.
19. Como JJ, Diaz JJ, Dunham CM, Chiu WC, Duane TM, Capella JM, Holevar MR, Khwaja KA, Mayglothling JA, Shapiro MB, Winston ES. Practice management guidelines for identification of cervical spine injuries following trauma: update from the eastern association for the surgery of trauma Practice Management Guidelines Committee. J Trauma. 2009;67:651–9.
20. Tuckett JW, Lynham A, Lee GA, Perry M, Harrington U. Maxillofacial trauma in the emergency department: a review. Surgeon. 2014;12:106–14.
21. Winterton JV, Patel K, Mizen KD. Review of management options for a retrobulbar hemorrhage. J Oral Maxillofac Surg. 2007;65:296–9.
22. Vidya B, Cariappa KM, Kamath AT. Current perspectives in intra operative airway management in maxillofacial trauma. J Maxillofac Oral Surg. 2012;11:138–43.
23. 4th and National Audit Project of the Royal College of Anaesthetists and The Difficult Airway Society. Major complications of airway management in the United Kingdom. Report and findings.
24. Mort TC. Complications of emergency tracheal intubation: immediate airway-related consequences: part II. J Intensive Care Med. 2007;22:208–15.
25. Mort TC. Complications of emergency tracheal intubation: hemodynamic alterations–part I. J Intensive Care Med. 2007;22:157–65.
26. Apfelbaum JL, Hagberg CA, Caplan RA, Blitt CD, Connis RT, Nickinovich DG, Hagberg CA, Caplan RA, Benumof JL, Berry FA, Blitt CD, Bode RH, Cheney FW, Connis RT, Guidry OF, Nickinovich DG, Ovassapian A, American Society of Anesthesiologists Task Force on Management of the Difficult Airway. Practice guidelines for management of the difficult airway: an updated report by the American Society of Anesthesiologists Task Force on Management of the Difficult Airway. Anesthesiology. 2013;118:251–70.
27. Law JA, Broemling N, Cooper RM, Drolet P, Duggan LV, Griesdale DE, Hung OR, Jones PM, Kovacs G, Massey S, Morris IR, Mullen T, Murphy MF, Preston R, Naik VN, Scott J, Stacey S, Turkstra TP, Wong DT, Canadian Airway Focus Group. The difficult airway with recommendations for management–part 2–the anticipated difficult airway. Can J Anaesth. 2013;60:1119–38.

28. Lee SS, Huang SH, Wu SH, Sun IF, Chu KS, Lai CS, Chen YL. A review of intraoperative airway management for midface facial bone fracture patients. Ann Plast Surg. 2009;63:162–6.
29. Marlow TJ, Goltra DD Jr, Schabel SI. Intracranial placement of a nasotracheal tube after facial fracture: a rare complication. J Emerg Med. 1997;15:187–91.
30. Gataure PS, Vaughan RS, Latto IP. Simulated difficult intubation. Comparison of the gum elastic bougie and the stylet. Anaesthesia. 1996;51:935–8.
31. Henderson JJ, Popat MT, Latto IP, Pearce AC. Difficult Airway Society guidelines for management of the unanticipated difficult intubation. Anaesthesia. 2004;59:675–94.
32. Hung OR, Pytka S, Morris I, Murphy M, Stewart RD. Lightwand intubation: II–clinical trial of a new lightwand for tracheal intubation in patients with difficult airways. Can J Anaesth. 1995;42:826–30.
33. Hung OR, Stewart RD. Lightwand intubation: I–a new lightwand device. Can J Anaesth. 1995;42:820–5.
34. Verdile VP, Heller MB, Paris PM, Stewart RD. Nasotracheal intubation in traumatic craniofacial dislocation: use of the lighted stylet. Am J Emerg Med. 1988;6:39–41.
35. Jain A, Naithani M. Infant with unanticipated difficult airway–Trachlight™ to the rescue. J Anaesthesiol Clin Pharmacol. 2012;28(3):361–3.
36. Law JA, Broemling N, Cooper RM, Drolet P, Duggan LV, Griesdale DE, Hung OR, Jones PM, Kovacs G, Massey S, Morris IR, Mullen T, Murphy MF, Preston R, Naik VN, Scott J, Stacey S, Turkstra TP, Wong DT, Canadian Airway Focus Group. The difficult airway with recommendations for management–part 1–difficult tracheal intubation encountered in an unconscious/induced patient. Can J Anaesth. 2013;60:1089–118.
37. Smith CE, Pinchak AB, Sidhu TS, Radesic BP, Pinchak AC, Hagen JF. Evaluation of tracheal intubation difficulty in patients with cervical spine immobilization: fiberoptic (WuScope) versus conventional laryngoscopy. Anesthesiology. 1999;91:1253–9.
38. Watts AD, Gelb AW, Bach DB, Pelz DM. Comparison of the Bullard and Macintosh laryngoscopes for endotracheal intubation of patients with a potential cervical spine injury. Anesthesiology. 1997;87:1335–42.
39. Frova G. Do videolaryngoscopes have a new role in the SIAARTI difficult airway management algorithm? Minerva Anestesiol. 2010;76:637–40.
40. Healy DW, Maties O, Hovord D, Kheterpal S. A systematic review of the role of videolaryngoscopy in successful orotracheal intubation. BMC Anesthesiol. 2012;12:32.
41. Aziz M. Use of video-assisted intubation devices in the management of patients with trauma. Anesthesiol Clin. 2013;31:157–66.
42. Vezina MC, Trepanier CA, Nicole PC, Lessard MR. Complications associated with the Esophageal-Tracheal Combitube in the pre-hospital setting. Can J Anaesth. 2007;54:124–8.
43. Dillon JK, Christensen B, Fairbanks T, Jurkovich G, Moe KS. The emergent surgical airway: cricothyrotomy vs. tracheotomy. Int J Oral Maxillofac Surg. 2013;42:204–8.
44. Tidke AS, Borle RM, Madan RS, Bhola ND, Jadhav AA, Bhoyar AG. Transmylohoid/submental endotracheal intubation in pan-facial trauma: a paradigm shift in airway management with prospective study of 35 cases. Ind J Otolaryngol Head Neck Surg. 2013;65:255–9.
45. Perry M. Acute proptosis in trauma: retrobulbar hemorrhage or orbital compartment syndrome–does it really matter? J Oral Maxillofac Surg. 2008;66:1913–20.
46. Ballard SR, Enzenauer RW, O'Donnell T, Fleming JC, Risk G, Waite AN. Emergency lateral canthotomy and cantholysis: a simple procedure to preserve vision from sight threatening orbital hemorrhage. J Spec Oper Med. 2009;9:26–32.

The Assessment of the Risk for Cardiac Event After Noncardiac Surgery

2

Fabio Guarracino, Giulia Brizzi, and Rubia Baldassarri

2.1 Introduction

The anaesthesiologist has a key role in the preoperative clinical evaluation of the surgical patient. This evaluation considers the type of patient and the type of surgery the patient will undergo. Over the last 10 years, thanks to the progress of diagnostic and surgical techniques and to the technological implementation, surgery has undergone significant changes that can be summarized in a particular boost towards less invasive techniques, such as robotic surgery, and wider indications than in the past. But even the surgical patient has changed over time. In fact, the population is getting older, and the physiology of aging is accompanied by an increase in morbidity, with many older patients who are candidates for surgery and often with cardiovascular disease. Each year an increasing number of elderly patients with cardiovascular disease undergo noncardiac surgery.

Improved cardiovascular disease treatment has determined a better quality of life for cardiopathic patients over the last 10 years, and even heart failure with severe ventricular dysfunction allows a better quality of life when treated according to good practice. However, perioperative cardiovascular complications are the strongest predictors of morbidity and mortality after major noncardiac surgery, and for this reason the patients with cardiovascular disease undergoing surgery often cause concern in the preoperative evaluation and require instrumental examinations. We can also estimate that approximately 30 million patients die every year within 30 days of noncardiac surgery [1] and that myocardial ischemia is frequently the cause of death.

For these reasons periodically, scientific societies publish recommendations on the management of the cardiopathic patient undergoing noncardiac surgery. The recent ESC/ESA Guidelines [2] of 2014 provide the context for conducting an

F. Guarracino (✉) • G. Brizzi • R. Baldassarri
Department of Anaesthesia and Critical Care Medicine, Cardiothoracic and Vascular
Anaesthesia and Intensive Care, Azienda Ospedaliero Universitaria Pisana, Pisa, Italy
e-mail: fabiodoc64@hotmail.com

© Springer International Publishing AG 2018
D. Chiumello (ed.), *Practical Trends in Anesthesia and Intensive Care 2017*,
http://doi.org/10.1007/978-3-319-61325-3_2

Table 2.1 Cardiovascular risk and surgery

Low risk: <1%	Intermediate risk: 1–5%	High risk: >5%
Superficial surgery	Intraperitoneal: splenectomy, hiatal hernia repair, cholecystectomy	Aortic and major vascular surgery
Breast	Carotid symptomatic (CEA or CAS)	Open lower limb revascularization or amputation or thromboembolectomy
Dental	Peripheral arterial angioplasty	Duodeno-pancreatic surgery
Endocrine: thyroid	Endovascular aneurysm repair	Liver resection, bile duct surgery
Eye	Head and neck surgery	Oesophagectomy
Reconstructive	Neurological or orthopaedic: major (hip and spine surgery)	Repair of perforated bowel
Carotid asymptomatic (CEA or CAS)	Urological or gynaecological: major	Adrenal resection
Gynaecology: minor	Renal transplant	Total cystectomy
Orthopaedic: minor (meniscectomy)	Intra-thoracic: nonmajor	Pneumonectomy
Urological: minor (transurethral resection of the prostate)		Pulmonary or liver transplant

effective preoperative evaluation of the cardiopathic patient candidate for noncardiac surgery. This must include preoperative risk stratification based on assessment of the patient's functional capacity, cardiac risk factors and cardiovascular function and type of surgery (Table 2.1) the patient will undergo.

The approach must be tailored to the individual patient so that some preoperative testing will be performed independently of the type of surgery and urgency of the operation and only in patients who are likely to benefit from it. In fact the aim of the preoperative evaluation of the surgical patient is not a screening for cardiovascular disease but rather a risk stratification and an implementation of perioperative strategies that can minimize it. Therefore it should be emphasized that not every patient with cardiovascular disease requires detailed preoperative cardiac evaluation. For example, patients with stable cardiovascular disease undergoing low- or intermediate-risk surgery do not require an additional preoperative cardiac assessment, while cardiopathic patients scheduled for high-risk noncardiac surgery should undergo cardiac assessment by a multidisciplinary expert team that includes anaesthesiologists, surgeons, and cardiologists, as well as other specialists if necessary.

2.2   The Issue of Perioperative Myocardial Ischemia

Perioperative myocardial ischemia represents the most feared event of the surgical team.

Myocardial ischemia in the surgical period has its own peculiarities from a pathogenetic and physiopathological point of view. In fact, the classification of myocardial ischemia is based on five different types of mechanism inducing ischemia, where the perioperative event is included in type 1 and type 2 [3]. Type 1 is represented by a classic acute event in which an endothelial lesion on an unstable coronary plaque leads to coronary thrombosis with vessel occlusion and arterial flow interruption. In this situation after a few minutes, we can see the typical ST elevation on the electrocardiogram (STEMI). In type 2, the mechanism does not involve endothelial lesion and platelet activation but an acute imbalance in O_2 demand/O_2 delivery at myocardial level, resulting in myocardial ischemia. In this case the electrocardiogram typically does not show the elevation of ST segment (NSTEMI).

The two above-mentioned mechanisms are both responsible for perioperative myocardial ischemic events in approximately 50% of cases. This means that half and possibly more of myocardial ischemia in the surgical patient are not related to coronary occlusion but to a coronary mismatch caused by a reduction of O_2 delivery (e.g., during hypoxemia, anaemia, haemorrhage, hypotension) or by an increased demand (e.g., due to tachycardia, hypertension, inadequate anaesthesia, postoperative pain, and suspension of beta-blocker therapy). It is interesting to notice that the two types of myocardial ischemia have different presentation times. The mismatch type has usually an early presentation, and if it causes death, it will be between the first and the third day; the ischemia due to coronary occlusion occurs later, and mortality is shifted to a few days after surgery.

It is easy to understand that the scenario of perioperative myocardial ischemia causes important perioperative issues. In particular, the consequences are relevant to the preoperative evaluation and management of the patient at risk of myocardial ischemia. Indeed, knowledge of pathophysiology helps to understand that at least half of patients do not have coronary occlusion as a mechanism of ischemia, and so, for example, they are not protected by antiplatelet agents. On the other hand, the other half of the problem makes clear that preoperative provocative cardiac tests can be completely negative without excluding the patient in question from the risk of having a myocardial ischemic event. There are also implications on postoperative monitoring. We should ask ourselves if it is worthwhile admitting the patient to intensive care on the day of surgery, as we know that the event, if it occurs, will happen after the patient is out of our observation.

Knowledge of the problem should lead to the creation of organizational models in which intensive care units are not unnecessarily occupied during the night after surgery but where there is a very careful alert system that allows the early detection of possible ischemic events [4]. Obviously, this requires a multidisciplinary approach involving anaesthesiologists, cardiologists and surgeons.

The aspects that we have discussed here regarding the mechanisms of myocardial ischemia are the basis of the knowledge necessary to understand why guidelines recommend much selectivity in requesting preoperative examinations: often the sensitivity and specificity of a provocative cardiac test are not very different from tossing a coin; often resting cardiac tests are not adequate to explore the complex world of the intraoperative period with all its possible acute physiological variations.

Table 2.2 Clinical risk factors

Ischemic heart disease (angina pectoris, myocardial infarction)
Heart failure
Stroke or transient ischemic attack (TIA)
Renal dysfunction (serum creatinine concentration >170 µmol/L or 2 mg/dL or a creatinine clearance <60 mL/min/1.73 m^2)
Diabetes mellitus requiring insulin therapy

2.3 Preoperative Risk Stratification

Preoperative risk stratification should be performed considering the presence of risk factors in the patient for the occurrence of cardiovascular complications. Clinical risk factors, listed in Table 2.2, are derived from clinical history and clinical examination and allow risk stratification using the Revised Lee Cardiac Risk Index.

In addition to the traditional Lee cardiac risk index [5], for the preoperative evaluation, the model of the American College of Surgeons National Surgical Quality Improvement Program (NSQIP) Myocardial Infarction Cardiac Arrest (MICA) can be used, a model based on the 2007 NSQIP database. In this model, type of surgery, functional status, creatinine concentration, ASA physical status classification, and age were found to be independent predictors of perioperative myocardial infarction or cardiac arrest. The prognostic information provided by the two models is complementary. However, the predictive ability of the NSQIP MICA model was superior to the Revised Lee Cardiac Risk Index, and the risk [6] can easily be calculated at the bedside (http://www.surgicalriskcalculator.com/miorcardiacarrest).

Assessment of preoperative functional capacity must take into account the metabolic equivalent tasks (METs) or exercise testing when needed.

2.4 Preoperative Testing: Which Exams in Which Patient [2]

2.4.1 Preoperative ECG

Every day, thousands of patients scheduled for noncardiac surgery are routinely submitted to resting ECG during the preoperative evaluation. The resting ECG has no sufficient specificity and sensitivity to diagnose congenital or acquired heart disease. For this reason, ECG is only recommended in cases where the presence of risk factors requires further investigation.

Preoperative resting ECG is not recommended in asymptomatic patients without risk factors undergoing low-risk surgery. Instead it could be performed in patients without risk factors who are about to undergo intermediate-or high-risk surgery if they are over 65.

A resting ECG should be performed only *in patients with risk factors* (Table 2.3) undergoing *intermediate- or high-risk surgery*.

Table 2.3 Recommendations for preoperative resting ECG

Patient population	2014 ESC/ESA Guidelines
Patients with risk factors scheduled for intermediate- or high-risk surgery	Recommended (I,C)
Patients with risk factors scheduled for low-risk surgery	May be considered (IIb,C)
Patients without risk factors scheduled for intermediate-risk surgery	May be considered (IIb,C)
Patients without risk factors scheduled for low-risk surgery	Not recommended (III,B)

Risk factors as listed in Table 2.5. Types of surgery as listed in Table 2.1

Table 2.4 Recommendations for preoperative resting echocardiography

Patient population	2014 ESC/ESA Guidelines
	Class of recommendation (Latin number) and level of evidence (second letter)
Asymptomatic patients	Not recommended (III)
Patients scheduled for high-risk surgery	May be considered (IIb,C)
Patients scheduled for intermediate- or low-risk surgery	Not recommended (III,C)
Patients with severe valvular heart disease	–
Patients with known or suspected valvular heart disease scheduled for intermediate- or high-risk surgery	Recommended (I,C)

Types of surgery as listed in Table 2.1

2.4.2   Preoperative Echocardiography

A routine echocardiography in a cardiopathic but clinically asymptomatic and stable patient is not necessary in the preoperative evaluation.

Routine preoperative echocardiography is only recommended in patients with known or suspected valvular heart disease scheduled for intermediate- or high-risk surgery. The Guidelines suggest that it may also be considered in patients undergoing high-risk surgery (Table 2.4).

2.4.3   Imaging Stress Testing

The Guidelines recommend preoperative cardiac stress testing only if the results are likely to modify the perioperative management. It is recommended only in patients with poor functional capacity and more than two clinical risk factors before high-risk surgery. It may be considered in patients with one or two clinical risk factors and poor functional capacity before intermediate- or high-risk surgery. Imaging stress testing is generally not recommended before low-risk surgery.

In clinically stable patients who have undergone surgical myocardial revascularization in the previous 6 years, no preoperative cardiac stress tests should be performed. These are, however, recommended in patients with high cardiac risk scheduled for surgery in the first year after surgical myocardial revascularization.

2.4.4   Serum Biomarkers

Routine preoperative determination of serum biomarkers (brain natriuretic peptide [BNP], NT-proBNP, cardiac troponin) for risk stratification before surgery is not recommended in patients undergoing noncardiac surgery. It may be considered in high-risk patients. In particular, in these patients, the determination of cardiac troponins at 48–72 hours after major surgery may be considered, in order to monitor the possible onset of perioperative myocardial ischemia.

2.4.5   Preoperative Coronary Angiography and Myocardial Revascularization

Although many patients undergoing noncardiac surgery suffer from coronary artery disease, preoperative coronary angiography is rarely indicated. Considering the procedure-associated risk and lack of evidence that preoperative coronary revascularization improves perioperative outcome, the indications for preoperative coronary angiography are identical to those in the non-surgical setting.

There is no evidence that preoperative coronary revascularization improves perioperative outcome in asymptomatic patients or in patients with stable coronary artery disease (CAD). In general, recommendations for perioperative coronary revascularization are identical to those used in the medical field and follow the ESC Guidelines on the management of stable CAD. In accordance with these Guidelines, a routine prophylactic preoperative coronary revascularization is not recommended in patients with documented CAD scheduled for low- or intermediate-risk surgery. Prophylactic preoperative coronary revascularization could be considered in the presence of a significant stress-induced myocardial perfusion defect.

2.5   Preoperative Pharmacological Management: Medications for Heart Failure

The management of cardiac therapies in the preoperative evaluation of cardiopathic patients is an aspect of particular interest. More and more patients are taking cardiovasoactive drugs and anticoagulant and antiplatelet agents.

Considering the most commonly used drugs such as beta blockers, ACE inhibitors (ACEIs) and angiotensin II (ARBs) receptor antagonists and statins, it is generally recommended to continue the home therapy in the perioperative period.

The Guidelines [2] recommend the continuation of beta-blocker therapy in the perioperative period in patients currently receiving this medication. However, regarding preoperative initiation of beta-blocker therapy in patient in non-chronic treatment, the ESC/ESA Guidelines suggest that the preoperative start of beta blockers may be considered in patients: 1) scheduled for high-risk surgery, 2) with ≥2 clinical risk factors or ASA physical status ≥3, and 3) with known ischemic heart disease or myocardial ischemia.

Atenolol or bisoprolol may be considered first-choice drugs if the decision for preoperative initiation of oral beta-blocker therapy is made. Neither the initiation of beta blockers in patients undergoing low-risk surgery nor the initiation of high-dose beta-blocker therapy without titration is recommended.

Therapy with ACEI and ARBs should be kept under close control in patients with chronic heart failure and left ventricular dysfunction. If necessary this therapy should be started at least a week before surgery.

A temporary interruption of ACEI or ARBs for the increased risk of severe hypotension during anaesthesia associated with this therapy may be considered in patients with arterial hypertension.

Regarding statins, Guidelines recommend perioperative continuation of chronic statin therapy with preference to statins with a long half-life or extended-release formulation. Initiation of statin therapy should be considered before vascular surgery, ideally at least 2 weeks before surgery.

2.6   Preoperative Pharmacological Management: Antiplatelet Agents and Anticoagulant Therapy

2.6.1   Antiplatelet Agents

2.6.1.1 Aspirin

The decision for or against low-dose aspirin in patients undergoing noncardiac surgery must be based on individual weighing of the perioperative risk of bleeding against that of thrombotic complications. Continuation of chronic aspirin therapy for secondary cardiovascular prevention may be considered. Its discontinuation should be considered when difficult intraoperative haemostasis is anticipated. Following percutaneous coronary intervention, aspirin should be continued for 4 weeks after bare-metal stent (BMS) implantation and for 3–12 months after drug-eluting stent (DES) implantation, unless the risk of life-threatening surgical bleeding is considered unacceptably high.

2.6.1.2 Dual Antiplatelet Therapy

More and more patients are now treated with dual antiplatelet therapy, often posing problems on management of therapy and surgical timing.

In postcoronary angioplasty patients, maintenance of P2Y12 receptor antagonists should be considered for 4 weeks after the BMS implantation and 6–12 months after the DES implant (6 months in the case of a new generation stent). In a patient subjected to coronary angioplasty without a stent implant, surgery should be scheduled at least two weeks after the beginning of antiplatelet therapy.

Table 2.5 Risk factors for thromboembolic events

* Atrial fibrillation associated with heart failure, hypertension, age ≥75 years, diabetes, stroke, vascular disease
* Advanced age
* Female sex
* Mechanical prosthetic heart valves, recently inserted biological prosthetic heart valve
* Mitral valvular repair within the past 3 months
* Recent venous thromboembolism within past 3 months
* Thrombophilia

2.6.1.3 Anticoagulant Therapy

Before deciding for or against the perioperative administration of oral anticoagulants, the risk of life-threatening perioperative bleeding must be weighed against the potential thromboembolic risk. Discontinuation of therapy is recommended a few days before surgery in patients at low risk of thrombosis. Patients on oral vitamin K antagonists can undergo noncardiac surgery when the international normalized ratio (INR) is <1.5.

Patients with risk factors for thromboembolic events (Table 2.5) require preoperative bridging therapy with unfractionated heparin (HFU) or low-molecular-weight heparin (LMWH). The last dose of LMWH should be administered no later than 12 hours before surgery. Depending on the type of oral vitamin K antagonists, it is recommended to stop therapy 3–5 days before surgery. For patients receiving non-vitamin K antagonist direct oral anticoagulants (NOACs), it is recommended to discontinue NOACs for 2–3 times their respective half-lives before surgery with average risk of bleeding and for 4–5 times their biological half-lives before surgery with high risk of bleeding. Due to their well-defined "on" and "off" action, preoperative bridging therapy with UFH or LMWH is usually not required.

2.7 How to Deal with Arrhythmia [2]

Changes in heart rhythm and conduction disorders can already be present and treated at home, or they can develop as a perioperative complication.

Ventricular rate control is essential in the management of perioperative atrial fibrillation and supraventricular arrhythmias. Drugs of choice are beta-blockers and calcium-channel blockers. The administration of beta-blockers is associated with an increased rate of conversion of atrial fibrillation to sinus rhythm in patients undergoing noncardiac surgery. In patients with heart failure, amiodarone represents an effective alternative.

In the case of ventricular arrhythmias, the continuation of anti-arrhythmic home therapy is always recommended.

When the ventricular tachycardia (VT) arises in the perioperative period, it needs to be promptly treated with electric cardioversion. Anti-arrhythmic drugs are recommended in patients with sustained VT.

2.7.1   Management of Patients with Pacemaker/Implantable Cardioverter Defibrillator

Patients with permanent pacemakers require increased perioperative attention because of the possible interference between device and electrocautery. Special precautions should be taken to reduce the risk of the interferences. In patients who are pacemaker dependent, the device should be set in an asynchronous or non-sensing mode by placing a magnet on the skin over the pacemaker. In patients with an implantable cardioverter defibrillator (ICD), the device should be deactivated by the arrhythmologist before surgery and adequately reactivated after the operation.

During the period of deactivation, the patient's ECG must to be continuously monitored, and an external defibrillator must be available.

2.7.2   Temporary Cardiac Pacing: When and How

The indications for perioperative temporary cardiac pacing are usually the same as for permanent cardiac pacing. Temporary perioperative pacing in noncardiac surgery is recommended [2] in patients with complete heart block and in those with symptomatic asystolic episodes. Temporary perioperative pacing is not recommended in asymptomatic patients with bifascicular block, independently of the presence of first-degree atrioventricular block.

These recommendations should recall how many useless requests for temporary pacemaker positioning are made due to the lack of knowledge of evidence-based literature and Guidelines. The availability of pads for emergency transcutaneous pacing should avoid even more inappropriate requests for arrhytmological consultation.

2.8   Cardiological Consultation: A Laissez-Passer?

The need for cardiological consultation is an important aspect of the preoperative evaluation. However, this rarely modifies patient management, which means that too many are requested.

The cardiological consultation should not be considered a laissez-passer for cardiopathic patients either by the anaesthesiologist or the surgeons. It should only be requested in the case of known cardiopathic patients with instable clinical conditions evaluated during clinical examination or specific situations (presence of ICD or pacemaker; management of the dual antiplatelet therapy in a patient after a recent coronary revascularization) which can be significantly affected by the cardiologist's opinion. The consultation should not be requested only because the patient is cardiopathic. In most cases a cardiopathic patient undergoes a yearly follow-up with a cardiologist. In the absence of conditions of recent instability, a cardiopathic patient should be considered less problematic. On the other hand, a patient with a silent clinical history may need a more careful preoperative evaluation to identify possible risk factors and a clinical evaluation to detect conditions needing further investigations.

The Guidelines [2] put the cardiological evaluation request of the cardiopathic patient scheduled for low- or intermediate-risk surgery in Class IIb, proving that in most cases the request is inappropriate.

Conclusions

Preoperative evaluation of patients with cardiovascular disease undergoing noncardiac surgery must be based on a careful clinical evaluation.

Indiscriminate use of routine preoperative cardiac testing is not justified in the evidence of literature, and it is not recommended by the Guidelines, because it is resource limiting and does not improve perioperative outcome [7]. Fewer exam requests should not be considered as an underestimation of the issue; rather they should give more consideration to the capability of identifying, during the clinical evaluation, risk factors and unstable conditions which need further investigation. This can only improve the evaluation of those patients who really deserve more attention and avoid the need for inappropriate examinations and consultations.

References

1. The Vascular events In noncardiac Surgery patIents cOhort evaluatioN (VISION) Writing Group, The Vascular events In noncardiac Surgery patIents cOhort evaluatioN (VISION) Investigators. Myocardial injury after non cardiac surgery. A large, international, prospective cohort study establishing diagnostic criteria, characteristics, predictors, and 30-day outcomes. Anesthesiology. 2014;120:564–78.
2. Kristensen SD, Knuuti J, Saraste A, Anker S, Bøtker HE, De Hert S, et al. AuthorsTask Force Members. 2014 ESC/ESA Guidelines on non-cardiac surgery: cardiovascular assessment and management: The Joint Task Force on non-cardiac surgery: cardiovascular assessment and management of the European Society of Cardiology (ESC) and the European Society of Anaesthesiology (ESA). European Heart Journal. 2014;35:2383–431.
3. Landesberg G, Beattie WS, Mosseri M, Jaffe AS, Alpert JS. Perioperative Myocardial Infarction. Circulation. 2009;119:2936–44.
4. Biccard BM. Detection and management of perioperative myocardial ischemia. Curr Opin Anestesiol. 2014;27:336–43.
5. Lee TH, Marcantonio ER, Mangione CM, Thomas EJ, Polanczyc CA, Cook EF, et al. Derivation and prospective validation of a simple index for prediction of cardiac risk of major noncardiac surgery. Circulation. 1999;100:1043–9.
6. Gupta PK, Gupta H, Sundaram A, Kaushik M, Fang X, Weldon J, et al. Development and validation of a risk calculator for prediction of cardiac risk after surgery. Circulation. 2011;124:381–7.
7. Guarracino F, Baldassarri R, Priebe HJ. Revised ESC/ESA Guidelines on non-cardiac surgery: cardiovascular assessment and management. Implications for preoperative clinical evaluation. Minerva Anestesiol. 2015;8:226–33.

Ultrasound in Intensive Care Unit: What to Ask, What to Expect

3

Manlio Prosperi, Maxim Neganov, and Andrea De Gasperi

3.1 Introduction

The treatment of the ICU patient ("critically ill" by definition) has witnessed in the last three decades a continuous improvement, both for the expanding of knowledge and the availability/development of a wide range of rapidly evolving technologies. This led the ICU provider to deepen and master several areas previously considered to be of exclusive competence of other specialists (cardiologist, radiologist, surgeons, etc.). Where dedicated resources and specific expertise exist, they represent a high added value: in order to be effective, the approach of individual specialists to the critically ill patient must be focused and coordinated. Aided by well-defined protocols, the multidisciplinary of the ICU physician has as main goal the treatment of the failing organs, the most consistent tract of the critically ill patient; together with urgent treatments, the steady "everyday clinical pursuit" is added and consists of diagnosing, treating, and monitoring the evolution of the ongoing illness. Fields of application of ultrasounds (US) are extremely wide when treating the critically ill: this is one of the reasons intensive care treatment deserves subspecialists with different skills to guarantee the quality of care. The use of POCUS is one of the areas in rapid, continuous development over the past few years: initially used and implemented to assess the respiratory system, it has been introduced into the daily clinical practice for the perioperative assessment of the hemodynamic profile and for a fine-tuning of the invasive maneuvers, both in and outside intensive care units. The POCUS is in some sense the physician's phonendoscope of the third millennium. The further development of training programs stems from the need to have advanced expertise in different specialistic areas, such as the initial approach of the major trauma patient, the neuro-cardiac or general surgical patients, the complex

M. Prosperi • M. Neganov • A. De Gasperi (✉)
2° Servizio Anestesia e Rianimazione, ASST Ospedale Niguarda Ca Granda, Milan, Italy
e-mail: andrea.degasperi@ospedaleniguarda.it

© Springer International Publishing AG 2018
D. Chiumello (ed.), *Practical Trends in Anesthesia and Intensive Care 2017*,
http://doi.org/10.1007/978-3-319-61325-3_3

medical patients, and the solid organ-transplanted patients. The benefit of the point-of-care examination is evident, for example, in the decision-making algorithms of the dyspneic patients while managing hemodynamic instability in the acute patient in the prehospital setting, in the emergency department, or in medical or surgical wards. However, the initial stabilization of the critically ill and the treatment of the progressive multi-organ failure development proceed as a continuum during the entire ICU stay, US being one of the best tools to guide into differential diagnosis algorithms and to help in defining the severity of organ(s) failure. Examples of US applications (among many others) in acute care both in ED and in the ICU (but also in the wards) are optic nerve measurements and transcranial Doppler (central nervous system); A, B, and C lung profiles and diaphragm mobility/width (chest and pulmonary medicine); transthoracic echocardiography (TTE) for both heart and large vessel assessment; evaluation of renal function and causes of renal failure (mechanical causes and measurement of intraparenchymal renal resistances); and hepatic assessment (parenchymal and vascularization: echo Doppler of hepatic artery, portal vein, suprahepatic veins). The FAST (Focused Assessment Sonography for Trauma) and CA-FAST (Chest Abdominal-Focused Assessment Sonography for Trauma) [1] exams provide the evaluation of intra-abdominal collections in abdominal spaces (such as hepatorenal, splenorenal, and Douglas spaces), relevant for abdominal screening in case of perforation or acalculous cholecystitis, together with an evaluation of intestinal peristalsis. Finally, the examination also includes the evaluation of the compressibility of the femoral vein axes in case of suspected deep venous thrombosis (CUS).

One of the first protocols used to create a systematic screening in the dyspneic patient was proposed by Lichtenstein along with the basic principles of pulmonary ultrasound: the BLUE (Bedside Lung Ultrasound Evaluation) protocol [2] is a fast, focused protocol (3 min evaluation) when performed with appropriate devices and standardized points of analysis scan. It has six different profiles with a step-by-step approach, and, considering pathophysiological aspects, it helps in the diagnosis of most pulmonary pathologies encountered in the emergency room.

If the large variety of ED and ICU applications are of the utmost importance, even more relevant is the definition of the relationship between these domains and the level of the required training. Ultrasound in the ICU may in some cases have a high specificity and a reduced sensitivity, and since this involves some risk, the diagnostic test should always be integrated with all the available clinical data. A key aspect of the problem is therefore to standardize the degree of expertise and the training needed to gain basic and advanced competences. There are many coding levels which allow a correct way of operating while reducing the chance of errors/misinterpretation: for example, in case of the US examination, the American Heart Association in agreement with the American Cardiology Association provides 12-h training classes to achieve a basic skill level in detecting pericardial effusion, severe left and right ventricular dysfunction, regional dysfunction in case of severe coronary syndrome, broad evaluation of valvular apparatus defects, and vena cava collapsibility related to the respiratory activity. In the same line, WINFOCUS [3] provides certified training pathways for ICU providers, combining expertise and levels of recommendations in the ICU diagnostics. These levels of recommendation have recently been endorsed by the Critical Care Medicine Society, which has issued recommendations (1A-1B-1C-2A-2B-2C) to define guidelines for the use of US in the ICU, both for general US examination [4] and for echocardiographic evaluation [5]. The shift from evidence to recommendation came not only from the level of evidence but also from the judgment of a large group of experts, who focused on the ultrasound use by intensivists looking at a broad spectrum of skills (such as the brain, chest, lung, heart, abdomen) rather than by single-field specialists, taking into consideration all the possible bias. Therefore, 1C is a strong recommendation, although the quality of evidence is poor (C); on the contrary, 2A, while having a lesser degree of recommendation (2), is supported by high-quality evidence (A) (see Tables 3.1 and 3.2).

Table 3.1 Summary of recommendation of US in critically ill patient [4]

General ultrasound in ICU	Overall grade
Diagnosis of pleural effusion (ruling in)	1A
Guidance of small pleural effusion drainage	1-B
Diagnosis of pneumothorax	1-A
Interstitial and parenchymal lung pathology	2-B
Ascites (nontrauma setting)	2-B
Acalculous cholecystitis (by intensivist)	2-B
Renal failure (mechanical causes)	2-C
DVT by intensivist	1-B
Central venous access general	1-A
Access location internal jugular	1-A

Table 3.2 Recommendation for the use of echocardiographic examination in critical patient [5]

Echocardiographic examination in ICU	Overall grade
Preload responsiveness, ventilated	1-B
Sepsis resuscitation	1-C
Left ventricle systolic function	1-C
Diastolic function	2-C
Acute cor pulmonale	1-C
Pulmonary hypertension	1-B
Right ventricle infarction	1-C
Pulseless electrical activity	2-C
Symptomatic pulmonary embolism	1-C
Ventricular tachycardia/fibrillation	1-B/C
Acute coronary syndrome	1-C
Cardiac tamponade	1-B
Valvular dysfunction	1-C
Native/prosthetic valve endocarditis	2-B/1-C

3.2   Pulmonary Ultrasound

A systematic pulmonary ultrasound approach is recommended as a primary procedure in patients with respiratory failure (1B). However, this approach also belongs to the daily assessment of pulmonary disease, to assist and guide invasive procedures related to the respiratory tract and finally for the integration of clinical data during ventilation and respiratory weaning process, including the estimation of diaphragm dynamic function [6, 7]. Pulmonary ultrasound is largely based on the analysis of artifacts that are generated by the interaction of air and water in the pulmonary parenchyma [2, 6, 7]. All the profiles of artifacts originate from the pleural line: pneumothorax and interstitial syndrome appear more evident in upper and anterior fields, while pulmonary effusions and consolidations are best detected at the lower and posterior areas in supine position. The involvement of the pulmonary surface by the vast majority of acute diseases allows a correlation between the artifacts and the pulmonary alteration by using the US. In fact, only lesions reaching the pleural line can be detected by lung ultrasound.

3.3   Pulmonary Ultrasound Examination

Pulmonary examination is performed on a patient in the supine position by a longitudinal scanning of four lung zones with a convex or microconvex probe for deeper structures or linear probe for superficial structures (pleura and ribs):

L1: second, third, and fourth anterior intercostal space
L2: fifth and eighth anterior intercostal space
L3: fourth and tenth mid axillary intercostal space
L4: posterior chest wall (mainly for US-guided thoracentesis)

The image outlining the longitudinal scan B-mode is the first sign, *bat sign*, where the wings indicate the rib's shadow cones. The pleural line is hyperechoic and located in the middle of the image below the two adjacent ribs, whose sliding interface of the visceral over the parietal *layer gives origin* to the underlying movement and allows the vision of the "lung sliding." Through the M-mode examination, the sliding sign is depicted as the *seashore sign* where the upper (still) and lower portions (created by lung inflation/deflation) of the screen are divided by the pleural line itself (Fig. 3.1).

3.4   Nomenclature of Pulmonary Artifacts

The *A line* is repetitive, horizontal artifact originating from the pleural reverberation. This is a transversal hyperechoic line in the intercostal space, placed 1 or half centimeter below the outer surface of the ribs, the so-called

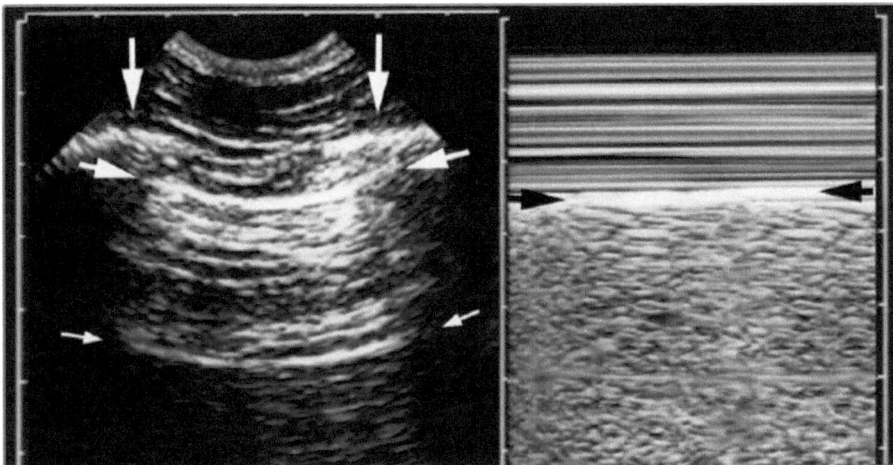

Fig. 3.1 Normal lung surface. (*Left*) Scan of the intercostal space. The ribs (*vertical arrows*). Rib shadows are displayed below. The pleural line (*upper, horizontal arrows*), a horizontal hyperechoic line, half a centimeter below the rib line in adults. The proportions are the same in neonates. The association of ribs and pleural line make a solid landmark called the bat sign. The pleural line indicates the parietal pleura in all cases. Below the pleural line, this horizontal repetition artifact of the pleural line has been called the A line (*lower, small horizontal arrows*). The A line indicates that air (gas more precisely) is the component visible below pleural line. (*Right*) M-mode reveals the seashore sign, which indicates that the lung moves at the chest wall. The seashore sign therefore indicates that the pleural line also is the visceral pleura. Above the pleural line, the motionless chest wall displays a stratified pattern. Below the pleural line, dynamics of lung sliding show this sandy pattern. Note that both images are strictly aligned, of importance in critical settings. Both images, i.e., lung sliding plus A lines, make the A-profile (when found at the anterior chest wall). The given basic information on the level of capacity pressure

pleural line (this is the physical site of the tissue-air interface, represented by the parietal and visceral pleura in touch).

The *B lines* are *comet tail*-like vertical artifacts originating from the pleural line; they are long, hyperechoic, well defined, and dynamic; they delete lines A at the intersection. Comet-tail artifacts are due to multiple reflections of the beam between an object and its surroundings when there is a marked difference in acoustic impedance. Small water-rich structures surrounded by air are at the origin of these artifacts. They could be found, as an example, in the case of aerated lung with abnormally thickened interlobular septa and extravascular water. Detection of multiple and diffuse vertical artifact B lines in lung ultrasound is usually associated with a diagnosis of radiological and clinical alveolar-interstitial syndrome. It has to be underlined that B lines can also be seen in the latero-basal scans in close to 25% of the patients with normal lungs. The *Z lines* are longitudinal artifacts and originate from the subcutaneous tissue.

3.5 Definition of Lung Profiles According to the BLUE Protocol [2]

The *A-profile* associates anterior lung sliding with bilateral A lines.
The *A'-profile* is an A-profile with abolished lung sliding.
The *B-profile* associates anterior lung sliding with bilateral B lines.
The *B'-profile* is a B-profile with abolished lung sliding.
The *A/B profile* is a half A-profile at one lung, a half B-profile at another.
The *C-profile* indicates anterior lung consolidation (a thickened, irregular pleural line is an equivalent).
The *PLAPS-profile* indicates posterolateral alveolar and/or pleural syndrome.

3.6 Syndromes Visualized on Lung Ultrasound

Pleural disease: effusion, hemothorax, and pneumothorax
Interstitial syndrome: mono or bilateral
Lung consolidation: pneumonia, atelectasis due to hypoventilation, atelectasis due to extrinsic compression, atelectasis related to endoluminal obstruction, abscess, pulmonary thromboembolism

3.7 Pneumothorax

The ultrasound features of pneumothorax are the following: the absence of lung sliding, absence of B lines, absence of pulmonary pulse, presence of lung consolidation, lung point and stratosphere sign (M-mode)

Sensitivity and specificity are 79–100% for pneumothorax not visible at thoracic X-ray and 96–100% with a complete pneumothorax: a pneumothorax may rule out in the presence of lung sliding and B lines, but in the absence of such signs, it can be confirmed only by the presence of a "lung point" which is the respirophasic re-appearing of the lung in touch with the chest wall in the lung region explored (Fig. 3.2).

The absence of sliding with M-mode appears as aligned dots next to the other on the time scale, hence straight lines, such as the representation of the pre-pleural tissues. This M-mode appearance has been named as *stratosphere sign*.

3.8 B Profile: Interstitial Syndrome

Echographic signs: multiple B lines (anterior B line + sliding).
Positive B line: the B lines can be counted ideally by defining the percentage of the hyperechogenic field and dividing it by ten (Fig. 3.3).

Fig. 3.2 Lung point
(abrupt shore appearance
of ventilated lung)

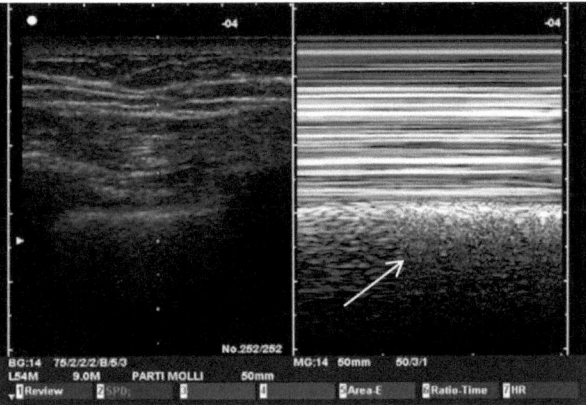

Fig. 3.3 B lines

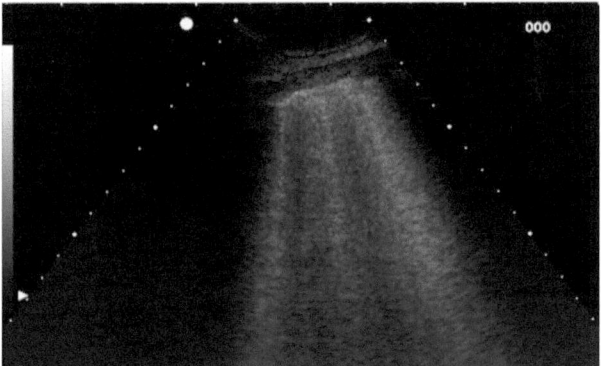

3.9   Characteristics of Pulmonary Consolidation

The main signs of consolidation are the well-defined superficial boundaries and subpleural echo-poor region or one with tissue-like echotexture. Additional signs in the static and dynamic images of a consolidation include bronchogram, thickening and irregularity of the pleural line, the presence of *shred sign* (irregular deep boundaries), vascular features, lung pulse, and associated effusion.

The *air bronchogram* is represented by light branching bands within pulmonary densities; the bronchogram is *dynamic* if air inside such ramifications is displaced by respiratory acts; on the contrary, if there is no motion related to respiratory movements, the air bronchogram is defined as *static*. The bronchogram is instead *fluid* if the bronchial branching contains liquid which is hypoechoic. The *shred sign* is a static sonographic sign observed in lung consolidation. The deeper border of consolidated lung tissue that makes contact with the aerated lung is "shredded" and irregular. There is no effusion inside. This sign is not seen in massive translobar consolidation where it is more difficult to appreciate the deeper border of the lung.

Fig. 3.4 Shred sign

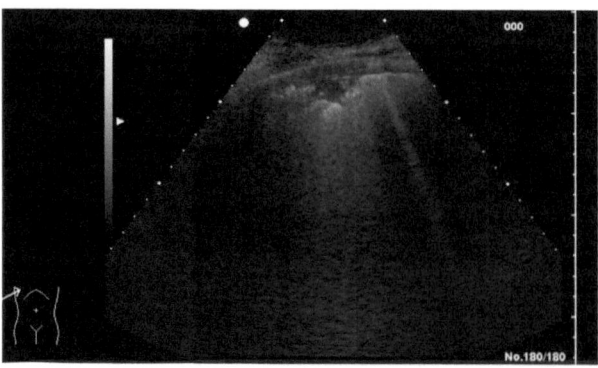

The vascular features within the pulmonary parenchyma may exhibit a mediastinal ipsilateral retraction.

The lung pulse is the evidence of cardiac activity on the pleural line when the compliance is low or the lung is not/poorly ventilated.

Atelectasis may have different echogenicity characteristics depending on their origin and nature: flogistic consolidation, extrinsic compression, bronchial obstruction, bronchial exclusion, and hypoventilation.

The *lung pulse* is an indirect sign of complete atelectasis, observed in bronchial obstruction and selective intubation. Among the patients with pulmonary consolidation with an air bronchogram, a dynamic bronchogram may indicate the presence of pneumonia (differential diagnosis with an atelectasis). A static bronchogram is instead observed in many cases of atelectasis related to absorption and in one third of pneumonia's cases. This finding increases the understanding of the physiopathology of pulmonary disease within a given clinical condition, addressing to bronchoscopy procedure for a bronchoalveolar lavage or to remove bronchial obstruction. Flogistic subpleural consolidation has generally well-defined, thick, and irregular pleural margins, a poor echogenic structure beneath the pleural line, and a presence of *shred sign* (Fig. 3.4). The air bronchogram is dynamic and sometimes may have fluid characteristics; there are no vascular abnormalities. In case of differential diagnosis between pneumonia and atelectasis, a dynamic bronchogram has sensitivity of 61% and a specificity of 94%. Onset of subpleural or lobar consolidation and dynamic arborescent linear air bronchogram is a reliable tool to detect early VAP in the ventilated patient, positive predictive value being 94% [8].

3.10   Pleural Effusion

The ultrasound examination is strongly recommended (1A) to diagnose and locate a pleural effusion (84% sensitivity and 100% specificity). The accuracy is also high, quantifying and qualitatively defining the fluid present in the pleural cavity. The US-assisted/-guided drainage procedure of pleural effusion is recommended (1B); in addition, significant reduction of complications (failure to drain large amounts of

Fig. 3.5 Pleural effusion

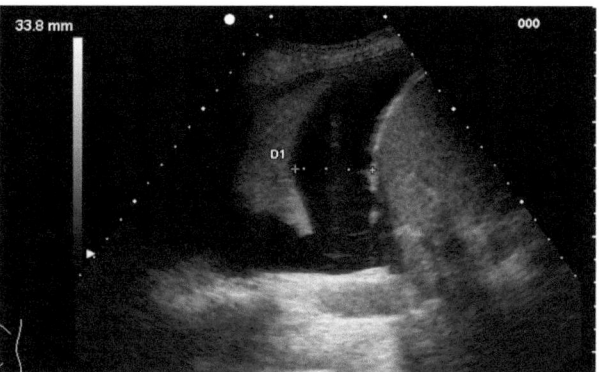

fluid or causing a pneumothorax) has been observed, compared to blind techniques. It should be noted that in cases of surgery-related increased intra-abdominal pressure, compartmental syndrome or dynamic/mechanical ileus, the hemi-diaphragms can be very high and that the phrenic nerve lesions can alter the localization of a pleural effusion (Fig. 3.5).

3.11   Pulmonary Embolism

Nazarian [9] conducted a prospective study including 357 patients with suspected pulmonary embolism (Wells score 4) using multi-organ ultrasound examination (the heart, lungs, and lower limbs). Compared with CT angiography, it resulted in sensitivity and specificity of 90 and 86%, respectively. Right ventricular size, filling, and function compared to left should always be looked in the presence of hemodynamic instability if a thromboembolic disease is suspected: CUS positivity will confirm diagnosis.

3.12   Diaphragm and Respiratory Weaning

Weaning from mechanical ventilation is a complex process involving on the one hand evaluation of pulmonary parenchyma, pleura and diaphragm, and volemic status and cardiac performance on the other [10–12]. The assessment of a diaphragmatic dysfunction is a contributing factor to the success of respiratory weaning among the ventilated patient in intensive care unit. It can be altered in case of neuromuscular diseases, phrenic nerve paralysis, after abdominal and cardiothoracic surgery, and in patients with prolonged periods of mechanical ventilation; the ultrasound assessment of diaphragm, together with the above described other elements, is a wise and efficient way of monitoring the weaning process of the critically ill in the ICU [13] (Fig. 3.6).

Di Nino [14] conducted a clinical trial among 63 patients during respiratory weaning with pressure support ventilation or spontaneous breathing. He found a

Fig. 3.6 The study
of diaphragmatic function
(from Matamis D)

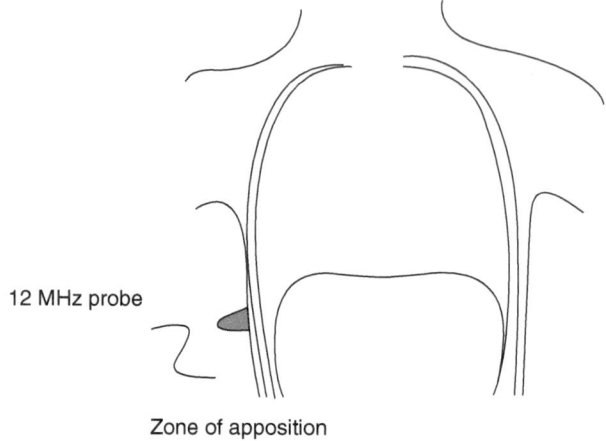

12 MHz probe

Zone of apposition

sensitivity and specificity of 88% and 71%, respectively, for successful extubation
within 48 h when a 30% of diaphragm thickness modification was documented.
Evaluation of diaphragmatic excursion can be performed during spontaneous respiratory activity, with noninvasive or invasive ventilation with pressure support, using
a high-resolution linear probe placed in the tenth intercostal space, over anterior or
mid-axillary lines. The US probe should be directed perpendicularly to the diaphragm, usually finding the area of interest ca. 5–20 mm below the costophrenic
recess. The lower edge of the costophrenic recess is identified at the end expiration
at the transition zone between the appearances of the *curtain sign*, given by lung
caudal displacement during the following inspiration, preventing the visualization
of the diaphragm and the liver (or spleen) because of the lung air content.
Diaphragmatic thickness can be observed and measured in M-mode. Normal values, measured at residual functional capacity volumes, can range from 1.8 to 3 mm,
with an average thickening of 54% (42–78%), when forced vital capacity is reached.
Diaphragmatic function can also be evaluated by measuring the diaphragmatic
excursion through a subcostal window, applying a convex probe directed toward the
diaphragmatic dome always in *time-motion mode* [15]. During the respiratory
weaning phase with pressure support ventilation, Kim [16] suggested a cutoff value
of 18 ± 3 mm for weaning trial and 7.8 cm during forced exhalation.

3.13 Airway Management

There are several aspects that should be considered while managing the airway
using US (linear probe 7–11 MHz) [17]:

1. Preliminary evaluation of the anterior region of the neck for pharyngeal and
   laryngeal abnormalities and in case of an obese patient, control of the adipose
   tissue located anteriorly to the trachea (its quantification might be predictive of
   difficult intubation).

2. Determination of the transverse width of the trachea, because of its relationship with the size of the double-lumen tube: 18 mm for 41 Fr tube, 16 mm for 39 Fr, 15 mm for 37 Fr, and 14 mm for 35 Fr [18].
3. Check of the tracheal tube position by looking for lung sliding and diaphragmatic movement (pulmonary expansion) or lung pulse detection, which is associated with a not collapsed, not ventilated lung (main stem intubation).

3.14 Percutaneous Tracheotomy

The ultrasound evaluation of the anterolateral neck region may precisely detect thyroid, cricoid, and tracheal rings by a very quick longitudinal scan using a linear probe. These findings may be very useful during preliminary evaluation of the percutaneous tracheotomy in the ICU. First step of this examination includes the evaluation of blood vessels and flow in the anterior region of the neck to detect and rule out any abnormalities about arterial or venous anatomy [19], which may result in immediate or post-procedural bleeding complications. The second part, using the same probe performing a transversal scan, has the main goal of evaluating the precise position of the tracheal rings, their centrality, and the transverse tracheal diameter at subglottic level (Fig. 3.7).

Once tracheal position and size of the thyroid lobes and the isthmus are identified, the physician proceeds marking the site of the puncture for subsequent guide wire insertion (as an alternative, the puncture could be US guided). Concomitant fiberoptical vision confirms the correct positioning of the guide wire before the passage of the cannula [20, 21].

3.15 Echocardiographic Diagnostics in Intensive Care

The transthoracic echocardiogram (TTE) of the patient with cardiovascular instability [22–24] has a 1B degree of recommendation and depends on the operator skill. This examination should not be confined to cardiothoracic ICUs, where this technique is normally implemented together with transesophageal echocardiography (TEE). The latter offers better image quality compared to the TTE, particularly of

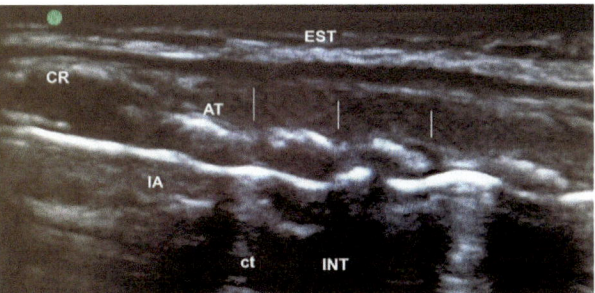

Fig. 3.7 Ultrasound image of the trachea. *CR* cricoid, *AT* tracheal rings, *IA* air interface, *CT* artifacts "comet tail," *white arrows*: tracheal spaces

the posterior structures, such as the pulmonary veins, the left atrium, the mitral valve, and otherwise non-visible structures during the TTE such as the aortic isthmus.

3.16   Fluid Responsiveness

Very often preload static parameters such as central venous pressure (CVP), wedge pressure, and ventricular volumes do not predict fluid responsiveness, and this is because every patient might actually have his own Frank-Starling response, which depends on heart contractility, venous return, and afterload. Furthermore, right atrial (RA) pressure is related to venous return, which in turn depends on venous capacitance gradient. Cyclic changes of ventricular filling induced by increased intra-thoracic pressure variations and heart-lung interaction during mechanically ventilation lead to delta-up and delta-down variations of stroke volume and IVC size. Fluid responder is usually defined the patient whose stroke volume increases by 10–15% following a 3 mL/kg (usually 250 mL) crystalloid or colloid fluid bolus [25]. According to some, close to half of the fluid challenges in ICU could be useless if not, in some cases, even harmful. The correct B-mode measurement of IVC must be performed 1–2 cm from its junction with the RA in a patient well adapted to the ventilation (tidal volume 6–8 mL/kg); mechanically ventilated patients with positive end-expiratory pressure in which the distensibility of the inferior vena cava (IVC) during the inspiratory phase is greater than 12% compared to the expiratory phase can be considered fluid responders (grade 1B). There are no rigid recommendations about the fluid responsiveness based on IVC collapse measurement during spontaneous ventilation or intra-abdominal compartment syndrome. Nevertheless, during spontaneous ventilation, an IVC diameter of less than 10 mm indicates fluid tolerance, while in case of mechanically ventilated patients, there is a poor correlation between IVC diameter and CVP. Passive leg-raising technique may be performed both during mechanical and spontaneous ventilation; it transiently increases venous return, allowing the physician with advanced echocardiographic training to predict the fluid responsiveness through the visualization of 10% increase in stroke volume or simply VTI (velocity time integral). In the presence of small hyperdynamic ventricles with critical variation of IVC size, hypovolemia has always to be considered and a fluid challenge warranted. Among hypotensive conditions in which hypovolemia has to be immediately ruled out, worth to be mentioned is the dynamic obstruction of left ventricular outflow tract, usually associated with hypertrophic cardiomyopathy and associated with the systolic anterior movement (SAM) of the mitral valve (Table 3.3). Pressors or inotropes in such a setting would be deleterious, volume optimization being instead even lifesaving.

3.17   Septic Shock

The evaluation of left ventricular contractility in patients with pre-existing or ICU-acquired vascular and heart abnormalities improves volume management and inotrope or pressor administration (1C). The association between systolic and diastolic

Table 3.3 Echocardiographic fluid response (FR) prediction

Dynamic parameter	Signs and values	FR prediction	Considered variable and pitfalls
Left ventricular size (PSAx)	LV area <10 cm2	+/−	Hypertrophy, inotropic drugs, vasodilatation
	Kissing wall		
LV size variation	>16%	+	Detection on beat to beat during ventilation cycle
Dynamic outflow tract obstruction	Systolic narrowing of outflow tract	+	Hypovolemia accentuates obstruction specially in hypertrophic obstructive cardiomyopathy (SAM)
Mitral valve (MV) flow	Pattern E/A	+/−	Diastolic dysfunction
Stroke volume variation (AV)	>12%	+	Arrhythmia, spontaneous respiratory efforts
			TV >8 mL/kg, compartment syndrome
IVC size	<10 mm	+	Low correlation with RAP in ventilated points
IVC diameter variation	>12% (>18% DI)	+	distensibility index DI
RV	Increased size	+	High negative predictive value
	Paradoxical septal motion		
Passive leg raising	SV o VTI >10%	+	Can be used in spontaneous breathing or arrhythmic points

dysfunction and septic shock is very high and can reach 50% according to some authors, particularly in case of Gram-negative bacterial infection. Moreover, left ventricular outflow dynamic tract obstruction can be observed during hypovolemic status if (inappropriately) treated with catecholamine infusion (hyperdynamic state of the septic shock). Chauvet et al. demonstrated a mechanical outflow tract obstruction together with a small, hyperdynamic, and pseudohypertrophic left ventricle in 22% of patients admitted to the ICU with a diagnosis of septic shock [26]. The use of echocardiography is supported by 2C quality of evidence during the vasoactive therapy and in the diagnosis of specific medical conditions, such as the Takotsubo syndrome, characterized by dilation and apical dyskinesia with a preserved function of the remaining cardiac segments.

Clinical studies demonstrate that up to 23% of the ICU patients have pure diastolic dysfunction, while 40% have variable systolic and diastolic dysfunction. Diastolic function assessment requires advanced training: nevertheless, a global heart dysfunction should be sought in patients with unstable hemodynamic status. Diastolic function is influenced by many variables (among them age, respiratory rate, heart rate, and P-R interval), along with non-diastolic physiological factors (e.g., preload, blood flow, systolic function of the left ventricle and contractile function of the left atrium); however, in the presence of normal contractility and size and thickness of the left ventricle's walls, diastolic function can be estimated using the E/A ratio, the ratio of peak velocity flow in early diastole (the E wave) to peak velocity flow in late diastole caused by atrial contraction (the A wave) [27].

3.18   Cor Pulmonale

In certain clinical conditions, the signs of the right ventricular dysfunction due to the pressure or fluid overload should be sought (1C). The acute cor pulmonale is caused by a sharp increase in the afterload of the right ventricle with a consequent flattening and paradoxical septal movement, diastolic dysfunction, and increased RV/LV diameter ratio (>0.6). Estimation of pulmonary artery systolic pressure (PASP) could add to the interpretation of the origin of the dysfunction (myocardial or valvular causes) (1B). Tricuspid annular plane excursion (TAPSE) measurement has low prognostic utility without any level of recommendations. In case of hemodynamic instability associated with suspected pulmonary embolism, the functional assessment of the right ventricle (1C) should be followed by lower extremities compression ultrasonography (CUS), if deep venous thrombosis is suspected, before considering angiographic CT, even if the former test results are negative. If myocardial infarction is suspected, an estimation of the telediastolic volumes, the contractility of both ventricles, and the abnormal movement of the interatrial septum toward left atrium can be obtained through the subcostal short-axis US approach (1C).

Clinical conditions such as ARDS and VILI require careful evaluation of the hemodynamic status and right ventricular function, which might be reduced in 20–25% of patients. Increased right ventricular strain is proportional to the increase in lung resistance, which in turn is conditioned by the mean airway pressure. Simultaneously, mechanical ventilation interacts with the patient's hemodynamic status since pleural pressure affects venous return and transpulmonary pressure interacts with right ventricular filling. Usually, the ratio between the right and left ventricle area at the end of the diastole should be less than 0.6; a value between 0.6 and 1 indicates a moderate dilation of the right ventricle, which becomes severe for values greater than 1. Although transthoracic examination is limited due to the high pulmonary expansion and a narrow ultrasound window of the four-chamber view, it is still useful in a decision-making algorithm for hemodynamic control and protective ventilation; assessment can take place, where possible, through TEE examination or by using a subdiaphragmatic approach [28].

3.19   Deep Venous Thrombosis

Among the major concerns of intensivists are venous thrombosis and pulmonary embolism. Many are the factors able to promote these conditions: sedation, muscle paralysis, indwelling intravascular devices, major surgery, and malignancies. Since a consistent part of the pulmonary emboli originates from the common femoral and popliteal veins, the initial approach to the patient with suspected pulmonary embolism starts with ultrasound evaluation of the lower district. Using high-frequency linear probe (5–10 MHz), intensivists have a powerful tool for a high-sensitivity and high-specificity diagnosis; there are two main techniques, which can be used alone or combined for a more accurate diagnosis. The first one is the compression ultrasound (CUS), which uses B-mode to obtain a cross-sectional visualization of the vessel. The detection of the vessel is followed by an external gentle compression by the probe, which normally should lead to the collapse of the vein, being minimal the deformation of the artery. Inability to compress the veins and the presence of echogenic intravascular material are the diagnostic signs of deep venous thrombosis [29]. The second technique is Duplex and combines CUS with pulse wave Doppler imaging.

3.20   Cardiopulmonary Resuscitation

American Heart Association (AHA) Advanced Cardiac Life Support (ACLS) and the European Resuscitation Council (ERC) and International Liaison Committee on Resuscitation (ILCOR) guidelines clearly emphasize to seek and treat any potentially reversible causes of cardiac arrest during the resuscitation manoeuvers. Recently updated ERC guidelines introduce cardiac US as a potential tool for detection of these conditions [30]. Considering that the diagnostic procedure and the intervention must yield quick results with minimal impact on CPR maneuvers and minimal impact on no flow intervals, ALS-conformed echocardiography could have an important role in this scenario. The use of focused ultrasound became widely used in emergency setting both in prehospital and hospital setting, leading to the development of various echocardiographic protocols. Among them, focused echocardiography evaluation in life support (FEEL) algorithm is a quick ten-step/four-phase approach, which may help intensivists during CPR [31]. Using subcostal window, which provides a better cardiac visualization during resuscitation, the FEEL algorithm enables to distinguish between pseudo-PEA (pulseless electrical activity) and true-PEA, influencing the actual management of the patient. Of the utmost importance is to underline that FEEL must not delay for any reason CPR and should not take more than ten seconds. Although there are no precise indications for timing of cardiac US, it is usually performed immediately after the ECG analysis and at the end of CPR cycle [32].

Cardiac US may be additionally applied following the return of spontaneous circulation (ROSC) after ventricular tachycardia/fibrillation resolution. The echocardiographic examination allows the detection of segmental hypokinesia and a possible ischemic origin of the cardiac event (1B), thus allowing to anticipate the possible indication of an early revascularization procedure [5].

Several studies have examined the use of ultrasound during cardiac arrest to detect potentially reversible causes. Although no documentation exists able to document improved outcomes using cardiac US, there is no doubt that echocardiography has the potential to detect reversible causes of cardiac arrest. The integration of ultrasound into ALS algorithm requires considerable training in order to limit a minimum the interruption of chest wall compressions.

3.21   Acute Myocardial Infarction

In case of cardiogenic shock, the TTE as point of care helps to save time when acute myocardial infarction is suspected, allowing visualization of segmental kinesis, ventricular function, transient mitral dysfunction, and papillary muscle rupture and, in the case of inferior myocardial infarction, to exclude the right ventricular involvement.

3.22 Pericardial Effusion and Cardiac Tamponade

The classical clinical picture of Beck's triad (hypotension, jugular distension, and soft or absent heart sounds) is not always present during cardiac tamponade. Echocardiography can help intensivist not only to diagnose this condition but also to guide pericardiocentesis. The pericardial effusion is considered minor if the separation between parietal and visceral pericardium is <0.5 cm, moderate if the width is >0.5, but <2 cm and large if >2 cm; moreover, its hemodynamic impact is related not only on the amount of pericardial fluid accumulation but specifically on the speed of fluid accumulation. A parasternal approach helps to differentiate between pericardial effusion and left pleural effusion, the latter being localized posteriorly to the descending aorta, the former anterior to it. Cardiac tamponade is characterized by systolic collapse of right atrium, right ventricle diastolic collapse, and a paradoxical respiratory modification of left and right ventricular filling, along with inferior vena cava distension. Using apical four-chamber view, there is a visible increase in right ventricle width during the inspiratory phase, with displacement of the septum toward the left ventricle in diastole and toward the right ventricular in systole. The patient with aortic dissection (90% of the cases at isthmus area, which is not detectable with the classic transthoracic echo) may develop pericardial effusion.

3.23 Valvular Dysfunction

Every patient with a newly diagnosed heart murmur at ICU admission should undergo an echocardiographic assessment to evaluate the presence of clinically significant valvular lesions, such as aortic stenosis and aortic or mitral insufficiency/regurgitation. A physician with a basic training is able to recognize clear vegetation in a high-risk patient (2C).

3.24 Renal Function and Resistive Index

The color-Doppler is also used to calculate the renal resistive index (RRI) at the level of interlobular arteries (normal RI <0.7). It measures the changes in blood flow velocity in the renal vessels and provides indirect information of renal blood flow and microcirculation. RRI is a semiquantitative parameter related to the sensitivity and Doppler settings (gain, PRF, filter, depth of field) and related to the loss of cortical diastolic flow and to the trend of RRI. Although a variation of this index relies upon a wide variety of extrarenal mechanisms, it could be considered in ICU as a predictor of persistent renal failure, thus well beyond the evaluation of the "simple" renal response to a fluid challenge. An increase in renal vasculature resistance is associated with a reduced renal perfusion, likely turning into an acute tubular necrosis. Feedback mechanisms, such as the renin-angiotensin system and endothelin secretion by the renal endothelium, are involved in the renal vascular regulatory mechanism. Renal perfusion pressure relies upon a delicate balance of mean arterial blood pressure, venous pressure, and intra-abdominal pressure; taken together (or in some cases also alone), these factors are able to play a relevant role in jeopardizing oxygen transport to high-energy structures (as sodium pumps of kidney tubule are). Experimental studies showed a linear relationship between intra-abdominal pressure and RI correlating IAP of 25 mmHg to RRI of 0.81 [33]. According to Darmon et al., a RRI value of 0.80 also represents the cutoff for a non-transient AKI in the critical patient [34]. Dewitte et al. reported, in patients with sepsis and non-transient renal failure (inability to recover a satisfactory excretory function within 3 days), higher renal resistances when compared to subjects with transient renal failure (0.76 vs 0.72). This figure did not show any clear relationship with norepinephrine dose. In a recent meta-analysis, Ninet et al. performed a systematic review on nine randomized clinical trials. In their conclusions RRI >0.80 was able to predict the persistence of acute renal failure in critically ill patients. Although the limit of this meta-analysis is the heterogeneity of the patients (clinical condition of shock, sepsis, extracorporeal circulation after cardiac surgery), it might help to understand the pathogenetic mechanisms of the renal injury in critically ill patients, and it should play an interesting role when monitoring the evolution of acute kidney injury [35]. Currently, there is no evidence-based recommendation for the RRI, mainly because of the paucity of experimental studies on homogeneous groups of patients. However, this index might prove to be of extreme interest while treating the oliguric phase of shock or during renal replacement therapy, giving a sort of "marker" of the kidney response to the acute injury and whether or not renal perfusion is "defended" by the treatment.

3.25   Ultrasound Evaluation of Muscle Function and Strength Wasting in Intensive Care Patient

Critical ill patients in the ICU are exposed to a gradual muscle wasting and loss of function due to various concomitant factors (bed rest without passive or active movements, poor nutritional status, now defined "sarcopenia" and medications); this process starts immediately and has its peak in the first 10 days. The ultrasound can be used to determine and monitor this condition through qualitative and quantitative evaluation of different muscle groups. Parry and Puthucheary demonstrated how the muscle volumetric assessment, measured using ultrasounds and including thickness and cross-sectional area of quadriceps and of vastus intermedius, can express the loss of strength and muscular function of the critical patients [36, 37].

Conclusions

Ultrasound in the ICU setting allows a fast, accurate, reproducible bedside examinations of most of the acute disorders encountered in the critically ill. As emphasized by many, but championed by Lichtenstein since the beginning, US enables a pathophysiological approach to a large part of the "failures" found in the critically ill, respiratory and circulatory dysfunctions being the most common. Visual medicine, made easy by the versatility of ultrasound, has to become a priority for the intensivist in the everyday clinical practice in and out the intensive care units.

Acknowledgments We would like to express our gratitude to Enrico Storti MD, who reviewed the manuscript and gave us appropriate and useful suggestions.

References

1. Zanobetti M, Coppa A, Nazerian P, Grifoni S, et al. Chest abdominal focused assessment sonography for trauma during the primary survey in the emergency department: the CA FAST protocol. Eur J Trauma Emerg Surg. 2015. PMID:26683569. doi:10.1007/s00068-015-0620-y.
2. Lichtenstein DA, Mezière GA. Relevance of lung ultrasound in the diagnosis of acute respiratory failure: the BLUE protocol. Chest. 2008;134(1):117–25.
3. Storti E, Neri L. Lung ultrasound in the ICU: from diagnostic instrument to respiratory monitoring tool. Minerva Anestesiol. 2012;78:1282–96.
4. Frankel HL. Guidelines for the appropriate use of bedside general and cardiac ultrasonography in the evaluation of critically ill patients—part I: general ultrasonography. Crit Care Med. 2015;43(11):2479–502.
5. Levitov A, Frankel HL. Guidelines for the appropriate use of bedside general and cardiac ultrasonography in the evaluation of critically ill patients—part II: cardiac ultrasonography. Crit Care Med. 2016;44(6):1206–27.
6. Nazerian P. Accuracy of lung ultrasound for the diagnosis of consolidations when compared to chest computed tomography. Am J Emerg Med. 2015;33:620–5.
7. Gallard E. Diagnostic performance of cardiopulmonary ultrasound performed by the emergency physician in the management of acute dyspnea. Am J Emerg Med. 2015;33:352–8.
8. Mongodi S, Via G, Girard M, Rouquette I, Misset B, Braschi A, Mojoli F, Bouhemad B. Lung ultrasound for early diagnosis of ventilator associated pneumonia. Chest. 2016;149(4):969–80.
9. Nazerian P. Accuracy of point-of-care multiorgan ultrasonography for the diagnosis of pulmonary embolism. Chest. 2014;145:950–7.
10. Zanforlin A. Lung ultrasound in the ICU: from diagnostic instrument to respiratory monitoring tool. Minerva Anestesiol. 2014;78:1282–96.
11. Goligher EC. Measuring diaphragm thickness with ultrasound in mechanically ventilated patients: feasibility, reproducibility and validity. Intensive Care Med. 2015;41:642–9.
12. Mayo P. Ultrasonography evaluation during the weaning process: the heart, the diaphragm, the pleura and the lung. Intensive Care Med. 2016;42(7):1107–17.
13. Vivier E, Mekontso Dessap A, Dimassi S, Vargas F, Lyazidi A, Thille AW, Brochard L. Diaphragm ultrasonography to estimate the work of breathing during non-invasive ventilation. Intensive Care Med. 2012;38:796–803.
14. DiNino E. Diaphragm ultrasound as a predictor of successful extubation from mechanical ventilation. Thorax. 2014;69(5):423–7.
15. Matamis D, Soilemezi E, Tsagourias M, Akoumianaki E, Dimassi S, Boroli F, Richard JCM, Brochard L. Sonographic evaluation of the diaphragm in critically ill patients. Technique and clinical applications. Intensive Care Med. 2013;39:801–10.
16. Kim W. Young Diaphragm dysfunction assessed by ultrasonography: influence on weaning from mechanical ventilation. Crit Care Med. 2011;39(12):2627–30.
17. Sustic A. Role of ultrasound in the airway management of critically ill patients. Crit Care Med. 2007;35(5 Suppl):S173–7.
18. Brodsky JB. The relationship between tracheal width and left bronchial width: implication for left-sided double-lumen tube selection. J Cardiothorac Vasc Anesth. 2001;15:216–7.
19. Sooby P. An anterior jugular vein variant in a patient requiring tracheostomy, demonstrating the importance of preoperative/procedural ultrasound. BMJ Case Rep. 2016;31:1757–90.
20. Dinh VA, Farshidpanah S, Lu S, Sokes P, Chrissian A, Shah H, Hecht D, Nguyen B. Real time sonographically guided percutaneous dilatational tracheostomy using a long axis approach compared to the landmark technique. J Ultrasound Med. 2014;33:1407–15.

21. Alansari M, Alotair H, Al Zohair Z, et al. Use of ultrasound guidance to improve the safety of percutaneous dilatational tracheostomy: a literature review. Crit Care. 2015;18:19–229.
22. Volpicelli G. Point-of-care multiorgan ultrasonography for the evaluation of undifferentiated hypotension in the emergency department. Intensive Care Med. 2013;39(7):1290–8.
23. Via G, Tavazzi G, Price G. Ten situations where inferior vena cava ultrasound may fail to accurately predict fluid responsiveness: a physiologically based point of view. Intensive Care Med. 2016;42:1164–7.
24. Via G. International evidence-based recommendations for focused cardiac ultrasound. J Am Soc Echocardiogr. 2014;27(7):683.e1–683.e33.
25. Miller A, Mandeville J. Predicting and measuring fluid responsiveness with echocardiography echo research and practice. Guidelines and recommendations. Echo Res Pract. 2016;3(2): G1–12.
26. Chauvet JL, et al. Early dynamic left intraventricular obstruction is associated with hypovolemia and high mortality in septic shock patients. Crit Care. 2015;19:262.
27. Otto CM. Textbook of clinical ecocardiography. 5th ed. Philadelphia: Elsevier; 2013.
28. Vieillard-Baron A. Experts' opinion on management of hemodynamics in ARDS patients: focus on the effects of mechanical ventilation. Intensive Care Med. 2016;42:739–49.
29. Di Bello C. Diagnosis of deep venous thrombosis by critical care physician using CUS. Open Crit Care Med J. 2009;3:43–7.
30. Monsieurs KG, Nolan JP. ERC Guidelines 2015. Resuscitation. 2015;95:1–80.
31. Breitkreutz R. Focused echocardiographic evaluation in resuscitation management: concept of an advanced life support-conformed algorithm. Crit Care Med. 2007;35(5 Suppl):S150–61.
32. Breitkreutz R, Price S, Steiger HV, et al. Focused echocardiographic evaluation in life support and peri-resuscitation of emergency patients: a prospective trial. Resuscitation. 2010;81: 1527–33.
33. Andrew W, Kirkpatrick K, Laupland B. The higher the abdominal pressure, the less the secretion of urine: another target disease for renal ultrasonography? Crit Care Med. 2007; 35(5 suppl):S206–7.
34. Darmon M, Schortgen F. Diagnostic accuracy of Doppler renal resistive index for reversibility of acute kidney injury in critically ill patients. Intensive Care Med. 2011;37:68–76.
35. Ninet S, Schnell D, Dewitte A, et al. Doppler-based renal resistive index for prediction of renal dysfunction reversibility: a systematic review and meta-analysis. J Crit Care. 2015;30(3): 629–35.
36. Parry SM. Ultrasonography in the intensive care setting can be used to detect changes in the quality and quantity of muscle and is related to muscle strength and function. J Crit Care. 2015;30(5):1151–4.
37. Puthucheary ZA. Qualitative ultrasound in acute critical illness muscle wasting. Crit Care Med. 2015;43(8):1603–11.

Blood Coagulation During Sepsis and Septic Shock: Is There Still Room for Anticoagulants?

4

Giorgio Tulli

Up to nowadays, Sepsis has been considered as a dynamic and systemic host answer to a serious infection. In 2016, Sepsis has been redefined as a life-threatening organ dysfunction caused by a disorderly host answer to the infection.

The organ dysfunction can be detected when an acute change in the total SOFA scoring ≥2 points occurs as a consequence of an infection. The basic SOFA scoring can be equal to zero in patients that do not have pre-existent organ dysfunctions. A SOFA scoring ≥2 points reflects a mortality risk of approximately 10% in a population of a general hospital with an infection. Even patients with a modest dysfunction can get worse. This risk underlines the gravity of this condition and the need of a rapid and adequate intervention. In plain words, Sepsis is a life threatening organ dysfunction caused by a disregulated host response to infection.

The Septic Shock has been redefined as a type of Sepsis for which the circulatory and cellular/metabolic abnormalities substantially increase mortality. Patients with Septic Shock can be classified as patients affected by Sepsis with the particularity of showing: (1) a persistent hypotension that requires vasopressors to maintain an average arterial pressure ≥65 mmHg and (2) a serum lactate level ≥2 mmol/L (18 mg/dL) despite an adequate resuscitation with liquids. Considering these criteria, the hospital mortality is above 40% [1, 2].

For centuries, medical doctors had looked for solutions to prevent and cure infectious diseases. In 1841, the Austrian medical doctor Ignaz Semmelweis observed that: "medicine students and medical doctors fingers and hands, that got dirty during recent cadavers dissections, carried those specific infections in the pregnant women's genital organs."

G. Tulli
Department of Intensive Care Units and Postoperative Medicine, Azienda Sanitaria Fiorentina (ASL CENTRO Regione Toscana), Piazza Santa Maria Nuova 1, Florence, Italy
e-mail: giotulli@gmail.com

© Springer International Publishing AG 2018
D. Chiumello (ed.), *Practical Trends in Anesthesia and Intensive Care 2017*,
http://doi.org/10.1007/978-3-319-61325-3_4

Thanks to this observation, protocols for an appropriate hands hygiene were implemented in the obstetrical lane under study and the fetal dead from obstetrical Sepsis went down from 16 to 3% [3].

In the last decades, we assisted to continuous improvements in the understanding of this disease pathogenesis. However, Sepsis still causes a mortality of 25/30%, with an annual increase by 10% [4]. This mortality rate doubles if Sepsis is combined with an organ failure. Still nowadays, Sepsis remains one of the modern Medicine's main challenges [5]. In the third millennium, Sepsis is the main cause of death worldwide and it counts from 75 to 300 deaths over 100,000 inhabitants [6, 7]. In the United States almost $24 billion are yearly spent to cure septic patients and the trend is continuously upwards [8].

Today, the focus is the inflammatory response during Sepsis: the so-called SIRS (Systemic Inflammatory Response Syndrome). Septic patients show many biological markers due to inflammation. Often, these markers precede the organ failure, denoting a causal relationship between the two [9]. The inflammatory response to the infection is a protective mechanism against the microbial invasion. However, an exaggerated inflammatory response can lead to the Multiple Organ Dysfunction Syndrome (MODS) and death.

The host response to the invading pathogens determines the Sepsis-affected patient outcome [10]. This concept is based on the Sepsis antibiotic therapy limits and is supported by a continuously better knowledge of cell and molecules involved in the interaction host–pathogen [11]. All living being has developed sensor mechanisms to detect invading pathogens. In the human being, these sensors are the so-called Pattern Recognition Receptors (PRR).

These receptors recognize not only the pathogens molecular patterns (PAMPs), but also the Damage Associated Molecular Patterns (DAMPs) that reveal cellular stress in sterile inflammation condition [12, 13]. Receptors and ligands underwent a strong selective process throughout the human evolution [14, 15]; the pathogens played a key role in this selective process. To illustrate this concept, we take as example the Gipsy population living in the plague-affected Europe during the Middle Age. Their Toll-Like Receptors (TLR) genes evolved and came out to be more similar to the TLR genes of the European populations living in the same regions and in the same conditions (plague-affected Europe), than to the TLR genes of the Gipsy populations living in the north-west Indian regions, where the Gypsy populations came from [16]. Considering that the host answer to the pathogen influences the Sepsis gravity, it does not surprise that also these immuno-related genes variations play a role in determining the Sepsis gravity [17].

The inflammation and its disorder in the Coagulation are strongly related: one system is a positive feedback for the activation of the other one and vice versa. The Coagulation abnormalities are universal in septic patients and they probably play a key role in the MODS [18].

Coagulopathy in Sepsis varies from a thrombo-embolic disease clearly declared ("overt") to a microvascular dysfunction of fibrin ("non-overt"). In the most serious cases, the fulminant DIC shows up as both thrombosis and spread bleeding. Sepsis coagulopathy is probably generated by multiple alteration with respect to the single mediator. This is the reason why many therapies addressed to the single mediator had failed to improve Sepsis outcomes.

The cellular processes activated by the invading pathogens during Sepsis are not limited to the common immune-related genes, but also influence systems less intuitively linked to the immune system. Two important examples are (1) the system that regulates the endothelial barrier integrity and (2) the hemostasis (i.e., the activation of the coagulation). The first system (i.e., the system that regulated the endothelial barrier integrity) facilitates leukocytes access to the tissues through diapedesis, contributing in this way to the pathogens clearance. The second system—the coagulation's activation—is also linked to the pathogens' compartmentalization and eradication. It seems that intensity and regulation of the coagulation activation during Sepsis play an important role in the patient outcome, both in terms of pathogens clearance and relative infection treatment and in terms of development of tissue secondary damage (e.g., DIC o MOD [19])

Which is the most important coagulation monitoring to be done during Sepsis?

The coagulation disorders monitoring during Sepsis is complex and sensitive. It is better interpreted through serial measurements. The common coagulation laboratory tests—PT, PTT, and Fibrinogen—unfortunately have many limitations. Firstly, plasma coagulation tests eliminate the platelets contribution to thrombosis. Platelets actively contribute to thrombosis, giving a useful surface for the thrombin generation and for the coagulation factors recruitment that later propagate the coagulation system [20].

The common tests do not reflect in vivo blood coagulation and do not supply qualitative or functional data. The alternatives to the common tests (i.e., the natural anticoagulants measurement, fibrinolytic activity markers, DIC molecular markers) are not always available during the routine, are not completely validated for specific diseases paths, and cannot be practical in clinical practice. However, they remain of fundamental importance. The common coagulation laboratory tests have a high sensitivity and a low specificity. They are listed here below.

1. Platelet count
2. PT/PTT/INR
3. Fibrinogen
4. Fibrinolysis markers (D-dimer, FDP)
5. Anticoagulation markers (Protein C, Antithrombin)
6. Fibrinolytic activity (plasminogen, alfa 2 antiplasmin)
7. Antifibrinolytic activity (PAI-1)
8. DIC markers (fragment of prothrombin's activation F1+2, Factor IX, Factor X, activation's peptides)
9. Scoring composed system to monitor DIC dynamically (ISTH nonovert/overt DIC Score, JAAM Score and Revised JAAM Score).

The coagulation viscoelastic tests on whole blood are generally considered of importance for a dynamic monitoring. The viscoelastic measurements on whole blood give to medical doctors a deeper and more dynamic understanding of in vivo coagulation. The coagulopathy temporal evolution in septic patients could be well identified and used as a guide for therapy. These tests could also have a prognostic value for Sepsis-affected patients that show risk to develop MODS. Unfortunately, the evidence quality that supports thromboelastometry (TEM) in the routinely Sepsis monitoring is low or moderate [21]. There is a lack of studies that have used TEM in Sepsis to determine the institution of an appropriate therapy. The definition of hypercoagulation and hypocoagulation are not standardized and the internal validity of their usage in the clinical trials is often a problem.

The so-called hypocoagulable patients (i.e., those with prolonged reaction time, with reduced alfa angle or reduced maximum width) have a higher mortality and are more frequently associated with DIC. The patients with serious Sepsis with the highest SOFA and APACHE II present a reduced clot solidity and a prolonged Clot Formation Time [22]. TEM can be a useful negative predictor for the coagulopathy development.

About the TEM prognostic value in determining Sepsis mortality, the premature hypocoagulability represents an independent risk factor for mortality at 28 days in a group of serious Sepsis-affected patients [23].

Some researchers compared SAPS II and SOFA to ROTEM values (rotational thromboelastometry) and found a good correlation between these two systems; ROTEM pathologically altered values correlated with 58.7% of survival at 30 days in contrast to 87% when values were normal. In this study, ROTEM predicted a better survival than SAPS II and SOFA [24].

Other researchers [25] used thromboelastography (TEG) to monitor severe patients in intensive care. Patients were hypocoagulable (22%), normal (48%), and hypercoagulable (30%). The hypocoagulable patients more frequently showed MODS and died. Those patients that were normal at the entrance and then developed hypocoagulation showed a mortality of 80%. According to several studies, those patients that were hypercoagulable or normal at the entrance less likely developed MODS and died. This can help in the stratification of patients that are at risk of developing organ failure.

Platelet aggregometry offers another important viscoelastic measurement during Sepsis. The test utilizes platelet multiple agonists and electrical impedance through filaments to determine platelet function in a whole blood sample. Some researchers [26] conducted the test on 90 patients, comparing 30 patients with severe Sepsis to 30 post-surgical patients and to 30 healthy patients. The Sepsis-affected patients showed a reduced response to the standard agonists compared to healthy and post-surgical patients. Thrombocytopenia and dysfunction effects showed up in critical patients, with a significant increase of mortality when the dysfunction is prolonged during the recovery in Intensive Care [27].

A topic of high interest in the research is the utilization of combined data to predict patient's risk to develop MODS starting from a coagulopathy induced by Sepsis. The diagnostic algorithms, such as ISTH DIC SCORE, SAPS II, SOFA, and APACHE II, combined with more common viscoelastic measurements, can supply the most accurate prognostic values [28]. A 2005 study that utilizes a composite scoring for coagulopathy detected an evolution of coagulation disorders in the first

24 h of serious Sepsis. A coagulopathy that gets worse during the first day is associated with a higher 28 day-mortality [9]. Some Japanese researchers studied multiple platelet markers in Sepsis, such as the TAT complex, PC, and PAI-1, to estimate mortality and development of "overt" DIC.

When these markers appeared combined, the area below the curve—in a group of well-defined patients that were going to develop "overt" DIC—was 0.95. JAMM scoring is another step ahead in improving DIC diagnosis in Sepsis and specially its dynamic diagnosis in the temporal passage from "nonovert" DIC to "overt" DIC.

Many years ago, Japanese researchers were the first in developing scoring systems for DIC, utilizing the combination of easily obtainable coagulation tests, such as platelet count and routine clotting times. Only recently, the Japanese Association Acute Medicine (JAAM) updated the Japanese scoring system. Gando and his collaborators validated in a perspective manner the renewed Japanese scoring on 624 serious Sepsis-affected patients [29]. The JAAM scoring system for DIC seems to be a valid test to dynamically diagnosing DIC in Sepsis-affected patients and it can be useful to personalize anticoagulant strategies in these patients [30]. A DIC diagnosis utilizing this new scoring system is a strong predictor of adverse outcome.

4.1   Inflammation and Coagulation

In Sepsis, a non-controlled infection degenerates in a progressive and disordered inflammation that leads to SIRS. During SIRS, the multiple production of pro- and anti-inflammatory cytokine within the bloodstream is exacerbated [31]. The abnormal production of cytokine contributes both to the abundant activation of coagulation factors and platelet and to the vascular endothelial cellular damage that leads to vascular permeability and DIC. In addition to assuring thrombus generation after the coagulation system activation, an advanced DIC can lead to bleeding when platelets and coagulation factors are finished [8]. These conditions result in an extended cross-talk between inflammation and coagulation with a potential outcome of MODS and possible death [32, 33] (Figs. 4.1 and 4.2).

4.2   Pathogenesis of the Formation of Thrombus in Sepsis

During Sepsis, the coagulation activation is ubiquitarian and induced by PAMPs (Pathogens Associated Molecular Patterns), such as LPS and the exotoxins. The coagulation cascade—interpreted as an over-regulation of fibrinogen and factor V—is mediated by the TF expression on monocytes and macrophages and on the micro particles that express TF from platelets, monocytes, and macrophages [34, 35].

This pro-coagulative reaction is partially made reversible by the contextual fibrinolysis activation attributable to the increased expression of the endogen activator of tissue plasminogen. In turn, this reaction is rapidly inhibited by the increased synthesis of the Plasminogen activator inhibitor-1 (PAI-1) [36].

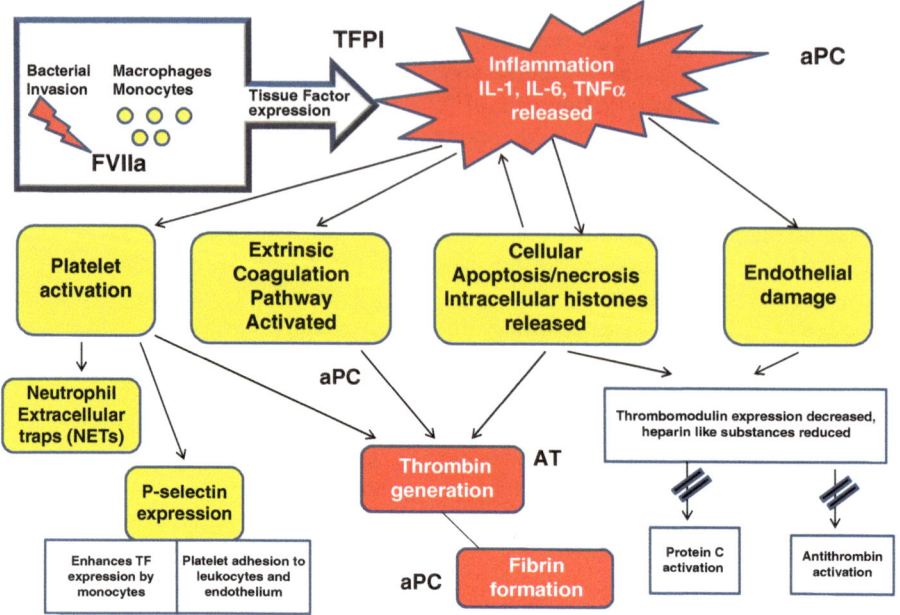

Fig. 4.1 Inflammation and coagulation

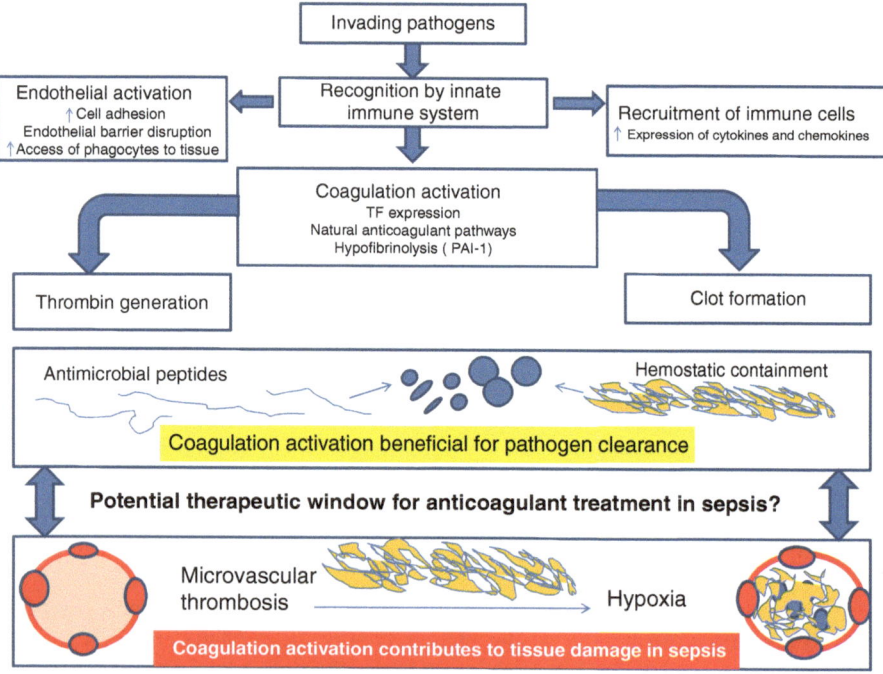

Fig. 4.2 Septic procoagulative state and Tissue Damage

In patients with DIC—that complicates serious Sepsis—TAFI levels increase and, in turn, TAFI activation increase further accelerates the thrombotic pathway [37]. In animals, this univocal sequence induces a pro-coagulative and anti-fibrinolytic state in less than three hours [38]. In human being, if the septic lesion is controlled by therapies, this hemostatic imbalance decreases in few days with a final progressive fibrinolytic phase. However, if the insult is explosive, the hemostatic sequence loses control and induces a spread thrombosis followed by hemorrhage—situation known as DIC.

The post-mortem autopsies of serious Sepsis-affected patients show a spread bleeding with micro-vascular thrombus formation and organ damage [39]. Studies on animals with endotoxemia demonstrated that endotoxemia causes the vascular deposition of fibrin, with the following result in organ failure. Stopping or getting coagulopathy slower in these animals has been demonstrated to be a regression of the same organ dysfunction [40, 41]. Lastly, studies on the clinical outcome of DIC patients show an increased mortality and they suggest that DIC prevention can be a key therapeutic objective [42].

As above mentioned, the inflammatory host response to an invading organism gives rapid starting to a pro-coagulative state in the septic patient. The thrombin generation can be detected within few hours in models where TNF and endotoxin are instilled in human beings [43, 44]. The endothelial damage, that damages the anticoagulative key mechanisms, is observed within 15 minutes since the LPS infusion in rabbits [45].

A key point in the formation of this pro-coagulative state is the interaction between TF and the inflammatory cytokine release. TF expression seems to be the event that detects the starting of coagulation in Sepsis. TF is responsible of the binding with and of the activation of factor VII on cellular surfaces, forming—in this way—the complex enzyme-cofactor and—afterwards—the amplified production of Factor Xa. Not only the tissue factor is prematurely incremented in septic patients, but also the alteration of the TF pathway can prevent the coagulative abnormalities in animals [46, 47].

The debate on which is the TF primary source is still ongoing since many cells are capable to express the Tissue Factor. Among them, we mention the endothelial cells and the mononuclear phagocytes—such as the macrophages and monocytes, the lungs, kidneys, brain astrocytes [35]. The microcyte microparticles that express TF are able to activate the coagulation system [48]. The pro-inflammatory cytokines such as TNF, IL-1, and IL-6 are over-regulated after the TF expression and play a strategic role in the anticoagulative natural suppression and in the endothelial damage [49].

Moreover, PAF is released after inflammation [50]. Platelet activation is present in many thrombosis accelerators. P-selection expression enhances TF expression by monocytes and platelet adhesion to leukocytes and endothelium [51, 52]. Once platelets adhere to leukocytes and endothelium, platelets become useful surface for thrombin formation and play as a cellular signal of other coagulation factors [20].

4.3   The Natural Anticoagulants in Sepsis

In physiological conditions, the surface of the endothelial cells expresses components of the anticoagulant pathways, which rapidly and significantly decrease in the DIC process induced by Sepsis [53]. This explains why reduced activities of AT, PC, or TFPI in Sepsis are often observed, even if coagulation appears activated only in moderation [54, 55]. A rapid depletion of AT and PC is associated with a more unlucky prognosis [47, 56]. Moreover, an increase of plasma thrombomodulin and of soluble PC endothelial receptor suggests that the endothelial activation damage by inflammatory mediators takes place in vivo [47].

The three main endogenous anticoagulants alterations are evident in serious Sepsis and they contribute to hypercoagulability in the premature inflammatory stage. TFPI is a premature regulator of the coagulative path activated by the interaction between TF and FVIIa. TFPI acts to prevent the initial coagulation in two different steps? In the first step, TFPI binds itself and inhibits FXa. In the second step, the complex TFPI-FXa binds itself and inhibits the complex TF-FVIIa, preventing in such a way the premature amplification of coagulation. TFPI is both consumed and degraded in Sepsis leading to a procoagulative state [57]. TFPI is rapidly consumed because of its relatively low concentration in plasma: approximatively 1.025 nM [58]. Vascular endothelial cells expression of TFPI is degraded by plasmin, which is over-regulated in premature Sepsis. This effect has been demonstrated in baboons in which *Escherichia coli* had been instilled, showing that TFPI activity diminished in coincidence with the maximum activity of TPA [55].

The Activated Protein C (APC) is a strong anticoagulant that has profibrinolytic and anti-inflammatory properties. An alteration in Sepsis significantly contributes to a premature hypercoagulability. PC is activated by thrombin once it binds to thrombomodulin. The PC endothelial receptor and the co-factor protein S strongly amplify its activation [59].

Once activated, PC proteolytically breaks Factor V and VIII—both factors are essential for thrombin generation. PC synthesis is damaged, while consumption and degradation by neutrophil elastase further contribute to decrease its concentration in plasma [49]. Thrombomodulin expression is drastically reduced by inflammatory cytokine such as TNF alfa, IL-1, and IL-6. Finally, the Endothelial Protein C Receptor (EPCR) is down-regulated in serious Sepsis, limiting PC activation. The scientific evidence shows that because of the endothelial damage, EPCR could be hidden and no more available for the activation of PC. This effect takes place prematurely, within 2 days in severe Sepsis [60].

The Serine-protease Antithrombin (AT) is a natural thrombin antagonist that is activated by circulating "heparin like" substances. In severe Sepsis, AT synthesis is down-regulated and its consumption is heavily increased because of a constant increase in thrombin generation [61]. Moreover, "heparin like" glycosaminoglycans (GAGs) on endothelial surface are reduced by pro-inflammatory cytokines. This reduction limits even more AT bioactivity [62].

4.4 Resistance to Fibrinolysis in Sepsis

In healthy human beings, endotoxin instillation produces a predictable and rapid change in the coagulative system. Within 120 min, inflammatory markers such as TNF and IL-6 are produced with a contemporary rise in plasminogen activators; this indicates an endothelial activation. Within 150 min, there is a counterbalance thanks to an even higher PAI increase, which sustains clot longevity [44].

Thrombin induces TAFI formation. TAFI is the prosthetic enzyme that reduces clot permeability and increases clot firmness. In Sepsis, thrombin formation—mediated by TF—together with the inflammatory state produce dense clots that are resistant to fibrinolysis. Probably, this phenomenon is mediated by both TAFI and by platelet secretion of polyphosphate that reduce TPA effectiveness [63, 64]. Moreover, elastase secretion by neutrophils degrades fibrinolytic proteases, contributing to the clot persistence. The production of such an aggregate clot could be the defensive mechanism against bacterial proteases that break clot integrity and allows for bacterial dissemination [65]. In patients with meningococcal infections, TAFI levels are strongly increased, and are correlated to the disease severity. They are both associated with a higher mortality [57].

4.5 Endothelial Damage in Sepsis

Vascular endothelial is an important hemostasis regulator and it is a site of immune cells interaction. Endothelial cells mediate pro-inflammatory and anti-inflammatory mechanisms; they regulate fibrinolysis, vasomotor tone, and they have signalling properties for immune cells [66].

Endothelium acts as an important defensive barrier against bacterial invasion. The endothelial cells' superficial layer is a thin layer negatively charged with glycosaminoglycans and glycoproteins called glycocalyx. The intact glycocalyx repels circulating platelets and it acts as an anticoagulant layer, since it is rich in heparan sulfate. Ideally, endothelium can balance pro-coagulant and anti-coagulant mechanisms which occur after the lesion, limiting thrombin formation when vascular reparation is completed. However, when the local lesion becomes systemic, as it happens in Sepsis, the scale moves to a pro-coagulant state [19].

The increased vascular permeability—that follows inflammation—is a Sepsis signal and it significantly contributes to organ dysfunction and to coagulation disorders. Since inflammation and coagulation are, as above-mentioned, strongly related, therapies get involved in the endothelial protection can benefit coagulation abnormalities. Multiple mechanisms are implicated in endothelial damage and they lead to an increased endothelial permeability [67, 68].

The premature transfer towards the pro-coagulative state in Sepsis is mediated by pro-inflammatory markers, which result in a decreased expression of proteins bond to the membrane, such as thrombomodulin [69].

The endothelial lesion can also cause loss and decreased expression of EPCR [70]. The EPCR down-regulation effect on PC pathway has been described above.

The endothelial cells apoptosis, following endotoxin or LPS exposition, causes a release of histones, which intensifies inflammation and induces thrombosis. The endothelial alteration in inflammatory syndromes—such as Sepsis—causes a rapid platelet adhesion that can also lead to micro-circulatory thrombosis. Cellular endothelial layer demolition importantly contributes to premature coagulopathy in Sepsis.

4.6   DIC in Sepsis

Clinically, DIC is defined as a diffuse thrombosis and bleeding. Coagulation factors consumption due to continuous thrombosis can lead to a hypo-coagulative state. In 50–70% of patients with serious infections, there are coagulation abnormalities, while 35% meet DIC criteria [71].

The main way to treat DIC is the eradication of the disease's underlying cause and the support to the occurring coagulative alterations. DIC needs to be faced rapidly, since it is associated with high mortality. DIC diagnostic criteria have been described and combine both laboratory and clinical criteria. Some criteria can be clinically utilized to distinguish OVERT DIC with diffuse bleeding from NON OVERT DIC, to better identify the anticoagulant therapeutic window.

4.7   Pathogenesis of Multiple Organ Dysfunction in Sepsis

Organ dysfunction associated with serious Sepsis takes place because of the multiple interactions between pro-inflammatory status and hyper-coagulation. The role played by DIC as causal factor in MODS is well proved. Alternatively, a recent study shows other MODS mediators, such as the release of intracellular proteins by necrotic and apoptotic cells. HMGB-1 proteins come from dying cells:they are released in the host circulation causing systemic inflammation and they propagate thrombosis [72]. Macrophages, endothelial cells, and monocytes are able to release HMGB-1 proteins. These proteins—which are activating cytokines—are high in septic patients and are associated with mortality in Sepsis model in rats.

There are also other intracellular proteins which are released in the blood stream, such as histones associated with NETs, that are highly toxic for the organs. They induce inflammation and thrombosis [52, 73, 74]. NETs are activated by inflammatory cytokines and by platelet activation, and are built by DNA fibers rich in histones and antimicrobiotic proteins (Fig. 4.3).

Histones (H3, H4) induce thrombin formation through multiple mechanisms (Fig. 4.4). Firstly, extracellular histones damage the activation of thrombomodulin-dependent PC in a dose-dependent way, therefore reducing the natural anticoagulant APC and eliminating its anti-inflammatory properties.

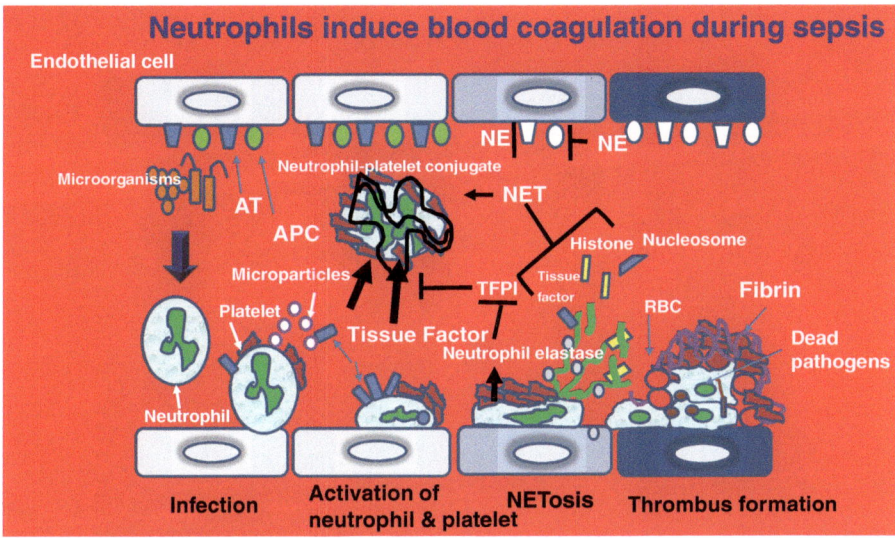

Fig. 4.3 Neutrophils accumulate and adhere to the vascular endothelium in collaboration with platelets during sepsis. There, neutrophils express Tissue Factor (*TF*), release TF-bearing neutrophil microparticles (*NMP*) and expel neutrophil extracellular traps (*NETs*) which initiate the coagulation cascade. In addition, neutrophil derived granule proteins, expecially neutrophil elastase (*NE*) participate in thrombus formation by inhibiting tissue factor pathway inhibitor (*TFPI*) and anticoagulants such as antithrombin (*AT*) and activated protein C (*APC*). Both thrombi formation and endothelial damage lead to substantial microcirculatory damage and organ dysfunction if they occur systematically

Secondly, thrombin formation is increased by histone mediated platelet activation and by p-selectin expression. P-selectin expression increases platelets adhesion to endothelial cells and leukocytes. HMGB-1 and histones released in the circulation increase inflammation and thrombosis, promote cellular death, and enhance MODS.

In contrast to the activation of coagulation as a host defensive mechanism, it has to be noticed that an excessive hemostasis de-regulation is associated with following organ failure and death. A high DIC score is strongly associated with mortality. Concerning fibrinolysis, several studies proved the correlation between a secondary increase in inhibitor-1 levels of the plasminogen activation and the organ failure. Similarly, sequential studies of natural inhibitors of coagulation AT and PC are consistent with a correlation between their plasmatic level reduction and death or organ failure. The continuous worsening of AT and PC decreasing activities within the first day of severe Sepsis is associated with the incremented development of new organ failure and 28th day mortality. This suggests that prolonged and disproportional coagulation and anti-fibrinolysis are a contribution to organ failure and death.

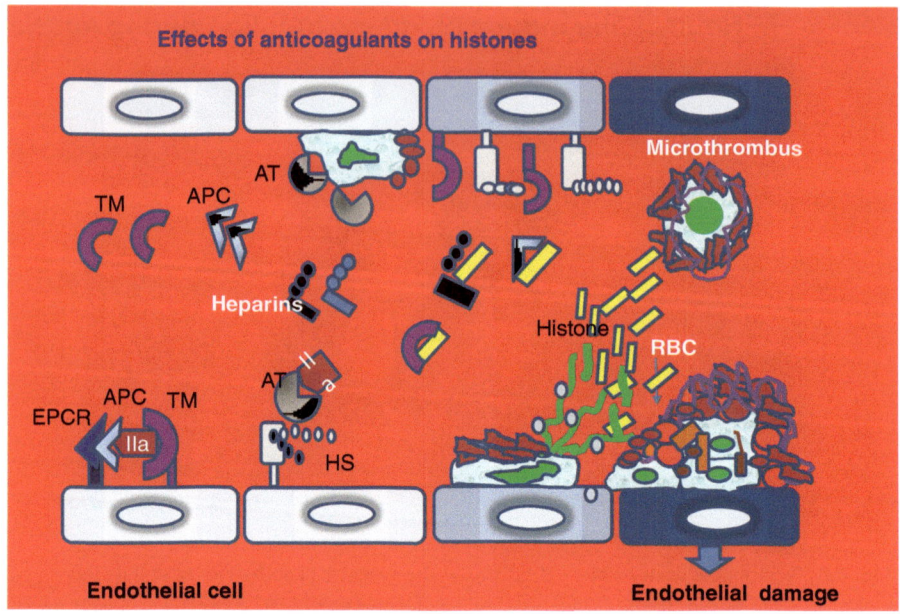

Fig. 4.4 Antithrombin attenuates the leukocyte adhesion to the endothelium and suppresses the expelling of damage associated molecular patterns (*DAMPs*). Activated protein C, recombinant throbomodulin and heparins bind to histones and neutralize their damaging effects *EPCR*: endothelial protein C receptor; *APC*: activated protein C; *Iia*: thrombin; *TM*: thrombomodulin; *HS*: heparin sulphate; *AT*: antithrombin

4.8   Diagnosis of DIC in Sepsis

Actual Sepsis diagnostic criteria include general variables such as hypo-hyperthermia, tachycardia, tachypnea, hypotension, hyperglycemia, edema, and altered mental status [75]. Moreover, a white blood abnormal count and high levels of PCR and Procalcitonin can aid in the diagnosis.

In 1983, Japanese Health and Welfare Ministry set the original diagnostic criteria for DIC. In 2001, the International Society of Thrombosis and Hemostasis proposed the diagnostic criteria for overt DIC [76]. Then, the Japanese Association for Acute Medicine introduced a new set of criteria, including SIRS score, platelet count, prothrombin time, and fibrin/fibrinogen degradation products to start the treatment in the appropriate time [77]. AT or APC treatment results in no improvement in outcome for patients with Sepsis at premature state. However, it can improve the outcome for those patients with DIC. It results clear that new diagnostic criteria are required to determine the appropriate time to start the anticoagulant treatment [78].

Thromboelastography (TEG) could give a credible and dynamic evaluation of the hemostatic state in Sepsis [79, 80]. TEG variables moderately correlate with the gravity of organ dysfunction and they can predict the survival of patients with severe

Sepsis [22, 24, 25]. TEG could be a potential instrument to evaluate the hepatic damage extension in endotoxemia and to evaluate the effectiveness of pharmacological intervention.

4.9   Why Is Coagulation Activated During Sepsis?

The fact that coagulation activation can be beneficial during infections was suggested many years ago [81] and it's proven by high quality data obtained in the last decade. Excellent critical revisions of studies that link coagulation to innate immunity have been recently published [10, 82, 83].

Many studies suggest that coagulative proteins are necessary for the eradication of invading pathogens. It is today known that tissue factor triggers pathways of coagulation-independent signals mediated by Protease Activated Receptors (PARs) on immune cells [84]. These PAR-dependent signals evocate pro- and anti-inflammatory pathways that regulate the migration and proliferation of immune cells, angiogenesis, endothelial adhesion, and many other components of the host response to infection [85, 86]. The PAR-dependent pathways are also activated by other hemostasis components such as Activated Protein C, Xa Factor and Thrombin, which increase the list of coagulative factors that regulate the immune function.

The contact system, formally known as initiator of coagulation intrinsic pathways, is also involved in the host response to pathogens. The kininogen, one of the contact system elements, is today recognized as an important source of antimicrobial peptides released when this protein recognizes many microorganisms [87]. A study intended to search for positive selection's genetic stigmata recently demonstrated that kininogen has been exposed to a strong selective pressure during the evolution [88]. Other hemostasis components, such as coagulation factors II, X, and fibrinogen, release antimicrobial peptides not necessarily involved in blood coagulation [82].

Coagulation activation contributes to the pathogen clearance through another mechanism. Precisely, coagulation activation forms a physical barrier that contains the infectious focus, facilitating pathogen clearance by immune cells. Today, this hypothesis [89] is supported by evidence indicating that the downregulation of hemostasis different components (such as fibrin and platelets) prevents pathogen clearance. A study on fibrinogen-deficient rats in a Listeria monocytogenes infection model demonstrated that fibrin can be protective during infections. The rats treated with warfarin—an anticoagulant that decreases fibrin formation—reproduced these results [90].

A similar strategy confirmed the thrombin and fibrin formation role in *Yersinia enterocolitica* [91]. Again, another study using an infection model with streptococcus group A suggested damaged pathogens clearance in the fibrinogen-deficient rats [92]. Factor XIII—the most preserved coagulation factor in the evolution line [93]—seems to be important for pathogens clearance, as suggested by a study demonstrating that pus-forming streptococci are immobilized and killed within the fibrin clots, in a factor XIII dependent modality [94]. In addition, the fibrinolytic system—which regulates the hemostasis function through fibrin thrombus degradation when they are no more necessary—seems to be involved in the pathogen clearance. It has been demonstrated that Sepsis is associated to an altered fibrinolysis, attributed to the fibrinolysis inhibitor's (PAI-1) rapid increase in plasma [44, 95].

For many years, the hypofibrinolytic status has been considered as a cause of microvascular thrombosis and tissue damage. As alternative explanation, downregulating fibrinolysis, host is able to limit invading pathogens diffusion through more resistant fibrin clots. Studies on genetically modified rats support this theory. Plasminogen "tissue type" activator deficient rats, which show an altered fibrinolysis, present a lower bacterial increase in the primary infectious site (lungs) in a gram-negative Sepsis model [96]. Accordingly, fibrinolysis and alfa-2 antiplasmin inhibitor deficiencies (PAI-1) [97–99], both associated with an increased fibrinolytic activity, result in an altered pathogen clearance in bacterial and viral infectious models.

As many other famous example show [100, 101], another significant evolutionary characteristic derives from examples of pathogens virulence factors on proteases that degrade fibrin clots and from plasminogen activator generated by Yersinia pestis.

A low platelet count has been recognized as an important prognostic factor in Sepsis; platelets are a true biomarker for Sepsis severity. In this regard, it has been recently demonstrated that platelet turnover—measured by platelet immature fraction—correlates with Sepsis severity [102]. However, recent studies indicate that platelets play an important role in host defense. Some researchers demonstrated that platelets interact with liver's Kupffer cells to encapsulate pathogens contained in blood [103].

In another interesting study concerning a pneumonia Sepsis model, thrombocytopenia induced by antibodies resulted in a worse survival and in a proportional increase in bacterial growth [104].

NETs (Neutrophil Extracellular Traps) participation in host defense [105, 106] and platelet activation role in NET formation [107] provide evidence to the relationship between hemostasis and innate immunity. In spite of all these evidences, we have to keep in mind the complexity of the interaction between hemostasis, innate immunity, and pathogens. For example, for reasons which are still unknown, factor XI deficiency in rats, associated to a reduced fibrin formation, demonstrated to improve, rather than impede, the host response in different infection models [108, 109].

However, survival advantages observed in the coagulation factor deficient rats studies have not been always observed when different infection models were used [110]. In some situations, the so-called arms race between pathogen and host seems to have changed fibrin as an advantage, rather than a limitation for some pathogens. This complexity is well illustrated in many animal models by the heterogeneous effect of downregulation of the generation/thrombin clot strength in Sepsis outcome.

Clinical data support the idea that one of the activation coagulation levels could be beneficial for the pathogen clearance. This is because the initial studies that suggested that coagulation inhibition would limit tissue damage during Sepsis were not proved in phase 3 clinical trial of anticoagulant agents [111–113]. Factor V Leiden

(FVL) impact—a procoagulative variant of coagulation factor V—in Sepsis mortality is still a matter of discussion. This has been analyzed in a phase 3 big population study. FVL-carrying participants presented a 28th day mortality significantly lower in respect of non-carrying participants [114]. Even if these data could not be confirmed by other studies [115], they question the concept of an effective coagulation activation damage during Sepsis.

Summarizing, from one side, the laboratory and clinical evidence goes towards a coagulation activation beneficial role during Sepsis. From the other side, new evidences support the classic paradigm that coagulation activation can contribute to tissue damage during Sepsis.

Studies on in-vivo microvasculature images showed tissue perfusion disorders in septic patients that could be strongly improved by activated protein C anticoagulant use [116, 117]. Moreover, the negative results of anticoagulant agents in Sepsis clinical randomized trials have been recently questioned by recent systematic reviews and clinical trials [118, 119]. These clinical trials suggested a beneficial effect of this treatment strategy in septic patients sub-groups. If future trials and larger meta-analysis will confirm it, these results indicate the existence of a threshold above which coagulation activation becomes damaging during Sepsis [120].

All these combined data suggest that coagulation activation is an important component of the comprehensive answer against invading pathogens, and that the invading pathogen eradication could be considered as the ultimate cause of coagulation activation during infection and Sepsis. From this point of view, it is possible to understand why many hemostasis individual components are harmonized towards the thrombin formation increase during Sepsis, based on fibrin and platelets importance in host answer to infection. From this new perspective of evolutionary medicine, coagulation activation analysis during Sepsis could also contribute to the explanation of why systemic anticoagulants usage has not been beneficial in large Sepsis trials, underlining the importance of identifying the precise moment during which the coagulation activation changes from being beneficial to being harmful during Sepsis. In this context, each treatment-target in Sepsis that limits coagulation activation should be oriented to preserve the function of host defense mechanisms that seems to exist from millions of years.

4.10   Thrombosis as Protective Mechanism During Sepsis (Immunothrombosis) (Fig. 4.5)

Our understanding of thrombosis and inflammation during Sepsis evolved during decades of research on animals and humans. The way the first studies on animals had been conducted help us understand our former erroneous reading of Sepsis. Rats model utilized intravenous administration of endotoxin or LPS or even live bacteria such as *E. coli*. Models of LPS and endotoxin infusion used to overestimate uniformly the pro-inflammatory response in host [121, 122]. The first efforts aimed to the mere inflammation as mediator during Sepsis and were not a success in the clinical setting.

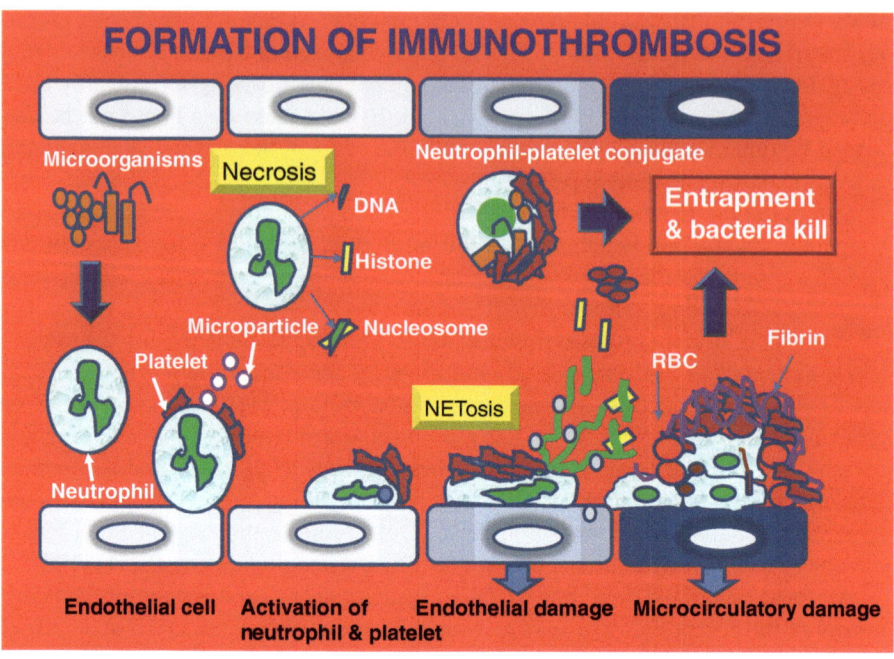

Fig. 4.5 Neutrophils accumulate and adhere to the vascular endothelium in collaboration with platelets during sepsis. There, neutrophils express Tissue Factor (*TF*), release TF-bearing neutrophil microparticles (*NMP*) and expel neutrophil extracellular traps (*NETs*) which initiate the coagulation cascade. In addition, neutrophil derived granule proteins, expecially neutrophil elastase (*NE*) participate in thrombus formation by inhibiting tissue factor pathway inhibitor (*TFPI*) and anticoagulants such as antitrombin (*AT*) and activated protein C (*APC*). Both thrombi formation and endothelial damage lead to substantial microcirculatory damage and organ dysfunction if they occur systematically

In the same way, the coagulation system inhibition had deleterious effects as showed by the highest mortality in patients that were hypocoagulant at the admission in Intensive Care and that show high tendency to bleeding [113]. These strategies totally ignored the protective compartmentalization mechanism. Compartmentalization involves the interaction of the acute phase of the proinflammatory response to the coagulation development, in an attempt to sequester invading bacteria or organisms.

Acute phase proteins, such as fibrinogen and Factor V, rapidly increase during acute Sepsis, determining the hyper-coagulant answer [123]. Simultaneously, two strong natural anticoagulants PC and AT are under-regulated. PC and AT could be seen as negative acute-phase proteins in these premature protective mechanism [124, 125]. The current Sepsis model is seen as both pro-inflammatory and anti-inflammatory or even as a mix (MARS). Following the bacterial invasion, we assist to the formation of extracellular chromatin strips as a fibrin net that contributes to host defense against microbial dissemination. They also facilitate platelet adhesion and platelet aggregation, damaging Protein C TM-dependent activation, and then ultimately they activate the coagulation process [91]. Coagulation activation contributes to bacterial compartmentalization and reduces bacterial invasion [92, 94, 126]. A premature inhibition of the fibrin formation by recombined AT or APC did not modify the inflammation and the increased pulmonary edema, and it exacerbated pathologic changes in lung in a model on rat with pulmonary injury induced by Pseudomonas aeruginosa [127, 128]. Therefore, the potential risk induced by coagulation inhibition in Sepsis premature stage should be always kept in mind.

4.11   The Problem of Anticoagulant Therapies Failure During Sepsis

Recombined Activated Protein C (rhaPC)—a natural anticoagulant used in Sepsis treatment—recent withdrawal from the market represents the last chapter of a story characterized by serial failures of large-scale clinical trials structured to test the generally accepted hypothesis that coagulation activation and microvascular thrombosis were the main determinants of tissue damage in Sepsis [129]. The first evidences on coagulation activation role during Sepsis included the histologic demonstration of microvascular thrombosis in septic patients' target organs and the progressive decreasing of platelet counts and of coagulation factors levels in tardive Sepsis stages, attributed to consumptive coagulopathy.

Indeed, in the previous years, the main experimental data indicated that Sepsis was associated to shift in hemostatic balance towards a pro-coagulative state. The most convincing data were the following: the demonstration that tissue factor expression in circulating leukocyte could be stimulated by pathogens; the acquired deficiency of endogenous anticoagulative proteins such as antithrombin and protein C in patients with Sepsis—with a strong increase in fibrinolysis inhibitors such as PAI-1–resulting in hypo-fibrinolysis [130]. All these data together supported the concept that coagulation activation was in case only partially responsible for organ failure observed in Sepsis. Coagulation manipulation in Sepsis animal models gave an additional support to this concept, demonstrating that organ failure and even mortality could be limited by hemostasis discrete elements block such as TF [131] and factor VII [132].

Built on this model, ambitious programs of clinical development of natural recombinant anticoagulants (AT, TFPI, and rhaPC) in septic patients have been carried on. All programs arrived at phase 3 trial and in the rhaPC case, it arrived to market approval. Unfortunately, benefits of this strategy were not confirmed by these trials results, even if additional clinical trials and meta-analysis are useful to confirm that a definitive conclusion can be reached [120]. The animal models and the clinical design limitations are both considered as a potential explanation for the dissociation between pre-clinical and clinical data. We can also debate for a more preventive point of view on the direct cause-effect relationship between coagulation activation and MOF in Sepsis.

Indeed, the presence of microvascular thrombosis in target organs in Sepsis has been demonstrated in studies with a limited number of patients that did not consider, in their analysis, the different phases in Sepsis [39, 133]. More recent studies on autopsies confirming these findings are unfortunately limited to few cases of patients with fulminant sepsis [134, 135]. Moreover, even if we do not want to debate against the presence of some grades of systemic hypercoagulable state in Sepsis—this concept is supported by the recent demonstration of Sepsis as independent predictor of venous and arterial thrombosis [136, 137]—the presence of this phenomenon in the premature stages of Sepsis has been challenged by data generated using global hemostasis tests. These tests indicated a consistent "downregulation" of thrombin generation in premature Sepsis stages [138, 139]. In this context, a critical review of previous and current data using an evolutionary medicine setting [140] can improve our understanding on last and coming causes of hemostasis activation during Sepsis.

4.12 Therapies Directed to Sepsis Mediators and Anticoagulant Therapies

Therapies directed to coagulation which is activated in Sepsis should ideally re-balance inflammation and coagulation without influencing negatively host response to infection. Many trials failed to recognize inflammation as an important protective mechanism or they used a uniform therapy for patients with different Sepsis stages. Antibodies directed against TNF alpha, IL-1 receptors, and endotoxin failed to demonstrate a reduction in mortality [141, 142]. Trials with anticoagulants failed to demonstrate their efficacy because: inclusion of patients without DIC; uncertainty on when to start the treatment; and tendency to underestimate the importance of developing specific diagnostic criteria for DIC that utilize composed score systems, advanced markers of DIC and TEM.

4.13 TFPI in Sepsis

TFPI is rapidly consumed in Sepsis. Former studies on TFPI replacement efficacy demonstrated that in patients with INR >1.2, mortality did not change and adverse bleeding increased [111]. However, the analysis of a sub-group of this study demonstrated that in patients with CAP there was a tendency towards survival. In 2011, Wunderink et al. [143] published the results of a controlled placebo study in patients with CAP treated with Recombinant TFPI. This study does not show benefit in survival, even if there is an evident biological activity in the improvement of coagulation parameters.

TFPI inhibits the activity of the complex TF/Factor VII and Factor X on the prothrombinase complex, then suppressing the initial stages of thrombin generation [34]. Moreover, the anti-inflammatory effects of TFPI depend on its capacity to suppress intracellular inflammatory signals of Thrombin that bonds to PAR-1 (Protease Activated Receptor–1). Many studies evaluated protective effects of

Recombinant TFPI (rTFPI Tifacogin) on Sepsis. These studies found out that rTFPI significantly decreases thrombin generation, but no conclusions had been verified by clinical trials of phase 1 or 2 [111, 144, 145]. A large scale randomized controlled trial—the trial OPTIMIST (Optimized phase 3 tifacogin in multicenter international sepsis trial)—demonstrated absence of any possible improvement on mortality at 28 days in serious Sepsis after rTFPI treatment [111]. However, the explorative analysis revealed that rTFPi treatment improved survival in patients with severe community acquired pneumonia that were not receiving heparin at the same time [145]. Moreover, in CAPTIVATE, the other placebo controlled trial, intravenous tifacogin administration trial for the efficacy has been stopped in advance because there was no validation of beneficial trend [143].

4.14 Antithrombin in Sepsis

AT inhibits thrombin at a 1:1 ratio and it is maximally activated after interaction with receptor on endothelial surface [146]. AT shows anti-inflammatory properties through its inhibition of the thrombin-Factor X complex, which stimulates IL-1 and IL-6. Recently, JAAM DIC Committee evaluated the AT usage in a RCT perspectival study. Patients with DIC with AT over a three-day treatment showed a more rapid recovery determined through DIC scores, while bleeding events did not increase [147]. Iba et al., in a larger non-randomized study, determined that in patients with low basal AT activity and sepsis, a therapy with high dose AT 3000 IU/day (AT 3000) was associated with an improved survival rate (AT 1500 65.2% vs. AT 3000 74.4%) [148]. These studies utilized DIC score systems to determine "overt DIC" disappearance and the appropriate time for anticoagulant therapy.

AT inhibits many serine proteases that induce FXa, IXa, XIa, and thrombin. It is a direct inhibitor 1:1 of thrombin that leads to thrombin/antithrombin complex formation and to its following elimination. Moreover, its activity is maximized after the bond with glycosaminoglycans that act as co-factors on endothelial surface [146]. AT anti-inflammatory effects inhibit rolling and adhesion of leukocyte partially activated due to prostacyclin release [149] and P-selectin suppression [150]. Moreover, after the bond to proteoglycan heparin sulfate on endothelial surface, AT impedes pro-inflammatory cytokine expression [151, 152].

AT levels decreased for consumption as a consequence of thrombin generation [153] and cytokine down-regulation induced of proteoglycans heparin endothelial sulfates in Sepsis [62]. Premature administration of strong doses of recombinant AT improves outcomes in experimental sepsis probably due to its combined anticoagulant and anti-inflammatory effects [154].

A national study demonstrated that AT administration can be associated to a reduced mortality at 28 days in patients with serous pneumonia and DIC associated to Sepsis [155]. In patients with severe Sepsis, a maintenance dose of AT 1500 UI/day induces a reduction in mortality, together with a strongly shorter recovery in Intensive Care and a lower incidence of new organ failure [156]. Moderate AT doses (30 UI/kg/day) improve DIC score, also incrementing recovery from DIC without any bleeding risk in septic patients with DIC [155]. Unfortunately, high AT doses (7500 UI/day) did not have any effect on mortality at 28 days in adult patients with severe sepsis and septic shock in Kybersept trial [112]. However, in phase 3 Kybersept trial, it has been demonstrated that a treatment with high dose of AT without concomitant heparin could result in a significant mortality reduction in septic patients with DIC [157].

Recently, results from a phase 4 study in septic patients with DIC indicate that a higher initial AT activity, a supplemental dose of 3000 UI/day and younger age are significant factors for a better survival without an increased bleeding risk [119, 148].

4.15   Activated Protein C in Sepsis

For many years, it has been recognized that a rapid PC decrease in Sepsis and low PC levels correlate with a worse prognosis. In 2001, PROWESS study showed promising results of lower mortality with APC usage (Xigris). However, Xigris has been later withdrawn from the market when the trial PROWESS SHOCK revealed that there was not any benefit in mortality at 28 and 90 days [113]. Since then, numerous clinical studies analyzed sub-groups of this population and determined that rAPC can be beneficial. Casserly et al. [158] evaluated 15,022 patients registered with Surviving Sepsis campaign and found out that groups treated with rAPC had a reduced morality (OR 0.76; $P < 0.001$). Even hospital mortality was significantly lower in patients with MOF in respect to those with a single organ failure (OR 0.82 versus 0.78). A meta-analysis carried out by Kalil in 2012 [118] demonstrated benefits in patients with the highest levels of diseases severity, but also higher percentages of adverse bleeding in respect to those reported in PROWESS trial.

The results of this study indicate that rAPC could be beneficial in appropriately selected populations of septic patients. PC is a vitamin K dependent protein. It is converted to its activated form (APC) by proteolysis on the thrombin–thrombomodulin complex. APC inactivates factors Va and VIIIa that further limit thrombin generation. As with thrombin, the main part of pro-fibrinolytic actions of APC are mediated by the bond with endothelial receptor of Protein C and inhibition of PAR1 [159].

In addition to this anticoagulant and profibrinolytic activity, APC has important anti-inflammatory effects: downregulation of proinflammatory cytokine and TF in activated leukocytes, antioxidant properties, antiapoptotic activity and stabilization of the endothelial barrier [160–163]. Moreover, APC puts in place additional cytoprotective functions through histones degradation released in fibrin nets [164].

Based on these observations, rAPC Drotrecogin alpha was produced and, in 2001 [165], this agent's efficacy was tested in a single big scale RCT with demonstrated benefits in a unique subgroup analysis. Since then, Drotrecogin alpha was strongly promoted in SSC guidelines [166] and it was applauded as the most promising therapy in Sepsis therapy. However, there are doubts on its cost-efficacy and inconsistent results observed in more recent studies [167]. In 2011, rAPC production and distribution was suspended after the PROWESS-SHOCK study revealed that mortality at 28 days did not have any significant improvement after treatment with rAPC in patients with septic shock [113]. Nevertheless, its analysis of sub-group reveals that the relative mortality risk is lower in patients with a more reduced activity in respect to PC at study entry.

However, more than one researcher felt unsatisfied with the withdrawal of rAPC from the market, given the results of a single RCT. Casserly et al. [158], analyzing the SSC database containing 15,022 registered cases, found out that the percentage of intra-hospital mortality was significantly lower in the group treated with rAPC with respect to the placebo group. The efficacy demonstrated by rAPC is statistically significant in cases complicated by multiple organ failure, but not in those with only a single organ dysfunction. The meta-analysis reported by Kalil and La Rosa [118] detects an 18% reduction in intra-hospital morality after rAPC treatment, even if serious bleeding incidence increases by 5.6%. The authors concluded that rAPC increases bleeding risk. Nevertheless, it improves outcome in serious Sepsis.

4.16 Thrombomodulin in Sepsis

Thrombomodulin (CD14) is a glycoprotein endothelial transmembrane that has many regulatory functions in hemostasis. Binding to thrombin, it prevents fibrinogen's conversion into fibrin and it prevents thrombin interaction with platelets. The thrombin-thrombomodulin complex activates PC, which has a 100 times-increase in its activity as result [69]. rTM has been studied in DIC and Sepsis models, and in clinical trials as well. Hoppenstead and its collaborators [168] studied rTM in DIC and noticed that markers of thrombin production—such as TAT complex and 1.2 fragment of Prothrombin—are sequentially reduced with rTM treatment. In a study on 234 patients that compared soluble thrombomodulin (ART 123) to heparin in treatment for DIC caused by tumor or infection, the percentage of DIC resolution was 66.1% with ART 123 versus 49.9% with heparin [169].

In this study, it was observed a statistically significant lower percentage of adverse bleeding events with ART 123. In another study of 86 patients with Sepsis induced DIC, lower mortality and better SOFA scores were associated with rTM infusion versus those who did not receive rTM (37% versus 58%, $p = 0.038$) [170]. This finding was later confirmed in a 750 septic and DIC patients study; patients treated with ART 123 were associated with better mortality at 28 days [171]. The definition of the optimal timing for this DIC treatment will be pivotal.

TM binds to thrombin and then it converts PC in APC, giving a critical negative feedback regulation of thrombin generation [172]. Independently from anticoagulant activity, its antinflammatory effect is considered through interference with the activation of complement, LPS neutralization and suppression of the interaction between leukocyte and endothelium [173, 174].

When compared with heparin therapy, a phase 3 study revealed that Recombinant TM therapy (ART 123) had more significant improvement in DIC recovery and bleeding symptoms alleviation in patients with DIC with hematological tumors or infections [169]. Moreover, phase 2b studies validated the hypothesis that TM downregulated the mediators/markers of thrombin generation in septic patients with associated DIC without a serious increase in hemorrhage risk [168, 171]. The subgroup analysis revealed that benefits on survival are higher in patients combined with respiratory or cardiac dysfunction and coagulopathy. According to these results, a phase 3 study is actually ongoing in the United States on patients suffering severe Sepsis with coagulopathy.

A significant number of adverse bleeding effects have been observed in randomized trials that tested all these anticoagulants. The bleeding events' frequency in the treatment group is 1.7 times higher in the PROWESS APC and in the Kybersept AT trials. This is not surprising, since anticoagulants suppress thrombin generation. However, at the same time, we learnt that the adverse event frequently counterbalances the anticoagulants beneficial effects.

It is important to know that many randomized trials of TFPI, AT, and APC were studied to include septic patients without any criteria of coagulation activation and without any concern on temporal sequence. For the most severe patients, the "overt DIC" criteria were already defined at the time of the inclusion in the study. Moreover, a significant reduction in mortality has been observed in the AT or Recombinant TM open trials, when "overt DIC" was required for inclusion [175, 176]. In contrast, the patients with less serious diseases and without an excessive coagulation activation do not show a beneficial effect or even show an increased mortality. It is suspected that a possible adverse effect of anticoagulants—when used in advance—deletes the favorable effect on DIC.

4.17   Heparin in Sepsis

We expect heparin to modulate hemostatic abnormalities through AT maximization effect in the septic DIC treatment. A retrospective analysis demonstrated that the mortality percentage tended to be lower in septic patients treated with low dose heparin compared to placebo patients [177]. Moreover, the low heparin dose improves the Sepsis hypercoagulative state, later reducing DIC or MODS incidence and decreasing Intensive Care recovery days [178]. However, the unfractionated heparin administration is not generally recommended for patients with bleeding tendency. A meta-analysis demonstrated that heparin can reduce mortality at 28 days in patients with severe Sepsis, while there is not increase in bleeding risk in the heparin treated group [179].

4.18   Apoptosis in Sepsis

Studies with IL-7 on septic rat models demonstrated a benefit in reduction of apoptosis of T cells CD4 and CD8, improving immune function. IL-7 seems to have anti-apoptotic functions essential for leukocytes survival [180, 181]. The programmed cellular death can play an important role in reducing inflammatory histones and HMGB-1, that are released in the systemic circulation of septic patients [182, 183]. Similar studies on immuno-modulation reinforce the strong linkage between coagulation and inflammation. Host defense to infectious invasion is a strongly regulated process that involves inflammatory and anti-inflammatory processes. In an attempt to compartmentalize the invasion, the host creates hemostatic barriers with thrombin and thick fibrin nets. Pathologically, these fibrin depositions can generate a microvascular thrombus and result in organ ischemia. The first step to build new therapeutic trials is to establish an operating definition of Sepsis and DIC that is announced by biological markers. To conclude, we have to improve patients stratification and staging to determine the optimal time for interventions [77].

4.19 Conclusions and Take Home Messages

Hemostasis activation induced by Sepsis is modulated by acute changes in inflammatory proteins synthesis and regulation. The excessive coagulation activation and the strong decrease in natural anticoagulants levels are correlated with mortality and organ failure. Unfortunately, the real possibility that coagulation activation and fibrinolysis inhibition could play a role in the host defense against microbial dissemination in the human body has not been taken into account into the design of the different therapeutic trials with anticoagulants.

Although, it had been universally accepted that coagulation inhibition should have been started as early as possible with sufficiently high doses of inhibitor to block fibrin formation, and then modulating inflammation. The anti-inflammatory properties of natural inhibitor were considered the highest benefit procured by these therapies. The high doses were justified by the will to make these properties even more evident. This was supported by studies on animals that demonstrated that only over normal plasmatic levels were able to modulate inflammation, leukocyte adhesion, micro-circular changes, and apoptosis [149].

Moreover, there was another justification for the high early doses: the three natural inhibitors were considered dysfunctional. More than for the synthesis adaptive downregulation—induced by Sepsis—the early and acute decreasing in AT plasmatic levels was explained by its consumption, by its inhibition induced by proteases and by extravascular loss due to endothelial incremented permeability [146, 184]. As far as Protein C system is concerned, TM expression downregulation was considered the main mechanism to explain the decreased synthesis of Activated Protein C [185].

Following the same paradigm, the same measurement was adapted to all situations no matter the septic process stage, the bacterial in action, or the coagulation activation stage; the same inhibitor, with the same high dose and during the same period of time, was administered to all patients. PC therapeutic usage was excluded since its endothelial activation was considered dysfunctional, insufficient or unpredictable, in absolute contrast with clinical evidences demonstrating that a significant PC activation level remained and it could have induced significant APC levels [186].

The possibility that hemorrhagic adverse effects could have been decreased by AT concentrates or by PC concentrates has never been taken into account. The association of AT with heparin was allowed to facilitate inclusion in studies of patients by medical doctors utilizing this preventive or even therapeutic anticoagulation. All randomized TFPI, AT, or APC trials were designed to include patients without any criteria on coagulation activation and no matter its temporal sequence. Except for the first study PROWESS, all these trials failed, but their critically reviewed results bring a strong support to the chance that coagulation inhibitors could remain a useful treatment.

In all documented studies, post hoc analysis demonstrated that overt coagulation activation was strongly associated with mortality or with organ failure, even with the best inhibitor therapeutic effect [157, 187–190]. An analysis following PROWESS and other APC trials demonstrated a relationship between the drug's effect and its administration. However, in most severe patients that benefited from the treatment, overt DIC criteria were already present at the inclusion. On the contrary, no effect or even a trend towards incremented mortality was documented in less serious patients that did not show an excessive coagulation activation. This is in line with a possible adverse effect of APC when it is preventively used in contrast with its favorable effect in DIC.

Even more interesting is the observed significant mortality reduction in open AT and recombinant TM trials when an overt DIC diagnosis for the inclusion in the trial was requested by protocol. Stopping fibrin generation in the early Sepsis phase impedes a strong innate defense host mechanism against bacterial dissemination. The initial coagulation activation and the transitory fibrinolysis inhibition should be respected to foster bacterial compartmentalization. The preventive treatment or the treatment on patients that do not show an excessive coagulation activation could worsen their situation. Specific studied should be conducted to document operative characteristics of methods that allow a biologic monitoring of coagulation and fibrinolysis.

Sequential measurements of thrombin generation and of plasmatic levels of fibrin monomers could better document the excessive coagulation activation. The new JAAM scoring system for DIC seems to be the most valid test to diagnostic DIC in septic patients and it can be useful in anticoagulation treatment strategies customized on the single patient [30] (Figs. 4.6–4.8). A DIC diagnosis with this new scoring system is a strong predictor of adverse outcome. A further improvement in DIC diagnosis can be related with the best evaluation hypercoagulability tests, preferably with instruments with critical care characteristics. As thromboelastography showed, hypercoagulability correlates with mortality in many studies [191, 192], although its superiority on conventional tests does not have all necessary evidence yet [193].

Thromboelastography could give a reliable evaluation of fibrinolytic state. Up to today, a reduced anticoagulant activity within two days could be used as an appropriate temporal window for the treatment. Since the fibrinolysis secondary recovery by plasminogen activators can induce high bleeding risk, DIC treatment should be primarily directed against overt coagulation. Since anti-inflammatory efficacy is not confirmed, supra-normal doses and activated anticoagulants should not be used to limit bleeding risk. Anticoagulant therapies should use the natural anticoagulant replace at daily-programmed doses to rebalance the excess of coagulation activation, together with JAAM DIC score monitoring [194] (Fig. 4.9).

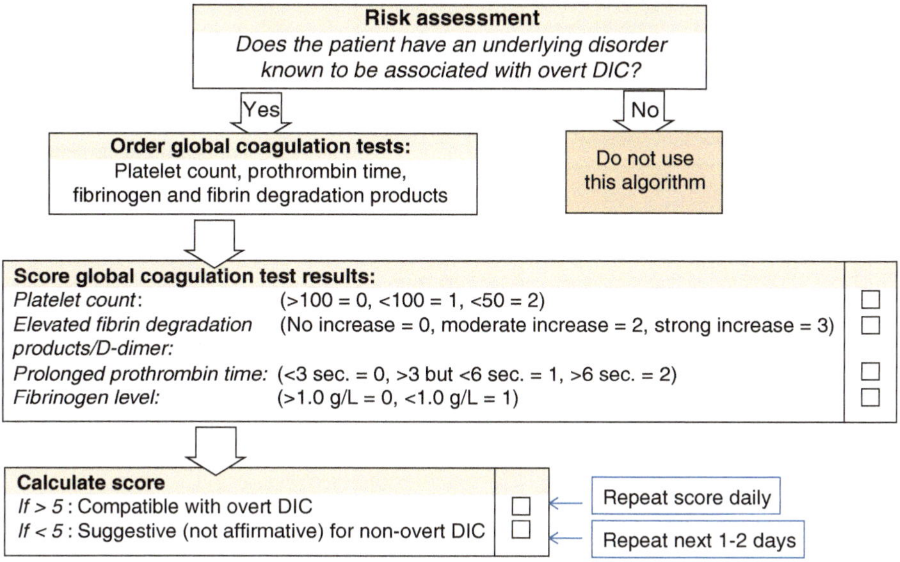

| **Risk assessment** |
| *Does the patient have an underlying disorder known to be associated with overt DIC?* |

Yes → **Order global coagulation tests:** Platelet count, prothrombin time, fibrinogen and fibrin degradation products

No → Do not use this algorithm

Score global coagulation test results:
Platelet count: (>100 = 0, <100 = 1, <50 = 2)   ☐
Elevated fibrin degradation   (No increase = 0, moderate increase = 2, strong increase = 3)   ☐
products/D-dimer:
Prolonged prothrombin time: (<3 sec. = 0, >3 but <6 sec. = 1, >6 sec. = 2)   ☐
Fibrinogen level: (>1.0 g/L = 0, <1.0 g/L = 1)   ☐

Calculate score
If > 5 : Compatible with overt DIC   ☐ ← Repeat score daily
If < 5 : Suggestive (not affirmative) for non-overt DIC   ☐ ← Repeat next 1-2 days

Fig. 4.6 HIST overt DIC scoring system

1. Risk assessment: does the patient have an underlying disorder known to be associated with DIC?
   yes = 2, no = 0   ☐

2. Major criteria

			Rising = −1	Stable = 0	Failling = 1
Platelet Count	>100×10⁹Γ⁻¹ = 0 ☐	<100×10⁹Γ⁻¹ = 1 ☐	☐	☐	☐
PT Prolongation	<3 s = 0 ☐	>3 s = 1 ☐	Failling = −1 ☐	Stable = 0 ☐	Rising = 1 ☐
Fibrin related-markers	Normal = 0 ☐	Raised = 1 ☐	Failling = −1 ☐	Stable = 0 ☐	Rising = 1 ☐

☐

3. Specific criteria

Antithrombin	Normal = −1 ☐	Low = 1 ☐
Protein C	Normal = −1 ☐	Low = 1 ☐
-----------	Normal = −1 ☐	Abnormal = 1 ☐

☐

4. Calculate score: ☐

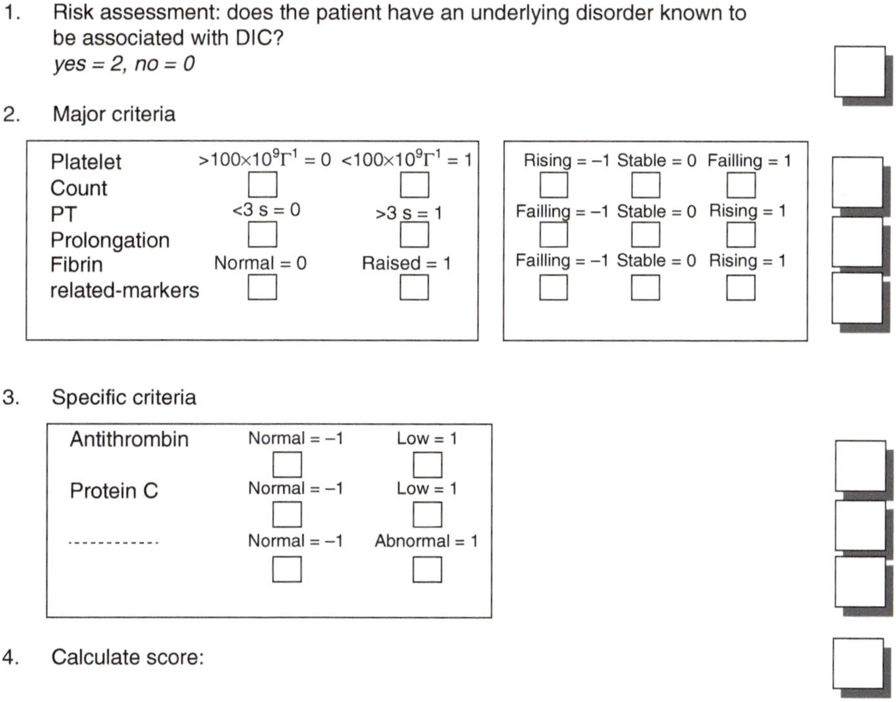

Fig. 4.7 HIST non overt DIC scoring system

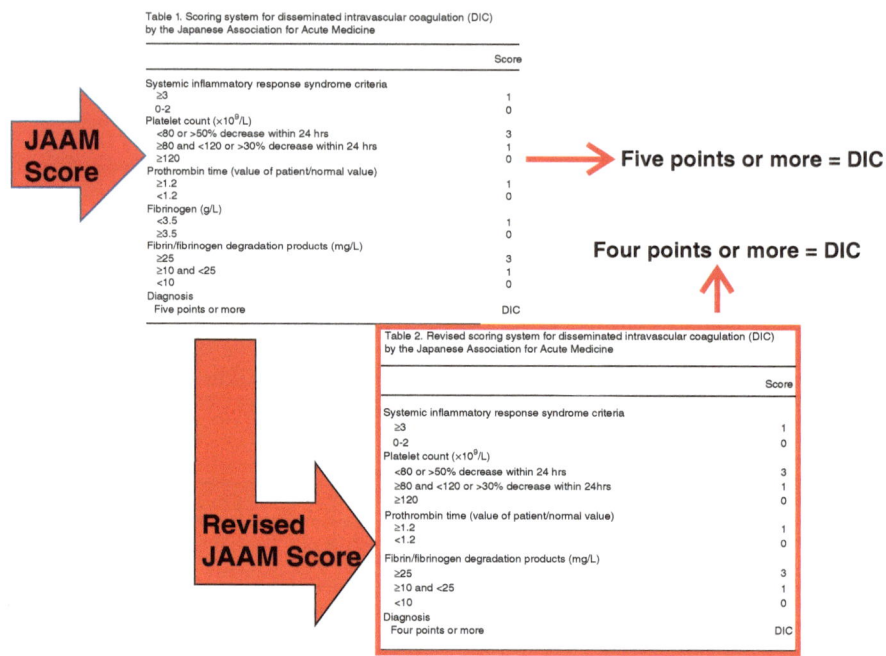

Fig. 4.8 JAAM score and revised JAAM score

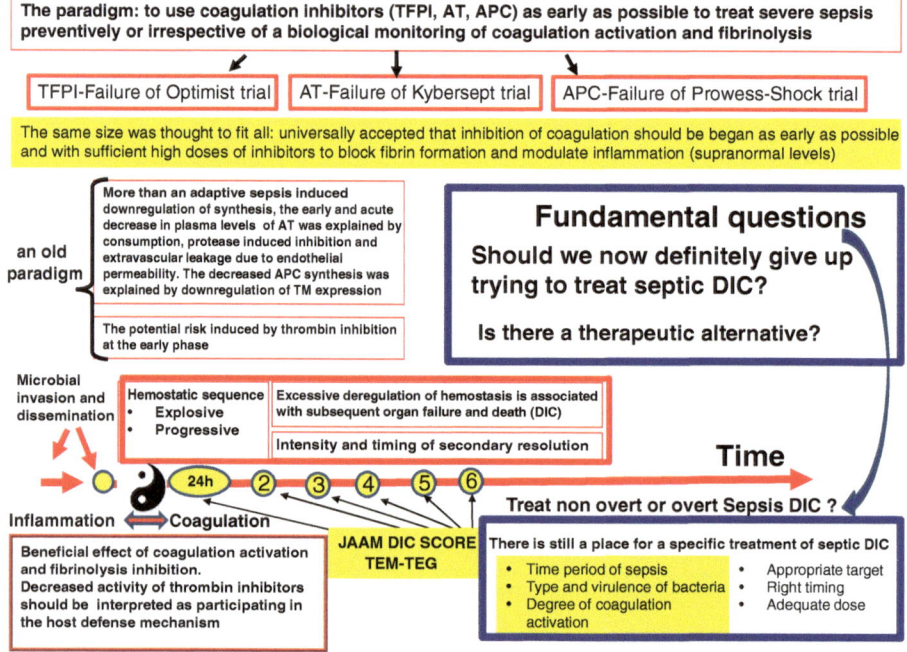

Fig. 4.9 Sepsis, coagulation and fibrolysis, dead end or one way? Is there still room for anticoagulants?

References

1. Vincent JL, et al. Sepsis definitions: time for change. Lancet. 2013;381:774–5.
2. Singer M, et al. The third international consensus definitions for sepsis and septic shock (Sepsis-3). JAMA. 2016;315:801–10.
3. Funk DJ, et al. Sepsis and septic shock: a history. Crit Care Clin. 2009;25:83–101.
4. Gaieski DF, et al. Benchmarking the incidence and mortality of severe sepsis in the United States. Crit Care Med. 2013;41:1167–74.
5. Angus DC, Van der Poll T. Severe sepsis and septic shock. N Engl J Med. 2013;369:840–51.
6. Mayr FB, et al. Epidemiology of severe sepsis. Virulence. 2014;5:4–11.
7. Brun-Buisson C, et al. EPISEPSIS: a reappraisal of the epidemiology and outcome of severe sepsis in French intensive care units. Intensive Care Med. 2004;30:580–8.
8. Iskander KN, et al. Sepsis: multiple abnormalities, heterogeneous responses and evolving understanding. Physiol Rev. 2013;93:1247–88.
9. Dhainaut JF, et al. Dynamic evolution of coagulopathy in the first day of severe sepsis: relationship with mortality and organ failure. Crit Care Med. 2005;33:341–8.
10. Wiersing WJ, et al. Host innate immune responses to sepsis. Virulence. 2014;5:36–44.
11. Salomao R, et al. Bacterial sensing, cell signaling and modulation of the immune response during sepsis. Shock. 2012;38:227–42.
12. Chen GY, Nunez G. Sterile inflammation: sensing and reacting to damage. Nat Rev Immunol. 2010;10:826–37.
13. Hansen JD, et al. Sensing disease and danger: a survey of vertebrate PRRs and their origins. Dev Comp Immunol. 2011;35:886–97.
14. Barreiro LB, Quintana-Murci L. From evolutionary genetics to human immunology: how selection shapes host defence genes. Nat Rev Genet. 2010;11:17–30.
15. Quach H, et al. Different selective pressures shapes the evolution of toll-like receptors in human and african great ape populations. Hum Mol Genet. 2013;22:4829–40.
16. Laayouni H, et al. Convergent evolution in European and Roma populations reveals pressure exerted by plague on toll-like receptors. Proc Natl Acad Sci U S A. 2014;111:2668–73.
17. Pino-Yanes M, et al. Common variants of TLR1 associate with organ dysfunction and sustained pro-inflammatory responses during sepsis. PLoS One. 2010;5:e13759.
18. Levi M, et al. Sepsis and thrombosis. Semin Thromb Hemost. 2013;39:559–66.
19. Seeley EJ, et al. Inflection points in sepsis biology: from local defense to sistemi organ injury. Am J Physiol Lung Cell Mol Physiol. 2012;303:L355–63.
20. Hoffman M, Monroe DM. A cell based model of hemostasis. Thromb Haemost. 2001;85:958–65.
21. Muller MC, et al. Utility of thromboelastography and/or thromboelastometry in adults with sepsis: a systematic review. Crit Care. 2014;18:R30.
22. Daudel F, et al. Thromboelastometry for the assessment of coagulation abnormalities in early and established adult sepsis: a prospective color study. Crit Care. 2009;13:R42.
23. Johansson PI, et al. Hypocoagulability, as evacuate by thromboelastrography, at admission to the ICU, is associated with increased 30 day mortality. Blood Coagul Fibrinolysis. 2010;21:168–74.
24. Adamzik M, et al. Comparison of thromboelastometry with SAPS II and SOFA scores for the prediction of 30 day serviva: a color study. Shock. 2011;35:339–42.
25. Ostrowski SR, et al. Consecutive Thromboelastography clot strength profiles in patients with severe sepsis and their association with 28 day mortality: a prospective study. J Crit Care. 2013;28:317.e1–317.e11.
26. Brenner T, et al. Viscoelastic and aggregometric point of care testing in patients with sepsis shock-cross links between inflammation and haemostasis. Acta Anaesthesiol Scand. 2012;56:1277–90.
27. Levi M, Lowenberg EC. Thrombocytopenia in critically ill patients. Semin Thromb Hemost. 2008;34:417–24.
28. Angstwurm MW, et al. New DIC score: a useful tool to predict mortality in comparison with APACHE II and LOD scores. Crit Care Med. 2006;34:314–20.

29. Gando S, et al. A multicenter prospective validation study of the Japanese Association for Acute Medicine disseminate intravascular coagulation scoring system in patients with severe sepsis. Crit Care. 2013;17:R111.
30. Tromp M, et al. The effects of implementation of the surviving sepsis campaign. Neth J Med. 2011;69:292–8.
31. Cavaillon JM, et al. Cytokine cascade in sepsis. Scand J Infect Dis. 2003;35:535–44.
32. Semeraro N, et al. Sepsis associated DIC and thromboembolic disease. Mediterr J Hematol Infect Dis. 2010;2:e2010024.
33. O'Brien M. The reciprocal relationship between inflammation and coagulation. Top Companion Anim Med. 2012;27:46–52.
34. Chu AJ. Tissue Factor, blood coagulation and beyond: an overview. Int J Inflamm. 2011;2011: 367284.
35. Pawlinski R, Mackman N. Cellular sources of tissue factor in endotoxemia and sepsis. Thromb Res. 2010;125:570–3.
36. Kidokoro A, et al. Role of DIC in multiple organ failure. Int J Surg Investig. 2000;2:73–80.
37. Emonts M, et al. Thombin activable fibrinolysis inhibitor is associated with severity and outcome severe meningococcal infection in children. J Thromb Haemost. 2008;6:268–76.
38. Jourdain M, et al. Effects of interalpha inhibitor in experimental endotoxic shock and DIC. Am J Respir Crit Care Med. 1997;156:1825–33.
39. Shimamura K, et al. Distribution patterns of microthrombiin DIC. Arch Pathol Lab Med. 1983;107:543–7.
40. Creasey AA, et al. Tissue factor pathway inhibitor reduces mortality from *Escherichia coli* septic shock. J Clin Invest. 1993;91:2850–60.
41. Taylor FB, et al. Lethal *E. coli* septic shock is prevented by blocking tissue factor with monoclonal antibody. Circ Shock. 1991;33:127–34.
42. Dahinaut JF, et al. Treatment effects of drotrecogin alpha activated in patients with severe sepsis with or without overt disseminated intravascular coagulation. J Thromb Haemost. 2004;2:1924–33.
43. Van der Poll T, et al. Attivation of coagulation after administration of TNF to normal subjects. N Engl J Med. 1990;322:1622–7.
44. Van Deventer SJ, et al. Experimental endotoxemia in humans: analysis of cytokine release and coagulation, fibrinolysis and complement pathways. Blood. 1990;76:2520–6.
45. Leclerc J, et al. A single enoli injection in the rabbit causes prolonged blood vessel dysfunction and a procoagulant state. Crit Care Med. 2000;28:3672–8.
46. Biemond BJ, et al. Complete inhibition of endotoxin induced coagulation activation in chimpanzees with a monoclonal Fab fragment against factor VII/VIIa. Thromb Haemost. 1995;73:223–30.
47. Levi M. The coagulant response in sepsis. Clin Chest Med. 2008;29:627–42.
48. Wang JG, et al. Levels of microparticle tissue factor activity correlate with coagulation activation in endotoxemic mice. J Thromb Haemost. 2009;7:1092–8.
49. Levi M. The coagulant response in sepsis and inflammation. Hemostaseologie. 2010;30:10–2. 14–16
50. Zimmerman GA, et al. The platelet-activating factor signaling system and its regulators in syndrome of inflammation and Thrombosis. Crit Care Med. 2002;30(5 Suppl):S294–301.
51. Mosad E, et al. Tissue factor pathway inhibitor and P-selectin as markers of sepsis induced nonovert disseminated intravascular coagulopathy. Clin Appl Thomb Hemost. 2011;17:80–7.
52. Semeraro F, et al. Extracellular histones promote thrombin generation through platelet-dependent mechnisms: involvement of platelet TLR 2 and TLR4. Blood. 2011;118:1952–61.
53. Aird WC. Sepsis and coagulation. Crit Care Clin. 2005;21:417–31.
54. Asakura H, et al. Decreased plasma activity of antithrombin or protein C is not due to consumption coagulopathy in septic patients with DIC. Eur J Haematol. 2001;67:170–5.
55. Tang H, et al. Sepsis induced coagulation in the baboon lung is associated with decreased tissue factor pathway inhibitor. Am J Pathol. 2007;171:1066–77.

56. Shorr AF, et al. Protein C concentrations in severe sepsis: an early directional change in plasma levels predicts outcome. Crit Care. 2006;10:R92.
57. Semeraro N, et al. Sepsis, thrombosis and organ dysfunction. Thromb Res. 2012;129:290–5.
58. Lwaleed BA, Bass PS. Tissue factor pathway inhibitor: structure, biology and involvment in disease. J Pathol. 2006;208:327–39.
59. Esmon CT. The endothelial cell protein C receptor. Thromb Haemost. 2000;83:639–43.
60. Guitton C, et al. Early rise in circulating endothelial protein C receptor correlates with poor outcome in severe sepsis. Intensive Care Med. 2011;37:950–6.
61. Levi M, et al. Bidirectional relation between inflammation and coagulation. Circulation. 2004;109:2698–704.
62. Kobayashi M, et al. Human recombinant interleukin-1 beta and tumor necrosis factor alpha mediated suppression of heparin like compounds on cultured porcine aortic endothelial cells. J Cell Physiol. 1990;144:383–90.
63. Mutch NJ, et al. Polyphosphate modifies the fibrin network and down regulates fibrinolysis by attenuating binding of tPA and plasminogen to fibrin. Blood. 2010;115:3980–8.
64. Campbell RA, et al. Contributions of extravascular and vascular cells to fibrin network formation, structure and stability. Blood. 2009;114:4886–96.
65. Dubin G, et al. Bacterial proteases in disease-role in intracellular survival, evasion of coagulation/fibrinolysis innate defenses, toxicoses and viral infections. Curr Pharmaceut Des. 2013;19:1090–113.
66. Ait-Oufella H, et al. The endothelium: physiological functions and role in microcirculatory failure during severe sepsis. Intensive Care Med. 2010;36:1286–98.
67. Lee WL, Slutsky AS. Sepsis and endothelial permeability. N Engl J Med. 2010;363:689–91.
68. David S, et al. Mending leaky blood vessels: the angiopoietin-Tie2 pathway in sepsis. J Pharmacol Exp Ther. 2013;345:2–6.
69. Levi M, Van der Poll T. Thrombomodulin in sepsis. Minerva Anestesiol. 2013;79:294–8.
70. Gleeson EM, et al. The endothelial cell protein C receptor: cell surface conductor of cytoprotective coagulation factor signaling. Cell Mol Life Sci. 2012;69:717–26.
71. Schouten M, et al. Effect of the factor V Leiden mutation on the incidence and outcome of severe infection and sepsis. Neth J Med. 2012;70:306–10.
72. Sunden-Cullberg J, et al. The role of high mobility group box 1 protein in severe sepsis. Curr Opin Infect Dis. 2006;19:231–6.
73. Ammollo CT, et al. Extracellular histones increase plasma thrombin generation by impairing thrombomodulin-dependent protein C activation. J Thromb Haemost. 2011;9:1795–803.
74. Fuchs TA, et al. Extracellular DNA traps promote thrombosis. Proc Natl Acad Sci U S A. 2010;107:15880–5.
75. Dellinger RP, et al. Surviving sepsis campaign: international guidelines for management of severe sepsis and sepsis shock 2012. Intensive Care Med. 2013;39:165–228.
76. Taylor FB Jr, et al. Scientific subcommittee on disseminated intravascular coagulation of the international society on thrombosis and haemostasis. Towards definition, clinical and laboratori criteria and a scoring system for disseminated intravascular coagulation. Thromb Haemost. 2001;86:1327–30.
77. Gando S, et al. Multicenter prospective validation of disseminated intravascular coagulation diagnostic criteria for critically ill patients: comparing current criteria. Crit Care Med. 2006;34:625–31.
78. Wada H, et al. Disseminated intravascular coagulation: testing and diagnosis. Clin Chim Acta. 2014;436:130–4.
79. Tsai HJ, et al. Application of thromboelastography in liver injury induced by endotoxin in rat. Blood Coagul Fibrinolysis. 2012;23:118–26.
80. Spiel AO, et al. Validation of rotation thromboelastrography in a model of sistemi activation of fibrinolysis and coagulation in humans. J Thromb Haemost. 2006;4:411–6.
81. Opal SM. Phylogenetic and functionionships between coagulation and innate immune response. Crit Care Med. 2000;28:577–80.

82. Van der Poll T, Herwald H. The coagulation system and its function in early immune defense. Thromb Haemost. 2014;112:640–8.
83. Engelmann B, Massberg S. Thrombosis as an intravascular effector of innate immunity. Nat Rev Immunol. 2013;13:34–45.
84. Ruf W. Protease activated receptor signaling in the regulation of inflammation. Crit Care Med. 2004;32:S287–92.
85. Coughlin SR. Protease activated receptors in hemostasis, trombosi and vascular biology. J Thromb Haemost. 2005;3:1800–14.
86. Mackman N. The many faces of tissue factor. J Thromb Haemost. 2009;7:136–9.
87. Nickel KF, Rennè T. Crosstalk of the plasma contact system with bacteria. Thromb Res. 2012;130(Suppl):S78–83.
88. Cagliani R, et al. Evolutionary analysis of the contact system indicates that kininogen evolved adaptively in mammals and in human populations. Mol Biol Evol. 2013;30:1397–408.
89. Alcock J, Brainard AH. Hemostatic containment – an evolutionary hypotesis of injury by innate immune cells. Med Hypoteses. 2004;62:861–7.
90. Mullarky IK, et al. Infection stimulated fibrin deposition controls hemorrhage and limits hepatic bacterial growth during listeriosis. Infect Immun. 2005;73:3888–95.
91. Luo D, et al. Protective roles for fibrin, tissue factor, plasminogen activator inhibitor-1 and thrombin activable fibrinolysis inhibitor, but not Factor XI, during defense against the gram-negative bacterium Yersinia enterocolitica. J Immunol. 2011;187:1866–76.
92. Sun H, et al. Reduced thrombin generation increases host susceptibility to group streptococcal infection. Blood. 2009;113:1358–64.
93. Loof TG, et al. Coagulation systems of invertebrates and vertebrates and their roles in innate immunity: the same side of two coins? J Innate Immun. 2011;3:34–40.
94. Loof TG, et al. Coagulation, an ancestral serine protease cascade, exerts a novel function in early immuno defense. Blood. 2011;118:2589–98.
95. Biemond BJ, et al. Plasminogen activator and plasminogen actor inhibitor release ng experimental endotoxaemia in chimpanzees: effect of interventions in the cytokine and coagulation cascades. Clin Sci. 1995;88:587–94.
96. Kager LM, et al. Endogenous tissue type plasminogen activator impairs host defence during severe experimental Gram negative sepsis (melioidosis). Crit Care Med. 2012;40:2168–75.
97. Kager LM, et al. Plasminogen activator inhibitor type 1 contributes to protective immunity during experimental gram negative sepsis (melioidosis). J Thromb Haemost. 2011;9:2020–8.
98. Lim JH, et al. Critical role of type one plasminogen activator inhibitor (PAI-1) in early host defense against non typeable Haemophilus influenzae (NTHi) infection. Biochem Biophys Res Commun. 2011;414:67–72.
99. Kager LM, et al. Endogenous alpha 2 antiplasmin is prove during severe gram negative sepsis (meliodosis). Am J Respir Crit Care Med. 2013;188:967–75.
100. Lathem WW, et al. A plasminogen activating protease spfically controls the development in primary pneumonic plague. Science. 2007;315:509–13.
101. Sodeinde OA, et al. A surface protease and the invasive character of plague. Science. 1992;258:1004–7.
102. Enz Hubert RM, et al. Association of immature platelet fraction with sepsis diagnosis and severity. Sci Rep. 2015;5:8019.
103. Wong CHY, et al. Nucleation of platelets with blood ne pathogens on Kupffer cells precedes other in immunity and contibutes to bacterial clearance. Nat Immunol. 2013;14:785–92.
104. De Stoppelaar SF, et al. Thrombocytopenia impairs host defense in gram negative pneumonia derived sepsis. Blood. 2014;124:3781–90.
105. Martinod K, Wagner DD, et al. Thrombosis: tanglet up in NETs. Blood. 2013;123:2768–76.
106. Yipp BG, Kubes P. NETosis: how vital is it? Blood. 2013;122:2784–94.
107. Clark SR, et al. Platelet-TLR4 activates neutrophil extracellular traps to ensnare bacteria in septic blood. Nat Med. 2007;13:463–9.

108. Luo D, et al. Factor XI deficient mice display reduced inflammation, coagulopathy and bacterial growth during listeriosis. Infect Immun. 2012;80:91–9.
109. Tucker EI, et al. Survival advantage of coagulation factor XI deficient mice during peritoneal sepsis. J Infect Dis. 2008;198:271–4.
110. Flick MJ, et al. Genetic elimination of the binding motif on fibrinogen for the *S. aureus* virulence factor ClfA improves host serviva in septicemia. Blood. 2013;121:1783–94.
111. Abraham E, et al. Efficacy and safety of tifacogin (recombinant tissue factor pathway inhibitor) in severe sepsis: a randomized controller trial. JAMA. 2003;290:238–47.
112. Warren BL, et al. Caring for the critically ill patients. High dose antithrombin III in severe sepsis: a randomized controller trial. JAMA. 2001;286:1869–78.
113. Ranieri VM, et al. Drotrecogin alpha activated in adults with septic shock. N Engl J Med. 2012;366:2055–64.
114. Kerlin BA, et al. Survival advantage associated with heterozygous factor V Leiden mutation in patients with severe sepsis and in mouse endotoxemia. Blood. 2003;102:3085–92.
115. Van Mens TE, et al. Evolution of factor V Leiden. Thromb Haemost. 2013;110:23–30.
116. De Backer D, et al. Effects of drotrecogin alfa activated on microcirculatory alterations in patients with severe sepsis. Crit Care Med. 2006;34:1918–24.
117. Donati A, et al. The aPC treatment improves microcirculation in severe sepsis/septic shock syndrome. BMC Anesthesiol. 2013;13:25.
118. Kalil AC, LaRosa SP. Effectiveness and safety of drotrecogin alfa activated for severe sepsis: a meta-analysis and meta-regression. Lancet Infect Dis. 2012;12:678–86.
119. Iba T, et al. Efficacy and bleeding risk of antithrombin supplementation in septic disseminated intravascular coagulation: a secondary survey. Crit Care. 2014;18:497.
120. Jiang L, et al. The efficacy and safety of different anticoagulant on patients with severe sepsis and derangment of coagulation: a protocol for network meta-analysis of randomized controlled trials. BMJ Open. 2014;4:e006770.
121. Copeland S, et al. Acute inflammatory response to endotoxin in mice and humans. Clin Diagn Lab Immunol. 2005;12:60–7.
122. Remik DG, Ward PA. Evaluation of endotoxin models for the study of sepsis. Shock. 2005;24(Suppl 1):7–11.
123. Levi M, et al. Factor V Leiden mutation in severe infection and sepsis. Semin Thromb Hemost. 2011;37:955–60.
124. Niessen RW, et al. Antithrombin acts as a negative acute phase protein as established with studies on HepG2 cells and in baboons. Thromb Haemost. 1997;78:1088–92.
125. Hayakawa M, et al. The response of antithrombin III activity after supplementation decreases in proportion to the severity of sepsis and liver dysfunction. Shock. 2008;30:649–52.
126. Bergmann S, Hammerschmidt S. Fibrinolysis and host response in bacterial infections. Thromb Haemost. 2007;98:512–20.
127. Kipnis E, et al. Massive alveolar thrombin activation in Pseudomonas aeruginosa induced acute lung injury. Shock. 2004;21:444–51.
128. Robriquet I, et al. Intravenous administration of activated protein C in Pseudomonas induced lung injury: impact on lung fluid balance and the inflammatory response. Respir Res. 2006;7:41.
129. Opal SM, et al. The next generation of sepsis clinical trial designs: what is next after the demise of recombinant human activated protein C? Crit Care Med. 2014;42:1714–21.
130. Levi M, et al. Infection and inflammation and the coagulation system. Cardiovasc Res. 2003;60:26–39.
131. Pawlinski R, et al. Role of tissue factor and protease activated receptors in a mouse model of endotoxemia. Blood. 2004;103:1342–7.
132. Xu H, et al. A coagulation factor VII deficiency protects against acute inflammatory responses in mice. J Pathol. 2006;210:488–96.
133. Kojima M, et al. A historical study on microthrombi in autopsy cases of DIC. Bibl Haematol. 1983;49:95–106.

134. Tajiri T, et al. Autopsy cases of fulminant bacterial infection in adults: clinical onset depends on the virulence of bacteria and patient immune status. J Infect Chemother. 2012;18:637–45.
135. Tajiri T, et al. Clinicopathological findings in fulminant type pneumococcal infection: report of three autopsy cases. Pathol Int. 2007;57:606–12.
136. Donzè JD, et al. Impact of sepsis on risk of postoperative arterial and venous thromboses: large prospective color study. BMJ. 2014;349:g5334.
137. Ribeiro DD, et al. Pneumonia and risk of venous thrombosis results from the MEGA study. J Thromb Haemost. 2012;10:1179–82.
138. Picoli-Quaino SK, et al. Impairment of thrombin generation in the early phases of the host response in sepsis. J Crit Care. 2014;29:31–6.
139. Massion PB, et al. Persistent hypocoagulability in patients with septic shock predicts greater hospital mortality: impact of impaired thrombin generation. Intensive Care Med. 2012;38:1326–35.
140. Brune M, Hochberg Z. Evolutionary medicine – the quest for a better under standing of health, disease and prevention. BMC Med. 2013;11:116.
141. Ziegler EJ, et al. Tretment of gram negative bacteremia and septic shock with HA-1° human monoclonal antibody against endotoxin. A randomized, double blind, placebo controller trial. The HA-1° Sepsis Study Group. N Engl J Med. 1991;324:429–36.
142. Fisher CJ, et al. Treatment of septic shock with the tumor necrosis factor receptor: Fc fusion protein. The soluble TNF Receptor Sepsis Study Group. N Engl J Med. 1996;334:1697–702.
143. Wunderink RG, et al. Recombinant tissue factor pathway inhibitor in severe community acquired pneumonia: a randomized trial. Am J Respir Crit Care Med. 2011;183:1561–8.
144. de Jonge E, et al. Tissue factor pathway inhibitor dose-dependently inhibits coagulation activation without influencing the fibrinolyrtic and cytokine response during human endotoxemia. Blood. 2000;95:1124–9.
145. Laterre PF, et al. A clinical evaluation committee assessment of recombinant human tissue factor pathway inhibitior (tifacogin) in patients with sevvere community acquired pneumonia. Crit Care. 2009;13:R36.
146. Roemisch J, et al. Antithrombin: a new look at the actions of a serine protease inhibitor. Blood Coagul Fibrinolysis. 2002;13:657–70.
147. Gando S, et al. A randomized controller multi center trial of the effects of antithrombin on DIC in patients with sepsis. Crit Care. 2013;17:R297.
148. Iba T, et al. Efficacy and bleeding risk of antithrombin supplement in septic DIC: a prospective multi center survey. Thromb Res. 2012;130:e129–33.
149. Neviere R, et al. Antithrombin reduces mesenteric venular leokocyte interaction and small intestine injury in endotoxemic rats. Shock. 2001;15:220–5.
150. Yamashiro K, et al. Inhibitory effects of antithrombin III agaist leukocyte rolling and infiltration during endotoxin induced uveitis in rats. Invest Ophtalmol Vis Sci. 2001;42:1553–60.
151. Oelschlager C, et al. Antithrombin III inhibits nuclear factor kB activation in human monocytes and vascular endothelial cells. Blood. 2002;99:4015–20.
152. Souter PJ, et al. Antithrombin inhibits lipopolysaccharide induced tissue factor and interleukin 6 production by mononuclear cells, human ombelical vein endothelial cells and whole blood. Crit Care Med. 2001;29:134–9.
153. van der Poll T, Opal SM. Host-pathogen interactions in sepsis. Lancet Infect Dis. 2008;8:32–43.
154. Minnema MC, et al. Recombinant human antithrombin III improves serviva and attenuates inflammatory responses in baboons lethally challenged with *Escherichia coli*. Blood. 2000;95:1117–23.
155. Tagami T, et al. Antithrombin and mortality in severe pneumonia patients with sepsis associated disseminated intravascular coagulation: an observational nationwide study. J Thromb Haemost. 2014;12:1470–9.
156. Eisele B, et al. Antithrombin III in patients with severe sepsis. A randomized, placebo controller, double blind multi center trial plus a meta-analysis on all randomized, placebo

controlled, double blind trials with antithrombin III in severe sepsis. Intensive Care Med. 1998;24:663–72.

157. Kienast J, et al. Treatment effects of high dose antithrombin without concomitant heparin in patients with severe sepsis with or without disseminated intravascular coagulation. J Thromb Haemost. 2006;4:90–7.

158. Casserly B, et al. Evaluating the use of recombinant human activated protein C in adult severe sepsis: results of the surviving sepsis campaign. Crit Care Med. 2012;40:1417–26.

159. Griffin JH, et al. Activated protein C. J Thromb Haemost. 2007;5:73–80.

160. Mosnier LO, et al. The cytoprotective protein C pathway. Blood. 2007;109:3161–72.

161. Feistritzer C, Riewald M. Endothelial barrier protection by activated protein C through PAR 1 dependent sphingosine 1-phosphatase receptor 1 cross activation. Blood. 2005;105:3178–84.

162. Joyce DE, et al. Leukocyte and endothelial cell interactions in sepsis: relevance of the protein C pathway. Crit Care Med. 2004;32:5280–6.

163. Rezaie AR. Regulation of the protein C anticoagulant and antiinflammatory pathways. Curr Med Chem. 2010;17:2059–69.

164. Chaput C, Zychlinsky A. The dark side of histones. Nat Med. 2009;15:1245–6.

165. Bernard GR, et al. Efficacy and safety of recombinant human activated protein C for severe sepsis. N Engl J Med. 2001;344:699–709.

166. Dellinger RP, et al. Surviving sepsis campaign guidelines for management of severe sepsis and septic shock. Crit Care Med. 2004;32:858–73.

167. Wiedermann CJ. When a single pivotal trial should be not enough- the case of drotrecogin alfa (activated). Intensive Care Med. 2006;32:604.

168. Hoppensteadt D, et al. Thrombin generation mediators and markers in sepsis associated coagulopathy and their modulation by recombinant thrombomodulin. Clin Appl Thromb Hemost. 2014;20:129–35.

169. Saito H, et al. Efficacy and safety of recombinant human soluble thrombomodulin (ART 123) in disseminated intravascular coagulation: results of phase III, randomized, double blind clinical trial. J Thromb Haemost. 2007;5:31–41.

170. Ogawa Y, et al. Recombinant human soluble thrombomodulin improves mortality and respiratory dysfunction in patients with severe sepsis. J Trauma Acute Care Surg. 2012;72:1150–7.

171. Vincent JL, et al. A randomized double blind placebo controlled phase 2b study to evaluate the safety and efficacy of recombinant human soluble thrombomodulin ART 123 in patients with severe sepsis and suspected disseminated intravascular coagulation. Crit Care Med. 2013; 41:2069–79.

172. Conway EM. Thrombomodulin and its role in inflammation. Semin Immunopathol. 2012; 34:107–25.

173. Iba T, et al. Recombinant thrombomodulin improves the microcirculation by attenuating the leukocyte-endothelial interaction in the rat LPS model. Thromb Res. 2013;131:295–9.

174. Shi CS, et al. The Lectin like domain of thrombomodulin binds to its specific ligand lewis y antigen and neutralizes lipopolysaccharide induced inflammatory response. Blood. 2008;112: 3661–70.

175. Fourrier F, et al. Double blind, placebo controller trial of antithrombin III concentrates in septic shock with disseminated intravascular coagulation. Chest. 1993;104:882–8.

176. Yamakawa K, et al. Treatment effects of recombinant human soluble thrombomodulin in patients with severe sepsis: a historical control study. Crit Care. 2011;15:R123.

177. Polderman KH, Girbes AR. Drug intervention trials in sepsis: divergent results. Lancet. 2004;363:1721–3.

178. Liu XL, et al. Low dose heparin as treatment for early disseminated intravascular coagulation during sepsis: a prospective clinical study. Exp Ther Med. 2014;7:604–8.

179. Wang C, et al. Heparin therapy reduces 28 day mortality in adults severe sepsis patients: a systematic review and meta-analysis. Crit Care. 2014;18:563.

180. Kasten KR, et al. Interleukin 7 (IL-7) treatment accelerates neutrophil recruitment through gamma delta T cell IL-7 production in a murine model of sepsis. Infect Immun. 2010;78: 4714–22.

181. Unsinger J, et al. Ipromotes cell viability trafficking, and functionality and improves surrvival in sepsis. J Immunol. 2010;184:3768–79.
182. Chang K, et al. Targeting the programmed cell death 1: programmed cell death ligand 1 pathway reverses T cell eustion in patients with sepsis. Crit Care. 2014;18:R3.
183. Venet F, et al. IL-7 restores lymphocytes functions in septic patients. J Immunol. 2012;189: 5073–81.
184. Schouten M, et al. Inflammation, endothelium and coagulation in sepsis. J Leukoc Biol. 2008;83:536–45.
185. Faust SN, et al. Dysfunction of endothelial protein C activation in severe meningococcal sepsis. N Engl J Med. 2001;345:408–16.
186. De Kleijn ED, et al. Activation of protein C following infusion of protein C concentrate in children with severe meningococcal sepsis and purpura fulminans: a randomized double blinded, placebo controller, dose-finding study. Crit Care Med. 2003;31:1839–47.
187. Dhainaut JF, et al. PROWESS study group: Drotrecogin alpha (activated) in the treatment of severe sepsis patients with multiple organ dysfunction: data fron the PROWESS trial. Intensive Care Med. 2003;29:894–903.
188. Ely EW, PROWESS Investigators, et al. Drotrecogin alpha (activated) administration across clinically important subgroups of patients with severe sepsis. Crit Care Med. 2003;31:12–9.
189. Wiederman CJ, Kaneider NC. A systematic review of antithrombin concentrate use in patients with disseminated intravascular coagulation of severe sepsis. Blood Coagul Fibrinolysis. 2006;17:521–6.
190. Nadel S, A global Perspective (RESOLVE) Study Group, et al. Drotrecogin alpha (activated) in children with severe sepsis: a multicentre phase III randomized controller trial. Lancet. 2007; 369:836–43.
191. Johanson PI, et al. Hypocoagulability, as evacuate by thromboelastography, at admission to the ICU is associated with increased 30 day mortality. Blood Coagul Fibrinolysis. 2010;21: 168–74.
192. Park MS, et al. Thromboelastography as a better indicator of hypercoagulable state after injury than prothrombin time or activated partial thromboplastin time. J Trauma. 2009;67: 266–75.
193. Collins PW, et al. Global tests of haemostasis in critically ill patients with severe sepsis syndrome compared to controls. Br J Haematol. 2006;135:220–7.
194. Levi M. Another step in improving the diagnosis of disseminated intravascular coagulation in sepsis. Crit Care. 2013;17:448.

Atrial Fibrillation in the Perioperative Period

5

Franco Cavaliere and Carlo Cavaliere

Atrial fibrillation (AF) is the most common cardiac arrhythmia in the general population. Its incidence increases with age so that in next years the number of subjects affected is likely to grow due to the elongation of average life expectancy. AF is an arrhythmia that poses major health problems because it is associated with greater incidence of arterial thromboembolism, stroke, heart failure, and higher overall mortality [1–6].

5.1 Epidemiology and Classification

A recent study has shown that AF has a prevalence of 1.8% in the Italian population over 15 years of age. Similar percentages, around 2%, were detected in England, Germany, and Sweden. In the USA, this arrhythmia affects 3–6% of hospitalized patients. Prevalence is higher in Caucasians and increases in the presence of congestive heart failure, valvulopathies, arterial hypertension, atrial tachyarrhythmias (returning nodal tachycardia, WPW syndrome), various thoracic diseases, sepsis, and conditions that increase the cardiovascular risk (diabetes mellitus, obesity, smoking).

AF is classified as: (a) persistent, if it lasts for longer than 7 days; (b) paroxysmal, if it reoccurs in less than seven days after being resolved, spontaneously or as a result of a therapeutic intervention; (c) long-standing persistent, if it lasts more than 12 months; (d) permanent, if the doctor and the patient decide to stop the attempts to resolve the arrhythmia. Valvular AF refers to patients with mitral stenosis or

F. Cavaliere (✉)
Department of Cardiovascular Sciences, Catholic University of the Sacred Heart, Rome, Italy
e-mail: fcavaliere54@gmail.com

C. Cavaliere
ENT Clinic, "Sapienza" University of Rome, Rome, Italy

© Springer International Publishing AG 2018
D. Chiumello (ed.), *Practical Trends in Anesthesia and Intensive Care 2017*,
http://doi.org/10.1007/978-3-319-61325-3_5

artificial heart valves; North American guidelines include valve repair in this group. In comparison with non-valvular ones, valvular AF may be associated with a higher risk of stroke and needs a specific prophylactic approach.

5.2 Etiology and Pathogenesis

AF pathogenesis is complex and not yet completely clarified. At the basis of this arrhythmia, there are some electrical alterations of the atrial myocardium. They include inhomogeneities of the refractory period that facilitate the onset of re-entry mechanisms; after-depolarizations (oscillations) that intervene during early or late reuptake phases, promoting the onset of extrasystoles; ectopic focal depolarizations, which often originate from pulmonary vein confluence areas in the left atrium. Finally, some studies have shown a correlation between the incidence of postoperative AF and the duration of P wave on the ECG.

The abovementioned electrical alterations can be induced by different factors. Genetic abnormalities are often the basis of isolated AF that is not associated with other cardiac disorders and occurs in subjects less than 60 years old. In most cases, however, the onset of AF is the consequence of structural alterations of the atria, which include fibrosis, dilation, hypertrophy, ischemia, and infiltration. Fibrosis, which manifests itself with an increase in the amount of collagen, is a process that progresses with age and is considered to be the primary responsible for the high incidence of AF in the elderly. Atrial dilation occurs during the natural history of mitral valvulopathy and left ventricular dysfunction. In the intra- and post-operative period, the atria may dilate acutely, for fluid mobilization or excessive intake; in addition, atriotomy performed in cardiac surgery represents an important mechanism of stimulation. In the perioperative period, the hyperactivity of the autonomic nervous system and the increased levels of mediators of inflammation, and oxidizing agents have a marked influence on atrial activity, favoring the onset of AF. Sympathetic hyperactivity also facilitates the occurrence of ectopic outbreaks and re-entry circuits, and shortens the refractory period. As a result, pain, agitation, and in general all factors that stimulate sympathetic activity may favor the onset of AF. A similar effect may be caused by the reduction of parasympathetic tone, while parasympathomimetic drugs as opioids may have a protective action.

5.3 Presentation and Diagnosis

The onset of AF is often felt by the patient for heart rate irregularity. In some cases, the arrhythmia manifests itself directly with an embolic episode. At clinical examination, AF can be suspected for irregularities of the arterial pulse and cardiac tones. Diagnosis is confirmed by the electrocardiographic detection of an absolute irregularity of the RR intervals, of the absence of the P wave or of an atrial cycle duration (when visible) irregular and less than 200 ms (corresponding to a frequency higher than 300 bpm). In the case of paroxysmal AF, which alternates with sinus rhythm periods, it is often necessary to resort to Holter monitoring.

Predisposing causes should be recognized and, if possible, treated. Electrocardiogram can show the presence of various electrical abnormalities, left ventricular hypertrophy, branch blocks, signs of myocardial infarction. Ashman's phenomenon consists in an aberrant intraventricular conduction (broad QRS complexes) in beats associated with a short RR cycle preceded by a longer RR one; it originates from the prolongation of the refractory period that follows long RR cycles. Transthoracic echocardiography (TTE) allows to evaluate valve function, contractility, chamber dimensions and wall thickness; systolic pulmonary pressure can often be estimated and the presence of endocavitary thrombi assessed. On this purpose, however, transesophageal echocardiogram (TEE) is more effective. AF is sometimes associated with thoracic diseases that can be diagnosed or suspected based on chest X-ray. The presence of extra cardiac diseases associated with a higher incidence of AF, as hyper- or hypothyroidism, should also be investigated.

5.4   Treatment

5.4.1   Prevention of Atrial Thrombosis and Thromboembolism

Three classes of drugs are used: vitamin K inhibitors, new oral anticoagulants, and platelet antiaggregates [7–10]:

1. *Sodium warfarin* (Coumadin®) and *acenocoumarol* (Sintrom®), known as vitamin K inhibitors or dicumarolics, hinder the hepatic synthesis of coagulation factors II, VII, IX, and X, and of proteins C and S. Vitamin K inhibitors are the gold standard for prevention of thromboembolism, but their narrow therapeutic range requires frequent controls of coagulation parameters and entails a greater risk of hemorrhagic complications. Their anticoagulant effect is assessed with the International Normalized Ratio (INR), the ratio between the prothrombin time of the patient and that of standard plasma blends. INR should be maintained between 2 and 3 or between 2.5 and 3.5 depending on the thrombogenic risk that characterizes the patient. The activity of this class of drugs is influenced by liver function, but not by renal function; besides, it can be influenced by the intake of numerous drugs and certain foods. In the initial phase of the therapy, INR should be dosed at least once a week; successively, dosages can be performed once a month. In the case of overdose or of the need to restore normal coagulation, the anticoagulant effect can be inhibited by the administration of vitamin K (Konakion®, 5–25 mg intravenously, possible allergic reactions) or, in urgent cases, of fresh frozen plasma (15 mL/kg) or concentrated prothrombin complex (30–50 units/kg).
2. *New oral anticoagulants* are the direct thrombin inhibitor dabigatran (Pradaxa®), and the two factor X inhibitors, apixaban (Eliquis®) and rivaroxaban (Xarelto®). Dabigatran is a competitive thrombin inhibitor and prevents the conversion of fibrinogen to fibrin. Apixaban and rivaroxaban are selective inhibitors of factor Xa. This factor intervenes at the point of convergence between intrinsic and extrinsic pathways of coagulation; its inhibition blocks the conversion of prothrombin

Table 5.1 CHA2DS2-VASc score utilized to quantify the risk of thromboembolism in patients affected by AF

C	Congestive Heart Failure History	1
H	Arterial **Hypertension** History	1
A_2	**Age** ≥75 years	2
D	**Diabetes**	1
S_2	**Stroke**/TIA/Thromboembolism History	2
V	**Vascular** Diseases History (i.e., obliterating arteriopathy, myocardial infarctum, coronary artery disease)	1
A	**Age** 65–74 years	1
Sc	Female **Sex**	1

The final score is obtained by adding partial scores. The zero value corresponds to low-risk; the value of one corresponds to low-moderate risk; values of two or greater correspond to moderate-high risk (modified from [2])

into thrombin. Unlike vitamin K inhibitors, these drugs do not require routine monitoring of coagulation parameters. Their blood levels increase in the presence of kidney failure which, when severe, contraindicates their use. Moderate renal function impairment requires a reduction in dosage. The relatively short half-life, 12–17 h for dabigatran, 5–9 h for rivaroxaban, and 12 h for apixaban, is the basis of the risk of thromboembolic episodes shortly after the acute suspension of these drugs. If dabigatran is to be discontinued and substituted with vitamin K inhibitors, the latter should be initiated 3 days before the last dose of dabigatran. In case of severe bleeding, the suspension of these drugs is recommended as well as the administration of coagulation factors, in particular, prothrombin complex concentrates. Specific antidotes for this class of drugs are now available. Idarucizumab is a humanized mouse monoclonal antibody fragment that reverses the effects of dabigatran and Andexanet alfa is a recombinant modified human factor Xa decoy protein that binds factor X inhibitors.

3. *Platelet antiaggregants* like acetylsalicylic acid, ticlopidine, and clopidogrel are relatively safe drugs, but their efficacy on thromboembolism is definitely lower than that of anticoagulants.

Prophylaxis of thromboembolism should be performed regardless of the type of AF, paroxysmal, persistent or permanent, but does not eliminate the risk of thrombosis. Vitamin K inhibitors, which provide the greatest protection, assure a reduction in embolic episodes of 60–70%. Of note, not all patients with AF have the same degree of risk of thromboembolism. Numerous indices expressing the risk of thromboembolism are available; CHA2DS2-VASc is the one suggested by the American Heart Association guidelines (Table 5.1). The score obtained with this index varies from 1 to 10. A value of zero is associated with a very low-risk and requires no therapy or, at most, the administration of platelet antiaggregates. A value of one suggests the need of platelet antiaggregates. Scores of two or more indicate the use of new oral anticoagulants or dicumarolics. The choice of prophylaxis modalities also depends on which heart disease is associated to AF. In patients affected by valvulopathies, only dicumarolics are indicated for the particularly high risk of thromboembolism. In cases where dicumarolic therapy is indicated, anticoagulation should be initiated as soon as possible with unfractionated heparin (an initial bolus of 80 UI/kg, followed by the infusion of 18 UI/kg/h, titrated to obtain an aPTT of 45–60 s) or with low molecular weight heparin (100 UI to 1 mg/kg every 12 h).

5.4.2 Rate Control vs Rhythm Control Strategies

Apart from the thromboembolic risk, AF poses two main problems: the loss of the atrial pump to ventricular filling and the onset of too high or low ventricular rates. These alterations are particularly damaging in patients with left ventricle diastolic dysfunction or mitral stenosis. The therapeutic goal can be limited to maintain ventricular rate within an acceptable range (rate control) or aimed to restore sinus rhythm (rhythm control). Although the second approach may appear as the best one, it should be considered that 50% of recent-onset AFs spontaneously convert to the sinus rhythm and that from the point of view of survival and morbidity, no significant difference has been observed between the two strategies.

5.4.2.1 Rate Control
In AF, the average ventricular rate depends on the length of the refractory period of the atrioventricular node, which blocks most of the electrical impulses that arrive from the atria at a frequency greater than 300 bpm. A too high rate may compromise ventricular filling and cause myocardial ischemia. On the other hand, bradycardia can interfere with the function of the left ventricle both in systolic and diastolic dysfunction. In the former, tachycardia represents a compensation mechanism; in the latter, diastolic stiffness limits the volume of blood that the left ventricle can accept in diastole. The rate control strategy aims to keep the average ventricular rate at rest below 80 bpm. In acute cases with good hemodynamic compensation, an initial goal may be to maintain the rate below 110 bpm. In order to control ventricular rate, the refractory period of the atrioventricular node is increased to reduce the number of atrial excitations transmitted through the conduction system. For this purpose, some drugs can be used:

- Beta-blockers act by reducing the effects of sympathetic hyperactivity; furthermore, they are particularly effective to prevent myocardial ischemia. Their prophylactic activity against AF has been proved in at least two conditions: paroxysmal AF induced by sympathetic hyperactivity and postoperative AF that occurs in 30% of patients after cardiac surgery. Main contraindications are the severe systolic dysfunction of the left ventricle and bronchial obstruction. Several molecules are used, including atenolol, bisoprolol, carvedilol, metoprolol, nadolol, propranolol, and timolol. Metoprolol is administered acutely at the dosage of 2.5–5 mg every 5 min up to 10–15 mg; oral dosage varies from 25 to 100 mg every 12 h. A special role is played by esmolol, which is particularly valuable in critically ill patients because of its short half-life of about 10 min. The dosage is 0.05–0.2 mg/kg/min after an initial bolus of 0.5 mg/kg.
- Non-dihydropyridine calcium antagonists (verapamil, diltiazem) prolong atrioventricular node conduction and refractory period. They have negative inotropic

and vasodilator effects, which contraindicate their use in ventricular systolic dysfunction and in arterial hypotension. They should also be avoided in patients with Wolff–Parkinson–White (WPW) syndrome. Verapamil can be administered intravenously as a bolus, 5–20 mg, and in rare cases as an infusion, at a rate of 5–10 mg/h. Orally, the dosage is 40–80 mg every 8 h.

- Amiodarone is a class III antiarrhythmic drug (K channel blockers) according to Vaughan Williams classification, and is effective both to reduce mean ventricular rate and to restore sinus rhythm. This drug is particularly useful in patients with cardiovascular instability and/or systolic dysfunction because of its modest negative inotropic effect; the vasodilator effect is also mild and is clinically apparent only during rapid intravenous infusion. Amiodarone may cause phlebitis and prolongation of QT with potential induction of polymorphic ventricular tachycardia (torsades de pointes); it is also contraindicated in WPW syndrome. Intravenously, an initial injection of 300 mg is given as a slow injection in 10 min (risk of hypotension by vasodilatation) or as an infusion in 2 h, followed by a 5-h infusion at a rate of 75 mg/h, and finally by a constant-rate infusion at 18 mg/h. Orally, the dosage is 200–400 mg daily.
- Digitalis slows down the average ventricular rate in the presence of AF because it increases the parasympathetic tone. For this reason, it may be ineffective in conditions characterized by an increased activity of sympathetic hyperactivity, as is often the case in the perioperative period. Digoxin is contraindicated in WPW syndrome. In the attack phase, the loading dose is 0.5–1 mg iv, followed by a maintenance dose of 0.25 mg orally.

The choice of the drugs to be used for heart rate control is partly based on associated pathologies. For instance, beta-blockers and calcium antagonists are indicated for the presence of coronary heart disease and arterial hypertension, digitalis in the presence of heart failure. A particular case is that of patients with WPW syndrome. Drugs such as calcium antagonists, amiodarone, and digitalis increase the refractory period of the atrioventricular node. In case the refractory period of the accessory bundle is shorter than the atrioventricular node, electric impulses can be transmitted from the atria to the ventricles through the former and high ventricular rates can occur. In patients with WPW, rate control approach is therefore based on the administration of beta-blockers, but rhythm control is recommended.

5.4.2.2 Rhythm Control

The decision to pursue AF conversion to sinus rhythm in emergency conditions is generally based on the presence of hemodynamic instability, too high or low ventricular rates, and myocardial ischemia. Otherwise, it is reasonable to follow the rate control strategy and to shift to the rhythm control only after a few days, when a spontaneous cardioversion becomes unlikely. The sinus rhythm can be restored by an electrical or pharmacological cardioversion. The former is recommended in patients with WPW syndrome.

- Electrical cardioversion. Its main advantage is the very high percentage of success, even in persistent AFs. Disadvantages are the need for sedation, the risk of thromboembolism, the proarrhythmic effect, possible skin lesions, and potential interference with medical devices, such as pacemakers and Implantable Cardioverter Defibrillators.

In electrical cardioversion, a monophasic or biphasic, synchronous shock is applied with an initial current intensity of 100–200 J. The classic position of the plates is that the sternal one is placed to the right of the sternal margin and immediately below the collarbone, while the apex one is positioned at the height of the left nipple at the midaxillary line. In cases of failure, in addition to testing for greater current intensity, the plates can be positioned in the antero-posterior position (left parasternal, left subscapular), which would favor the passage of a larger amount of current through the atria. The success of cardioversion depends on the amount of current that crosses the heart. A high body mass index (BMI) reduces the chances of success. The contact between the plate and the skin is particularly important because the air is an electrical insulator. In addition to the use of conductive pastes, gels, or adhesive plates, it is useful to exert pressure on the plates themselves. Some authors suggest to reduce electrical impedance by performing a trichotomy in areas where plates will be applied. The shock should be administered during exhalation when the chest impedance is lower. Furthermore, a second electric shock has more chances of success after an ineffective result because the electric impedance is reduced; the optimum lapse of time would be around 3 min.

Administration of some antiarrhythmic drugs influences the success of the attempt of electric cardioversion. Atropine given immediately before the electric shock could increase the rate of success. Verapamil, amiodarone, quinidine, and propafenone may be effective in preventing a new onset of AF after efficacious cardioversion. The incidence of recurrences is greater in AFs that last for more than a year and in those associated with not well-controlled hyperthyroidism, mitral valve diseases, congestive heart failure, and generally with an enlargement of the left atrium (diameter greater than 5 cm).

- Pharmacological cardioversion does not require sedation and, in case of failure, can facilitate the success of electrical cardioversion. On the other hand, it may require hospitalization and cardiovascular monitoring; it is proarrhythmic, involves the risk of thromboembolism, and is characterized by limited success rates for long-term AFs. Pharmacological cardioversion is indeed more effective in recent atrial fibrillations. In those less than seven days old, the percentage of success within 24 h from the beginning of antiarrhythmic therapy varies from 34 to 95%. Over seven days, the percentage falls below 40%, and often it is necessary to resort to electrical cardioversion.

Various antiarrhythmics may be used, including flecainamide 2 mg iv or 200–300 mg/os, propafenone 2 mg iv or 450–600 mg/os, amiodarone at the dosage reported above, ibutilide, dofetilide. Flecainamide and propafenone can sometimes convert AF into flutter and therefore require calcium antagonists or beta-blockers to slow the pulse transmission at the atrioventricular node level. In the patient who develops AF after surgery, the classic choice is that of amiodarone, especially when there is a basic heart disease. Vernakalant is a new antiarrhythmic agent indicated for the treatment of AF that occurs in the postoperative period after cardiac surgery. Given within three days from the onset of arrhythmia, the drug is administered intravenously at a dose of 3 mg/kg over 10 min and has a 50% success rate within 90 min from the administration (far greater than that of amiodarone). It is contraindicated in case of bradycardia, hypotension, marked prolongation of QT, severe valvulopathies, congestive heart failure.

5.4.2.3 Anticoagulant Therapy and Cardioversion

Whether cardioversion is performed electrically or pharmacologically, it exposes the patient to the risk of mobilization of any thrombi formed within the atria. In addition, even after sinus rhythm restoration, there is a temporary risk of formation of thrombi due to the persistence of transient atrial dyskinesias and generally to the risk of AF recurrence. In accordance with current guidelines, the prevention of these complications should be based on the time elapsed from the onset of arrhythmia:

(a) Patients in AF for less than 48 h:
  • High embolic risk: cardioversion is followed by anticoagulation for at least 4 weeks, started with unfractionated heparin or low molecular weight heparin and continued with dicumarolics.
  • Low embolic risk: cardioversion is followed by one options among heparin, low molecular weight heparin, new oral anticoagulant (dabigatran, rivaroxaban, or apixaban), or no therapy.
(b) Patients in AF for 48 h or more or for an unknown time period:
  • Non-urgent cardioversion: anticoagulation with dicumarolics (INR from 2 to 3) is performed three weeks before and 4 weeks later; new oral anticoagulants (dabigatran, rivaroxaban, or apixaban) can also be utilized. Alternatively, it is reasonable to proceed to cardioversion if transesophageal echocardiography excludes the presence of thrombi in the left atrium (particularly in the auricula) provided that anticoagulation is achieved before cardioversion.
  • Urgent cardioversion: electrical cardioversion and anticoagulation for the next four weeks initiated as soon as possible (low molecular weight heparin or heparin followed by dicumarolics)

5.5   Some Further Points

During the perioperative period, the anesthetist is called, in collaboration with other specialists and in particular with the cardiologist, to handle three main issues.

In patients affected by AF, the anticoagulant treatment should be discontinued during surgery and in the immediate postoperative period. After the interruption of oral anticoagulants, the recovery of an INR <1.5 is expected after at least 4–5 days. In the case of dabigatran, suspension should occur 1 or 2 days before surgery in patients with normal renal function and up to 4 days before in patients with creatinine clearance between 30 and 50 mL/min and undergoing high-risk hemorrhagic surgery.

In the lapse of time from the end of oral anticoagulants to surgery, treatment depends on the degree of thromboembolic risk assessed by the above-described scores:

- In patients with high thromboembolic risk, non-fractionated heparin or low molecular weight heparin is administered at therapeutic doses up to 12 h before surgery
- In patients with moderate thromboembolic risk, non-fractionated heparin or low molecular weight heparin is administered at therapeutic or prophylactic doses
- In patients with low-thromboembolic risk, low-molecular-weight heparin is given at prophylactic doses or not at all.

In patients who develop AF during the perioperative period, the treatment is based on the choice between rate control and rhythm control strategies. In cardiac or thoracic surgery, where the incidence of AF in the postoperative period is around 30–40%, high ventricular frequency should be preferably treated with beta blockers, provided there are no contraindications to their use. If the ventricular rate is not adequately controlled, a non-dihydropyridine calcium antagonist (verapamil, diltiazem) should be associated. Sinus rhythm restorative attempts can be performed with ibutilide or with cardioversion if AF persists. Anticoagulant therapy should be initiated and maintained according to the criteria used in non-surgical patients. Some drugs have prophylactic action against perioperative AF, and their use should therefore be considered in high-risk subjects. Beta-blockers could reduce the incidence of AF to 19% in cardiac surgery. Other therapeutic options are amiodarone and sotalol; colchicine is used because of its anti-inflammatory action.

During trans-catheter ablation, anesthesia support for patient sedation/anesthesia is often required. The procedure involves electrical separation of the entry point of the pulmonary veins from the rest of the atrium. This separation is obtained by causing an atrial wall injury by application of low temperatures (cryoablation) or radiolabel, resulting into the formation of a fibrous scar. In last few years, radio anatomic mapping systems have been introduced to create a three-dimensional representation of the atrium and the areas under ablation during the procedure. Such systems have considerably increased the effectiveness of ablation procedures, but have also prolonged the duration. Moreover, they are extremely sensitive to patient movements. It is therefore generally necessary to perform the procedure under sedation (usually midazolam and fentanyl), deep sedation (usually propofol and fentanyl), or general anesthesia. Each technique has advantages and disadvantages. General anesthesia and deep sedation ensure the patient's immobility even for long periods, but may in part hinder the recognition of some complications. These include perforation of the atrial wall which results in hemopericardium, onset of conduction blocks, formation of atrio-esophageal fistulas, paralysis of the phrenic nerve. In the last case, for example, the use of myorelaxants inhibits the detection of diaphragmatic contractions, which result from nerve stimulation and precede nerve damage. Similarly, general anesthesia abolishes the feeling of intense pain that often precedes atrial wall perforation.

References

1. Chelazzi C, Villa G, De Gaudio AR. Postoperative atrial fibrillation. ISRN Cardiol. 2011; 2011:203179.
2. January CT, Wann LS, Alpert JS, Calkins H, Cigarroa JE, Cleveland JC Jr, ACC/AHA Task Force Members, et al. 2014 AHA/ACC/HRS guideline for the management of patients with atrial fibrillation: executive summary: a report of the American College of Cardiology/ American Heart Association Task Force on practice guidelines and the Heart Rhythm Society. Circulation. 2014;130(23):2071–104.
3. Liao HR, Poon KS, Chen KB. Atrial fibrillation: an anesthesiologist's perspective. Acta Anaesthesiol Taiwanica. 2013;51:34–6.
4. Lip GYH, Tse HF, Lane DA. Atrial fibrillation. Lancet. 2012;379:648–61.
5. Shingu Y, Kubota S, Wakasa S, Ooka T, Tachibana T, Matsui Y. Postoperative atrial fibrillation: mechanism, prevention, and future perspective. Surg Today. 2012;42:819–24.
6. Zoni-Berisso M, Filippi A, Landolina M, et al. Frequency, patient characteristics, treatment strategies, and resource usage of atrial fibrillation (from the Italian Survey of Atrial Fibrillation Management [ISAF] study). Am J Cardiol. 2013;111:705–11.
7. Crystal E, Connolly SJ, Sleik K, Ginger TJ, Yusuf S. Interventions on prevention of postoperative atrial fibrillation in patients undergoing heart surgery: a meta-analysis. Circulation. 2002;106:75–80.
8. Douketis JD, Berger PB, Dunn AS, et al. The perioperative management of antithrombotic therapy: American College of Chest Physicians evidence-based clinical practice guidelines (8th Edition). Chest. 2008;133(6 suppl):299S–339S.
9. O'Dell KM, Igawa D, Hsin J. New oral anticoagulants for atrial fibrillation: a review of clinical trials. Clin Ther. 2012;34:894–901.
10. Whalley D, Skappak C, Lang ES. The need to clot: a review of current management strategies for adverse bleeding events with new oral anticoagulants. Minerva Anestesiol. 2014;80:821–30.

Haemodynamic Monitoring During Anaesthesia

6

Giulia Frasacco and Luigi Tritapepe

Growing complexity of surgical and anaesthetic procedures requires a careful evaluation of the pre-operative patient status and an accurate intra-operative haemodynamic monitoring, considering the progressive increase of fragile and elderly population undergoing surgical procedures.

There are no doubts that intraoperative monitoring of heart rate, body temperature, pulse oximetry, end-tidal CO_2, depth of sedation (complicated to assess objectively through reliable tools), depth of neuromuscular blockade, systemic invasive and non-invasive blood pressure have led to increased safety in the operating room. However, anaesthesiologist's interpretation of these parameters is of great importance.

Modern monitoring system allows clinicians/anaesthesiologists to achieve therapeutic goals, minimizing complications and improving patient outcomes.

Haemodynamic monitoring is not only an alert system avoiding misunderstanding errors (passive monitoring), but also a decision-making instrument for haemodynamic disarrangement evaluation (targeted or active monitoring) which allows prompt action.

Haemodynamic monitoring is necessary for the global patient status assessment, both in the operating room and in intensive care unit.

Monitoring devices are employed in an increasingly invasive and complex steps based on clinical examination and on the patient's response to treatment. Obviously every device could lead to some adverse events (infection, bleeding, etc.).

Appropriate and early application of diagnostic information from haemodynamic monitoring has been shown to reduce mortality and to improve outcome. Data obtained by patient's monitoring are used to manage a clinical plan, according to specific algorithm like the Goal Directed Therapy strategy.

G. Frasacco • L. Tritapepe (✉)
"Sapienza" University of Rome, Rome, Italy
e-mail: luigi.tritapepe@uniroma1.it

© Springer International Publishing AG 2018
D. Chiumello (ed.), *Practical Trends in Anesthesia and Intensive Care 2017*,
http://doi.org/10.1007/978-3-319-61325-3_6

At the bedside, in the operating room and in intensive care unit, a rapid and easy way to assess fluid responsiveness is to give fluid, called a "fluid challenge". More recently, less invasive monitoring improved the assessment of fluid responsiveness (e.g. pulse pressure variation, PPV, systolic pressure variation, SPV, stroke volume variation SVV) rather than a more invasive pulmonary artery catheter monitoring.

Monitoring system devices are getting more and more innovative, with the use of new technologies and advanced assessment devices which can lead to a better comprehension of physiological evaluation in critically ill patients.

Haemodynamic monitoring is the cornerstone of the perioperative patient status evaluation. In an unconscious patient it could offer information regarding cardiac output, fluid challenge status, organ and tissue perfusion, with indirect information about depth of sedation and pain control (hyperdynamic status).

Actually, a new challenge for the anaesthesiologist is to select the appropriate monitoring system for that specific patient in that specific setting.

There are no monitoring systems which can provide a complete evaluation of the patient haemodynamic status, at the same time. On the other hand, it does not seem adequate using several monitoring systems simultaneously.

In this chapter we will focus on different types of haemodynamic monitoring systems in the operating room setting, evaluating different diagnostic information derived from every single system and providing tools to choose the most adequate one for a specific clinical situation.

6.1   Introduction

The SIAARTI Study Group for the security in anaesthesia has developed the document called "Standards for monitoring during Anaesthesia" (ed. 2012; a next publication actually in review) dealing with the haemodynamic monitoring (cardiovascular function monitoring). In this document there are some generic information regarding:

6.1.1   Cardiovascular Assessment

Rationale: to assess an adequate cardiovascular function during anaesthesia.

1. ECG (electrocardiographic) and HR (heart rate). All patients should have a continuous ECG and HR monitoring during anaesthesia (loco-regional or general), with low and high values alarmed.
2. Arterial blood pressure (AP). All patients must have a non-invasive systolic and diastolic blood pressure monitoring, every 5 min interval or more frequent, according to the attending physician. The time of measurements will sign on medical record.
3. According to the clinical patient condition and the type of surgical procedure, the anaesthesiologist could increase the level of monitoring system, using invasive or non-invasive techniques, completed by echocardiography. Invasive arterial

blood pressure, central venous pressure, cardiac output or myocardial function parameters could be recorded.

Our challenge is to achieve the most adequate haemodynamic monitoring for a specific setting, optimizing the cardiovascular function and improving patient outcome.

Haemodynamic monitoring provides dynamic measures of cardiovascular system changes, in real time.

During anaesthesia, monitoring target is to guarantee an adequate tissue perfusion and oxygen delivery; predict and correct all causes of instability, avoiding irreversible organ failure and formulate the next step of therapy.

Different conditions could lead to haemodynamic instability: heart failure, fluid shift, hypovolemia and vascular tone modification.

In simple terms, we use dynamic measures to determine if the cardiac output (CO) is adequate or not and if it will increase with specific treatments (fluid administration, vasoactive or inotropic drugs use). Timely an adequate therapeutic strategy is started, the monitoring tool can assess the answer to therapy.

A combination of clinical examination, prior assessment of therapeutic strategy and the treatment response is often called "dynamic or functional monitoring" [1].

Haemodynamic basic measures and CO monitoring can provide information regarding the depth of anaesthesia and the pain control adequacy (ex: sudden increase in blood pressure and heart rate). Perioperative dynamic monitoring (GDT) involves the optimization of tissue oxygen delivery and allows to decrease the incidence of complications, in-hospital length of stay and mortality [2–4].

Despite improvements in technologies, at the moment there is not a haemodynamic monitoring device which can quantify/measure the whole haemodynamic patient assessment.

Many different tools are available. Every system has its own features and also limitations.

Devices which measure systemic blood pressure, heart rate and cardiac output can be extremely basic and non-invasive, but less accurate for some critical setting (ex: poor peripheral perfusion and vasoconstriction).

Minimal invasive (arterial catheter) and more invasive (central venous line and pulmonary artery catheter) devices directly allow measuring cardiac output. They can require time for positioning and lead to some complications.

Between these two categories of devices there are some monitoring systems which indirectly measure the CO and the fluid responsiveness. They can be used in less critical patients providing cardiac output monitoring, during anaesthesia.

6.1.2 Non-Invasive Arterial Blood Pressure and Heart Rate Measurement

Measuring arterial blood pressure (AP) is a cornerstone of haemodynamic assessment.

Blood pressure may be measured non-invasively with a cuff placed around a limb and attached to a sphygmomanometer or an oscillometric device. The oscillometric device measures systolic and diastolic pressure and the mean arterial blood pressure (MAP) through an algorithm. These devices correlate with the old mercury column system. Oscillometric techniques are less accurate in patients with arrhythmia or if the limb cuff is not well positioned; too small or too tight cuff can overestimate pressure values, on the other hand too wide and too big cuff can underestimate it [5].

Despite being easy to perform, the arterial pressure and the heart rate measures are very difficult to examine. Even if a very low value of blood pressure is often matched with a tachycardia, a normal blood pressure value is not always a haemodynamic stability index [6].

Hypotension can be due to an autonomic nervous system inability to balance the decreased cardiac output and the anomalous oxygen delivery.

The degree of the hypotension value can be different according to patient age, depth of anaesthesia, anaesthetic drug effect on haemodynamic status, pain control, and patient comorbidities. Under general condition, if CO decreases, baroreceptor activity tries to increase the sympathetic tone, leading to an increase in heart rate and vascular tone to restore the mean arterial pressure. So patient could have a sudden haemodynamic instability with a low CO, before hypotension appears [7].

Arterial blood pressure alone is a late marker of haemodynamic instability; if we consider simultaneously the heart rate, we can have information of the haemodynamic status.

During low blood flow or fluid loss, HR and non-invasive AP can detect haemodynamic changes.

Recent clinical trials evaluated the accuracy of less invasive devices which can continuously monitor the non-invasive blood pressure [8] and the cardiac output measured by arterial waveform or plethysmography analysis, in the operating room during anaesthesia [9].

Clinical trials suggest that non-invasive devices with more complex algorithm have a better performance and can be used in selected cases [10].

The gold standard for the arterial blood pressure monitoring is the invasive measure, especially in patients with haemodynamic derangement, needing controlled hypotension or increased organ perfusion or multiple arterial blood gas analysis [11].

Radial artery is the most used for cannulation, because it is rapid to detect and it has lower complications. You need a 20 G artery cannula with Seldinger technique or ultrasound-guidance or direct cannulation.

Allen test can be performed to evaluate the collateral arterial circulation, but with low sensitivity. Complication of this procedure can be: thrombosis, arterial spasm, distal embolism, infection, blood loss, and accidental drug injection.

The arterial blood pressure measurement is done by a non-squeezable closed circuit with a pressure transducer which transforms mechanical pulse in electrical one, visible on monitor screen. The zero of the system is done with the transducer at atmosphere pressure, positioned at the right atrium level or at the Willis circle (surgical procedure in sitting position) [12].

6.1.3 Intravascular Catheter

Central venous catheter and especially the pulmonary artery catheter (PAC) are the most invasive system of monitoring. They provide characteristic haemodynamic information as no other system can do. PAC is inserted through a central venous access (generally right internal jugular or left subclavian vein) and air inflation into the cuff on the tip of the catheter let it sail through the right heart till the pulmonary artery.

Complications are due to attempt of venous punctures and the passage in the right heart sections. The correct positioning in a pulmonary arterial branch is confirmed by the waveform on the monitor (pulmonary capillary Wedge Pressure Waveform—Pcwp).

Although not perfect, the pulmonary artery catheter has long been considered the optimal form of haemodynamic monitoring. Recent clinical trials have not confirmed the clinical effectiveness of its use [13, 14].

However in these trials no clinical target was selected and data have been often misunderstood. It is important to emphasize that the PAC insertion did not affect patient mortality [15] and it is the unique system that can continuously monitor the cardiac output, the mixed venous oxygen saturation (SvO_2), the intra-thoracic vascular pressure and the oxygen delivery (DO_2).

Shoemaker proposed a pre-operative optimization of haemodynamic values to improve post-operative outcomes, based on DO_2 600 mL/min/m^2, haemoglobin 11 g/dL, Pcwp 12 mmHg and targeted inotropic drugs to maximize the oxygen delivery [16–19].

However elevation of DO_2 values to improve haemodynamic status is not always resolving strategy and it can also be harmful [20–22].

Assessing a peri-operative optimization, PAC has to answer the question: could cardiac output provide an adequate oxygen delivery to satisfy metabolic tissue demand? If DO_2 is inadequate, tissue oxygen extraction is increased, with a consequent SvO_2 reduction (<70%). In this setting, low SvO_2 and high intra-thoracic vascular resistances, the cardiac output detects the instability status, leading to a specific therapy. A high CO value with low MAP can show a distributive shock status. On the other hand, a low cardiac output shows: hypovolemic shock (low right atrial pressure CVP and low Pcwp), cardiogenic shock (high CVP and high Pcwp), obstructive shock (CVP > Pcwp and high main pulmonary artery pressure MPAP).

In the presence of haemodynamic instability, the key point is to determine if the cardiac output will increase with fluid administration (preload dependent patient).

The assessment of preload and fluid responsiveness is crucial also in cardiogenic shock [23].

Static pressure (CVP and Pcwp) traditionally have been used to guide fluid management, but they are a poor predictors of fluid responsiveness: low value shows a "poor fluid filling" and high value an "adequate fluid filling".

Since they were rigorously designed, pulmonary artery occlusion pressure and central venous pressure fail to predict ventricular filling volume or fluid responsiveness, with a 50% reliability [24, 25].

The authors suggest that intra-operative or intensive care unit monitoring, with a single measurements of CVP, is not predictive of the patient's volemic status and it should not be used [26].

Even if the pulmonary artery catheter can predict the relationship between cardiac output and metabolic demand, it cannot predict the fluid challenge response.

Dynamic measures such as Stroke Volume Variation (SVV) are more accurate than static measurements for assessing fluid responsiveness in mechanically ventilated patients, during anaesthesia.

Stroke volume is the difference between the maximum and the minimum stroke volume over the main stroke volume measured at the same time, over consecutive mechanical breath. During positive pressure inspiration, the increased intra-thoracic pressure is associated with decreased venous return to the right ventricle (RV) and consequent RV cardiac output reduction (RV is preload-dependent). After 2–3 beat time, left ventricle (LV) stroke volume decreases due to reduced RV filling. These changes in LV stroke volume are most marked when a patient is hypovolemic. Given that the pulse pressure variation (PPV) varies beat-to-beat according to the SVV, PVV measure reflects the stroke volume variation [27–29].

Stroke volume variation and pulse pressure variation are specific and sensitive predictor of fluid responsiveness.

An SVV>15% in patients during mechanically ventilation with tidal volume >8 mL/kg or >10% with tidal volume 6 mL/kg predicts a fluid responsiveness [30–32].

Pulmonary artery catheter cannot quantify the SVV, and in the operating room, clinicians can use two alternative devices to get these information: pulse contour analysis (arterial waveform analysis) and oesophageal-Doppler.

6.1.3.1 Pulse Contour Analysis

Pulse contour analysis requires positioning an arterial line/catheter, generally in the radial or femoral artery. There are five devices providing continuous CO measurement using the arterial pressure waveform. Three of these systems require calibration with the thermodilution method. These monitoring tools assume that the pulse pressure is linked to the stroke volume. However this relationship is not easy and the amplitude of the differential pressure, in a specific stroke volume, depends on the aortic compliance (which has not a linear trend).

After years of study, available data seem sufficient to characterize the relationship between the pressure and the aortic compliance, but only recent technologies have allowed the construction of functional devices that use complex algorithms to analyze the pulse pressure waveform which correlates to the stroke volume. Such algorithms are needed to explain the influence of the reflected waves from the periphery, the magnitude of which is influenced by the systemic vascular resistance [33].

Different monitoring tools, with different algorithms and with or without an initial calibration, use this technology for the measurement of CO, the SVV and PPV.

6.1.4 Calibrated Systems

The more experienced calibrated device uses the transpulmonary thermodilution. A bolus of 20 mL cold saline (<8 °C) is injected into the right atrium via a venous central line and the thermal profile is registered in a central artery (femoral). This calibration method does not recommend the use of the radial artery, so the catheter must be placed in the femoral, axillary or brachial artery.

This system provides the measurement of the CO, the global end-diastolic volume (GEVD), dynamic indices (PPV and SVV). Although some studies have shown that GEDV can be superior to other pressure static measurements in predicting response to preload [34, 35] other studies have however shown a lower correlation.

However, the effectiveness of SVV and PVV in the intraoperative fluid-management has been confirmed [36]. To ensure the accuracy of the continuous measurement of CO, it is important to calibrate the system every 8 hours or if changes in clinical status occur.

An alternative method to measure the cardiac output is using the lithium dilution to calibrate this device. Unlike the transpulmonary thermodilution techniques, the dilution with lithium does not require a central line. Strictly speaking, this method uses the analysis of the pulse oscillatory power to provide continuous cardiac output data.

The analysis of the pressure waves power converts the arterial wave form into a "volume-time wave" using an autocorrelation to determine the stroke volume [37]. The analysis of the pulse power is less influenced by the reflected waves and by the variations in the transducer set-up because it is less dependent on the pulse wave form.

The system needs a catheter in the radial artery, allowing for monitoring from more conventional arterial access site. As for transpulmonary system, you can measure the CO, the PPV and SVV and the system should/must be recalibrated after 8 h.

The last calibrated device based on the pulse contour analysis is a new hemodynamic platform that uses the transpulmonary thermodilution tool for calibration. It provides the same parameters than other devices, despite its greater precision in the measurement of some pulmonary hemodynamic parameters (extravascular lung water) [38].

6.1.5 Non-Calibrated System

Among non-calibrated systems, that achieved success for their easy use, a special mention is for the system provided by a transducer, easily and quickly connectable to any arterial line already placed, allowing the measurement of CO. It does not need calibration for calculating the CO, but it is necessary to insert patient's age, height, sex and weight into the system, to determine the cardiac output from the pulse contour analysis.

Not surprisingly, in critical situations/setting, a non-calibrated system is not so reliable [39], although the third generation software shows a marked improvement in performance [40]. The measurement of SVV and PPV does not depend on accurate calibration, but when it is used to guide the perioperative fluid administration, non-calibrated system reduces complications in major surgery [41, 42].

The second not-calibrated device records the pressure value with analytical method. It is a technique designed for the continuous CO monitoring, derived from the blood pressure without initial calibration or central venous catheterization. Therefore, the system requires only an arterial line without a dedicated pressure transducer.

The technology of this system is based on the principle that in a vessel the volume variations mainly occur due to the radial expansion of pressure variations; so alterations of the systolic portion of the area under the pressure curve reflect the stroke volume variations [43].

This technique calculates the CO by physical parameters, such as left ventricle ejection strain, arterial impedance opposing the blood flow pulsatility, arterial compliance and peripheral vascular resistances [44]. The sampling frequency of this system is 1000 Hz, compared to other methods that sample at 100 Hz. The system captures 1000 times/s, compared to other methods that capture 100 times/s. A higher sampling frequency should allow for a greater precision of the measured data (CO, SVV, PPV and SVR).

Overall, these devices are very effective in predicting the preload responsiveness and protocols guided by SVV or PVV for the haemodynamic optimization, all lead to improvements in surgical outcome [45, 46].

However, it is important to remember that the SVV and PPV require the chest to be closed, to predict the preload responsiveness, although the one-lung ventilation in thoracic surgery does not compromise the predictive ability of these techniques [47].

The presence of arrhythmias or atrial fibrillation is a bias in the measurement of SVV and PPV; in fact, they seem to be a result of cyclical changes in the ventricular filling, rather than a cyclical changes due to mechanical ventilation. In these situations, the dynamic indices/parameters are unable to predict the preload/fluid responsiveness. Unlike non-calibrated systems, calibrated monitoring tool provides CO measurements that correlate with PAC measures [48, 49].

6.1.6 Oesophageal Doppler

The oesophageal Doppler is an alternative technique capable of measuring the SVV and CO. The Doppler can measure the blood velocity in the descending aorta, which can be converted into a volume, if the aortic diameter is measured. Some devices use nomograms based on patient's age, height and weight, while others use 2D ultrasound to measure the aortic diameter. The small ultrasound probe is

advanced into the oesophagus of the anesthetized patient until mid-oesophageal level.

The waveform profile will indicate the correct position and orientation of the probe.

The variations of the Doppler-waveform during the ventilatory cycle can be used to determine the SVV, with the same value/meaning of that derived from the pulse contour analysis. Despite the sampling corner that may affect the measurement of CO, the Stroke Volume Variation will be able to predict the fluid response. Optimization strategies based on SVV measurements with oesophageal Doppler led to improved surgical outcomes, in a wide variety of procedures [50, 51].

6.1.7   Totally Non-Invasive Systems

A completely non-invasive system, providing a continuous cardiac output (CCO) measures, uses an inflatable cuff put on the patient's finger to measure the blood pressure and to determine the stroke volume through the systolic single-beat pulse, calculated on impedance. Some authors [52] have shown how this system provides a reliable method, when compared to invasive systems for the determination of cardiac output, absolutely to prefer in specific clinical setting (ex. Intermediate-risk pregnant).

Another non-invasive monitoring system is the plethysmographic variability index (PVI) used as a continuous measure of vascular reactivity volume, with the highest values corresponding to a greater reactivity. The examination of the plethysmographic trace, using a modified pulsossimetric probe, allows the determination of the perfusion index. The perfusion index (PI) is a numerical value determined by the strength of the detected infrared signal. The signal strength correlates with the amount of volume at the sampling site. Changes in that index may indicate regional changes of volume status.

It has been suggested as a non-invasive monitoring to evaluate the fluid responsiveness and as a measure of the volemic status, continuously sampled in the low output state, in severe peripheral vascular disease or in spontaneous ventilation. (Pleth Variability Index (PVI)% = $[(PI_{max} - PI_{min})/PI_{max}] \times 100\%$) [53, 54].

6.2   EtCO$_2$

Even often forgotten as a hemodynamic monitoring, the measurement of carbon dioxide at the end of exhalation (EtCO$_2$) represents a simple and effective haemodynamic monitoring. It is ubiquitously present as monitoring in all operating rooms. This parameter is normally used to ensure an adequate minute ventilation, but a change in the EtCO$_2$ without a corresponding change in the minute-ventilation implies a change in the pulmonary/lung hemodynamic status. An unexplained fall in EtCO$_2$ represents an increase of dead space as occurs in pulmonary embolism [55]. Therefore a reduction of EtCO$_2$, not explained by an increase in minute-ventilation should guide to a prompt assessment of the hemodynamic status.

On the contrary, an unexplained increase in EtCO$_2$ implies an increase in the transport of CO$_2$ to the lungs. This could occur as a result of the development of distributive shock in early sepsis.

6.2.1 Electrical Impedance Cardiography

This technology assumes that the impedance (or resistance) to a current flowing through a conductor is related to the volume of the conductor itself [56]. Impedance variations result in volume changes, therefore, applying a constant current through the thorax, we can determine the voltage variability through lower resistance way, determined by the great vessels in the thorax and to obtain information regarding the modification of their volume.

This volume variation in the thoracic aorta can be converted into stroke volume by impedance wave-form analysis, using a similar algorithm of/as the pulse contour. However, many problems have to be solved to make this technology useful in the operating room.

6.2.1.1 Bio-Reactance-Based Non-Invasive Monitoring

To overcome the limitations of a bio-impedance systems, alternative methods have been developed.

The Bio-reactance system is based on the analysis of relative phase shifts (frequency modulation) which occurs when an oscillating current goes through the thorax, by detecting the pulsatile flow, rather than the fluid volume in the chest, resulting in a better signal.

A receiving amplifier records the transthoracic voltage in response to the injected current and circuitry for determining the relative phase shift from which the stroke volume, heart rate and CO are derived. Signals are applied to and recorded from the left and the right sides of the thorax and these signals are processed separately and averaged after digital processing.

Recent studies evaluated the accuracy and reliability of this system compared to PAC for CO monitoring, also in the variations over time and in CO changes induced by passive leg raising [57–59].

Recently, the system was also validated in surgery [60], but data are still not consistent to draw conclusions.

6.2.2 Ultrasound

The transthoracic echocardiography easily allows to identify a pericardial or pleural effusion, to assess volume status, to assess right and left ventricles contractility and the presence of hypokinesia caused by ischemia, to identify any valve abnormalities or obstructive heart failure which lead to hemodynamic impairment. With more experience, clinicians can make a general assessment of the ejection fraction and the volume status.

It is a perioperative diagnostic system rather that an intraoperative monitoring tool. Nevertheless, the evaluation of the inferior vena cava (ICV) has been used, even during anaesthesia, as a measure of volume status and as a predictor of preload responsiveness.

The diameter of the ICV can be easily measured; measures less than 2 cm, with a greater inspiratory collapse of 50% are related to intravascular volume depletion, while measures greater than 2 cm, with a less than 50% inspiratory collapse suggest an adequate volume or the inability of the right heart to accept further volume [61].

A transient and reversible increase in preload (passive leg raising), demonstrated by the distensibility of the ICV, can be used as a surrogate of a fluid challenge. (Distensibility Index (DI): $(ICV_{max} - ICV_{min})/ICV_{(max)} = DI\% \times 100$).

A DI> 18% identifies patients responding to fluids challenge with a sensitivity and specificity of 90% [62].

Some limitations related to the echocardiographic technique include: the inability to obtain adequate projections because of patient habitus or positioning and because of the operator skills.

Transesophageal echocardiography (TEE) is not a conventional monitoring device. It needs to be performed by an experienced sonographer and it may require a specialized cardiologist evaluation.

A standard TEE examination is based on 20 tomograms for the assessment of the global ventricular function, the volume status, the valve evaluation, the aorta vessel, the pericardium and the pleura evaluation [63].

TEE assessment is crucial for routine intraoperative monitoring in cardiac surgery and it should be also used in high-risk patient with hemodynamic instability and undiagnosed pathology. However, the use of TEE may change with the routine use of a miniaturized transesophageal probe [64] which allows left ventricular function and filling status assessment, through the trans-gastric left ventricle short axis.

6.2.2.1 Goal-Directed Therapy

The Goal-directed therapy (GDT) is a strategy of hemodynamic management. This term describes a potentially effective method to determine the optimal dose of fluid-therapy, vasopressors and inotropic drugs to use. It is based on clinical algorithms to optimize the cardiac output (CO) and the tissue oxygen delivery, avoiding tissue hypoperfusion.

This setting involves the use of more-invasive or less-invasive hemodynamic monitoring, according to the severity of patient condition and the complexity and duration of surgical procedures. The main reason to perform this approach (targeted-therapy and target-control) is that it can improve outcomes in terms of survival and quality of life, as evidenced by recent meta-analysis [4] and by studies examining long-term complications [65].

The importance of perioperative hemodynamic optimization has increased over the past decade and it has developed with the evolution of hemodynamic monitoring technologies [66], relegating the use of pulmonary artery catheter only in cardiac surgery and rarely to high-risk patients. From the over-physiological hemodynamic targets (CO and DO_2) we moved to the evaluation of the so-called functional hemodynamic monitoring parameters (SVV, PPV)[1], although recently a meta-analysis showed doubts related to the GDT with targeted-DO_2 [67].

A recent meta-analysis has enrolled adult patients undergoing non-cardiac surgery (elective or emergency surgery) managed with intra-operative Gold Directed-Therapy and with an algorithm of post-operative GDT. It showed benefits in terms of complications and mortality [68].

Conclusions

There are several devices for hemodynamic monitoring in anaesthesia.

In low risk surgery, when brief cases without blood loss are scheduled, monitoring of non-invasive blood pressure, heart rate and $EtCO_2$ will be able to provide sufficient data to diagnose an unexpected hemodynamic instability. In high-risk patients or in intermediate-risk surgery it may be sufficient the SVV monitoring to guide the hemodynamic optimization and the patient's preload management. In major and complex surgical procedures, where "mixed shock" can occur (for example in abdominal emergency surgery or in a patient with pre-existing cardiomyopathy or valve disease or pulmonary hypertension), complete and more invasive hemodynamic assessment must be performed with a calibrated device for the cardiac output measurement or a combined PAC with an SVV measuring tool.

References

1. Pinsky MR, Payen D. Functional hemodynamic monitoring. Crit Care. 2005;9:566–72.
2. Gan TJ, Soppitt A, Maroof M, et al. Goal-directed intraoperative fluid administration reduces length of hospital stay after major surgery. Anesthesiology. 2002;97:820–6.
3. Pearse R, Dawson D, Fawcett J, et al. Early goal-directed therapy after major surgery reduces complications and duration of hospital stay. A randomised, controlled trial [ISRCTN38797445]. Crit Care. 2005;9:R687–93.
4. Hamilton MA, Cecconi M, Rhodes A. A systematic review and meta-analysis on the use of preemptive hemodynamic intervention to improve postoperative outcomes in moderate and high-risk surgical patients. Anesth Analg. 2011;112:1392–402.
5. Pickering TG. Principles and techniques of blood pressure measurement. Cardiol Clin. 2002;20:207–23.
6. Amoore JN. Oscillometric sphygmomanometers: a critical appraisal of current technology. Blood Press Monit. 2012;17:80–8.
7. Parks JK, Elliott AC, Gentilello LM, et al. Systemic hypotension is a late marker of shock after trauma: a validation study of advanced trauma life support principles in a large national sample. Am J Surg. 2006;192:727–31.
8. Akkermans J, Diepeveen M, Ganzevoort W, et al. Continuous non-invasive blood pressure monitoring, a validation study of Nexfin in a pregnant population. Hypertens Pregnancy. 2009;28:230–42.
9. Stover JF, Stocker R, Lenherr R, et al. Noninvasive cardiac output and blood pressure monitoring cannot replace an invasive monitoring system in critically ill patients. BMC Anesthesiol. 2009;9:6.
10. Van de Vijver K, Verstraeten A, Gillbert C, et al. Validation of non-invasive hemodynamic monitoring with Nexfin in critically ill patients. Crit Care. 2011;15:P75.
11. Bellomo R, Uchino S. Cardiovascular monitoring tools: use and misuse. Curr Opin Crit Care. 2003;9:225–9.
12. Cullen DJ, Kirby RR. Beach chair position may decrease cerebral perfusion; catastrophic outcomes have occurred. APSF Newsl. 2007;22:25–7.

13. Harvey S, Harrison DA, Singer M, et al. Assessment of the clinical effectiveness of pulmonary artery catheters in management of patients in intensive care (PAC-Man): a randomised controlled trial. Lancet. 2005;366:472–7.
14. Shah MR, Hasselblad V, Stevenson LW, et al. Impact of the pulmonary artery catheter in critically ill patients: meta-analysis of randomized clinical trials. JAMA. 2005;294:1664–70.
15. Vincent JL, Pinsky MR, Sprung CL, et al. The pulmonary artery catheter: in medio stat virtus. Crit Care Med. 2008;36:3093–6.
16. Wilson J, Woods I, Fawcett J, et al. Reducing the risk of major elective surgery: randomised controlled trial of preoperative optimisation of oxygen delivery. BMJ. 1999;318:1099–103.
17. Shoemaker WC, Appel PL, Kram HB, et al. Prospective trial of supranormal values of survivors as therapeutic goals in highrisk surgical patients. Chest. 1988;94:1176–86.
18. Boyd O, Grounds RM, Bennett ED. A randomized clinical trial of the effect of deliberate perioperative increase of oxygen delivery on mortality in high-risk surgical patients. JAMA. 1993;270:2699–707.
19. Lobo SM, Salgado PF, Castillo VG, et al. Effects of maximizing oxygen delivery on morbidity and mortality in high-risk surgical patients. Crit Care Med. 2000;28:3396–404.
20. Hayes MA, Timmins AC, Yau EH, et al. Elevation of systemic oxygen delivery in the treatment of critically ill patients. N Engl J Med. 1994;330:1717–22.
21. Gattinoni L, Brazzi L, Pelosi P, et al. A trial of goal-oriented hemodynamic therapy in critically ill patients. SvO2 Collaborative Group. N Engl J Med. 1995;333:1025–32.
22. Heyland DK, Cook DJ, King D, et al. Maximizing oxygen delivery in critically ill patients: a methodologic appraisal of the evidence. Crit Care Med. 1996;24:517–24.
23. Hollenberg SM, Kavinsky CJ, Parrillo JE. Cardiogenic shock. Ann Intern Med. 1999;131:47–59.
24. Kumar A, Anel R, Bunnell E, et al. Pulmonary artery occlusion pressure and central venous pressure fail to predict ventricular filling volume, cardiac performance, or the response to volume infusion in normal subjects. Crit Care Med. 2004;32:691–9.
25. Marik PE, Baram M, Vahid B. Does central venous pressure predict fluid responsiveness? A systematic review of the literature and the tale of seven mares. Chest. 2008;134:172–8.
26. Marik PE, Monnet X, Teboul JL. Hemodynamic parameters to guide fluid therapy. Ann Intensive Care. 2011;1:1.
27. Michard F, Boussat S, Chemla D, et al. Relation between respiratory changes in arterial pulse pressure and fluid responsiveness in septic patients with acute circulatory failure. Am J Respir Crit Care Med. 2000;162:134–8.
28. De Backer D, Heenen S, Piagnerelli M, et al. Pulse pressure variations to predict fluid responsiveness: influence of tidal volume. Intensive Care Med. 2005;31:517–23.
29. Kobayashi M, Koh M, Irinoda T, et al. Stroke volume variation as a predictor of intravascular volume depression and possible hypotension during the early postoperative period after esophagectomy. Ann Surg Oncol. 2009;16:1371–7.
30. Berkenstadt H, Margalit N, Hadani M, et al. Stroke volume variation as a predictor of fluid responsiveness in patients undergoing brain surgery. Anesth Analg. 2001;92:984–9.
31. Reuter DA, Felbinger TW, Schmidt C, et al. Stroke volume variations for assessment of cardiac responsiveness to volume loading in mechanically ventilated patients after cardiac surgery. Intensive Care Med. 2002;28:392–8.
32. Monnet X, Rienzo M, Osman D, et al. Esophageal Doppler monitoring predicts fluid responsiveness in critically ill ventilated patients. Intensive Care Med. 2005;31:1195–201.
33. Rhodes A, Sunderland R. Arterial pulse power analysis: the LiDCO plus system. In: Vincent JL, Pinksy MR, Payen D, editors. Functional hemodynamic monitoring. Berlin: Springer; 2004.
34. Michard F. Global end-diastolic volume as an indicator of cardiac preload in patients with septic shock. Chest. 2003;124:1900–8.
35. Hofer CK, Furrer L, Matter-Ensner S, et al. Volumetric preload measurement by thermodilution: a comparison with transoesophageal echocardiography. Br J Anaesth. 2005;94:748–55.
36. Hofer CK, Muller SM, Furrer L, et al. Stroke volume and pulse pressure variation for prediction of fluid responsiveness in patients undergoing off-pump coronary artery bypass grafting. Chest. 2005;128:848–54.

37. Hamilton TT, Huber LM, Jessen ME. PulseCO: a less-invasive method to monitor cardiac output from arterial pressure after cardiac surgery. Ann Thorac Surg. 2002;74:S1408–12.
38. Kiefer N, Hofer CK, Marx G, et al. Clinical validation of a new thermodilution system for the assessment of cardiac output and volumetric parameters. Crit Care. 2012;16:R98.
39. Marik PE. Noninvasive cardiac output monitors: a state-of the-art review. J Cardiothorac Vasc Anesth. 2012;27:121–34.
40. Biancofiore G, Critchley LA, Lee A, et al. Evaluation of a new software version of the FloTrac/Vigileo (version 3.02) and a comparison with previous data in cirrhotic patients undergoing liver transplant surgery. Anesth Analg. 2011;113:515–22.
41. Cecconi M, Fasano N, Langiano N, et al. Goal-directed haemodynamic therapy during elective total hip arthroplasty under regional anaesthesia. Crit Care. 2011;15:R132.
42. Benes J, Chytra I, Altmann P, et al. Intraoperative fluid optimization using stroke volume variation in high risk surgical patients: results of prospective randomized study. Crit Care. 2010;14:R118.
43. Romagnoli S, Bevilacqua S, Lazzeri C, Ciappi F, Dini D, Pratesi C, Gensini GF, Romano SM. Most care: a minimally invasive system for hemodynamic monitoring powered by the pressure recording analytical method (PRAM). HSR Pro Intensive Care Cardiovasc Anesth. 2009;1(2):20–7.
44. Romano SM, Pistolesi M. Assessment of cardiac output from systemic arterial pressure in humans. Crit Care Med. 2002;30:1834–41.
45. Kapoor PM, Kakani M, Chowdhury U, et al. Early goal-directed therapy in moderate to high-risk cardiac surgery patients. Ann Card Anaesth. 2008;11:27–34.
46. Lopes MR, Oliveira MA, Pereira VO, et al. Goal-directed fluid management based on pulse pressure variation monitoring during high-risk surgery: a pilot randomized controlled trial. Crit Care. 2007;11:R100.
47. Suehiro K, Okutani R. Stroke volume variation as a predictor of fluid responsiveness in patients undergoing one-lung ventilation. J Cardiothorac Vasc Anesth. 2010;24:772–5.
48. Kurita T, Morita K, Kato S, et al. Comparison of the accuracy of the lithium dilution technique with the thermodilution technique for measurement of cardiac output. Br J Anaesth. 1997;79:770–5.
49. Halvorsen PS, Espinoza A, Lundblad R, et al. Agreement between PiCCO pulse-contour analysis, pulmonal artery thermodilution and transthoracic thermodilution during off-pump coronary artery by-pass surgery. Acta Anaesthesiol Scand. 2006;50:1050–7.
50. Conway DH, Mayall R, Abdul-Latif MS, et al. Randomised controlled trial investigating the influence of intravenous fluid titration using oesophageal Doppler monitoring during bowel surgery. Anaesthesia. 2002;57:845–9.
51. Guinot PG, de Broca B, Abou Arab O, Diouf M, Badoux L, et al. Ability of stroke volume variation measured by oesophageal Doppler monitoring to predict fluid responsiveness during surgery. Br J Anaesth. 2013;110:28–33.
52. Broch O, Renner J, Gruenewald M, Meybohm P, Schöttler J, et al. A comparison of the Nexfin® and transcardiopulmonary thermodilution to estimate cardiac output during coronary artery surgery. Anaesthesia. 2012;67:377–83.
53. Yin JY, Ho KM. Use of plethysmographic variability index derived from the Massimo® pulse oximeter to predict fluid or preload responsiveness: a systematic review and meta-analysis. Anaesthesia. 2012;67:777–83.
54. Lima AP, Beelen P, Bakker J. Use of a peripheral perfusion index derived from the pulse oximetry signal as a noninvasive indicator of perfusion. Crit Care Med. 2002;30:1210–3.
55. Hemnes AR, Newman AL, Rosenbaum B, et al. Bedside end-tidal CO_2 tension as a screening tool to exclude pulmonary embolism. Eur Respir J. 2010;35:735–41.
56. Summers RL, Shoemaker WC, Peacock WF, et al. Bench to bedside: electrophysiologic and clinical principles of noninvasive hemodynamic monitoring using impedance cardiography. Acad Emerg Med. 2003;10:669–80.
57. Squara P, Denjean D, Estagnasie P, et al. Noninvasive cardiac output monitoring (NICOM): a clinical validation. Intensive Care Med. 2007;33:1191–4.

58. Keren H, Burkhoff D, Squara P. Evaluation of a noninvasive continuous cardiac output monitoring system based on thoracic bioreactance. Am J Physiol Heart Circ Physiol. 2007; 293:H583–9.
59. Benomar B, Ouattara A, Estagnasie P, et al. Fluid responsiveness predicted by noninvasive bioreactance-based passive leg raise test. Intensive Care Med. 2010;36:1875–81.
60. Waldron NH, Miller TE, Nardiello J et al. NICOM versus EDM guided goal directed fluid therapy in the perioperative period. ASA, 2011. P. A680.
61. Perera P, Mailhot T, Riley D, Mandavia D. The RUSH exam: rapid ultrasound in shock in the evaluation of the critically lll. Emerg Med Clin North Am. 2010;28:29–56.
62. Barbier C, Loubières Y, Schmit C, Hayon J, Ricôme JL, et al. Respiratory changes in inferior vena cava diameter are helpful in predicting fluid responsiveness in ventilated septic patients. Intensive Care Med. 2004;30:1740–6.
63. Reeves ST, Finley AC, Skubas NJ, Swaminathan M, Whitley WS, et al. Basic perioperative transesophageal echocardiography examination: a consensus statement of the American Society of Echocardiography and the Society of Cardiovascular Anesthesiologists. J Am Soc Echocardiogr. 2013;26:443–56.
64. Cioccari L, Baur HR, Berger D, Wiegand J, Takala J, et al. Hemodynamic assessment of critically ill patients using a miniaturized transesophageal echocardiography probe. Crit Care. 2013;17:R121.
65. Rhodes A, Cecconi M, Hamilton M, Poloniecki J, Woods J, Boyd O, et al. Grounds goal-directed therapy in high-risk surgical patients: a 15-year follow-up study. Intensive Care Med. 2010;36:1327–32.
66. Suehiro K, Joosten A, Alexander B, Cannesson M. Guiding goal directed therapy. Curr Anesthesiol Rep. 2014;4:360–75.
67. Arulkumaran N, Corredor C, Hamilton MA, Ball J, Grounds RM, Rhodes A, et al. Cardiac complications associated with goal-directed therapy in high-risk surgical patients: a meta-analysis. Br J Anaesth. 2014;112(4):648–59.
68. Gurgel S, do Nascimento P. Maintaining tissue perfusion in high risk surgical patients: a systematic review of randomized clinical trials. Anesth Analg. 2011;6:1384–91.

Assisted Ventilation in the ICU: When and to Whom?

Rosa Di Mussi and Salvatore Grasso

Mechanical ventilation is a life-saving therapy for most critically ill patients [1]. We can distinguish between:

Controlled mechanical ventilation: during controlled mechanical ventilation, the patient has no role in the gas delivery process. Spontaneous respiratory muscle activity needs to be abolished.

Assisted mechanical ventilation: assisted mechanical ventilation involves a deep interaction between the patient and the ventilator machine. During this process, the patient's spontaneous respiratory effort is recognized by the ventilator and assisted with positive pressure applied at the airway open. In this way, the work of breathing (WOB) is shared between the patient and the ventilator. Ventilator's assistance needs to be synchronized with the patient's inspiratory effort. Breathing pattern should ideally remain totally under the patient control. Respiratory rate (RR), tidal volume (VT), inspiratory time and inspiratory time/expiratory time ratio (I:E ratio) should be variable on a breath by breath basis.

7.1 When Do We Use Controlled Mechanical Ventilation in the Intensive Care Unit (ICU)?

During controlled mechanical ventilation, patient's spontaneous respiratory effort should be absent due to pathological conditions or pharmacologically abolished for clinical reasons. Controlled ventilation is often used to rest the exhausted

R. Di Mussi • S. Grasso (✉)
Dipartimento dell'Emergenza e Trapianti d'Organo (DETO), Sezione di
Anestesiologia e Rianimazione, Università degli Studi di Bari "Aldo Moro",
Piazza Giulio Cesare 11, Bari, Italy
e-mail: salvatore.grasso@uniba.it

© Springer International Publishing AG 2018   103
D. Chiumello (ed.), *Practical Trends in Anesthesia and Intensive Care 2017*,
http://doi.org/10.1007/978-3-319-61325-3_7

respiratory muscles immediately after the institution of invasive mechanical ventilation in dyspnoeic patients. It is mandatory in pathological conditions deeply affecting the chain of respiratory impulse transmission from the respiratory centres to the respiratory muscles. The need to use deep sedation and eventually paralysis (such as in brain-injured patients) is another classical indication for controlled mechanical ventilation.

The duration of the controlled mechanical ventilation period should be ideally to be as short as possible since it is hampered by several side effects:

- *Ventilator-induced diaphragm disfunction*: according to Levine and co-workers, diaphragm atrophy may occur after only 18–69 h of controlled mechanical ventilation. The resulting diaphragm dysfunction is one of the commonest causes of weaning failure [2–4].
- *Reduced aereation of lung tissue*: diaphragmatic inactivity affects alveolar aeration by generating actelectasis in the dependent lung regions. Abnormally high intra-abdominal pressures worsen this scenario [5].
- *Haemodynamic impact*: in general, positive pressure mechanical ventilation has a double haemodynamic impact [6], the "preload" and the "afterload" effect. The first one is due to the reduction of venous return (RV). During spontaneous inspiration the right atrial pressure falls, following the negative pleural pressure. The resulting pressure gradient favours the RV. On the contrary, during positive pressure mechanical ventilation, the continuous positive intrathoracic pressure increases the right atrial pressure, negatively affecting the RV. On the other hand, mechanical ventilation has the potential to increase pulmonary vascular resistance by compressing the alveolar vessels. Pulmonary vascular resistances are the main determinant of the right ventricle afterload (afterload effect). Finally, positive intrathoracic pressure causes a decrease in the transmural aortic pressure and therefore in left ventricle afterload. The interplay between the preload and the afterload effect with specific pathological conditions such as hypovolemia, ARDS, the use of high PEEP or VT levels, the effects of drugs acting on the cardiovascular system or pre-existing cardiac or pulmonary diseases, determines the overall impact of mechanical ventilation on cardiovascular function. The controlled mechanical ventilation mode specifically amplifies the "preload effect" because it implies the absence of diaphragm contraction.

By definition, since assisted ventilation preserves and promotes diaphragmatic contraction, as compared to controlled ventilation, it should improve aeration in the dependent regions, attenuate the haemodynamic impact and, obviously, decrease the risk of ventilator-induced diaphragm atrophy. This is true if one thinks to the myriad of physiological studies on the assisted ventilator modes [1, 7, 8]. However, we lack randomized controlled trials to demonstrate the impact of assisted ventilation on clinically meaningful outcome parameters. Nevertheless, assisted ventilation is extensively used in clinical practice to reduce mechanical ventilation duration, ICU length of stay, ventilator acquired pneumonia, improve patients comfort and decrease the need of sedation.

7.2   How Does Assisted Ventilation Work?

Pressure support ventilation (PSV) is the prototype mode of assisted mechanical ventilation [9]. The two newer assisted modes, neurally adjusted ventilator assist (NAVA) and proportional assist ventilation (PAV), that have been recently introduced in clinical practice are called "proportional modes". They deliver a support that is proportional, on a breath-by-breath basis, to the patient's inspiratory effort [10–12].

7.3   Pressure Support Ventilation (PSV)

During PSV, every breath is patient-started and patient-terminated. The support level (i.e. the amount of positive pressure that the ventilator will apply at the airway opening to assist the spontaneous inspiratory effort) is fixed. All the breathing pattern parameters (VT, RR, inspiratory and expiratory time) depend on patient's spontaneous respiratory activity.

Pressure support assistance is delivered throughout three different phases (see Figs. 7.1 and 7.2):

1. Recognition of the start of patient's spontaneous inspiration (inspiratory trigger): during this phase, the ventilator shifts from the expiratory to the inspiratory phase.

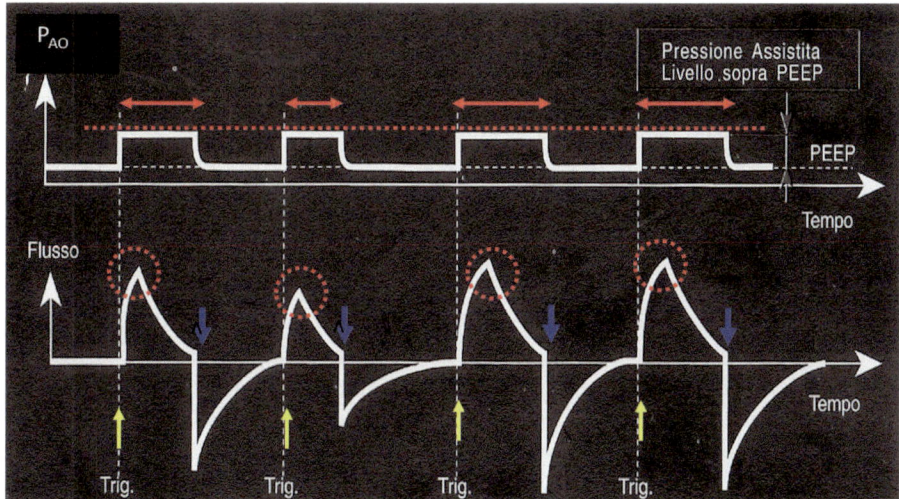

Fig. 7.1 Pressure support ventilation (PSV) algorithm: each patient's effore troggers the ventilator (*yellow arrows*). The ventilator assists the spontaneous inspiratory effort with a pre-set constant level of pressure (*dotted red line*). The interplay between the ventilator assistance and the spontaneous effort generates an ispiratory flow peak (*dotted red circles*) that ts different on a breth by breath basis. Once the inspiratory flow decays below a prefixed threshold (*expiratory trigger*, *blue arrows*) the ventilator cycles off into the expiratory phase

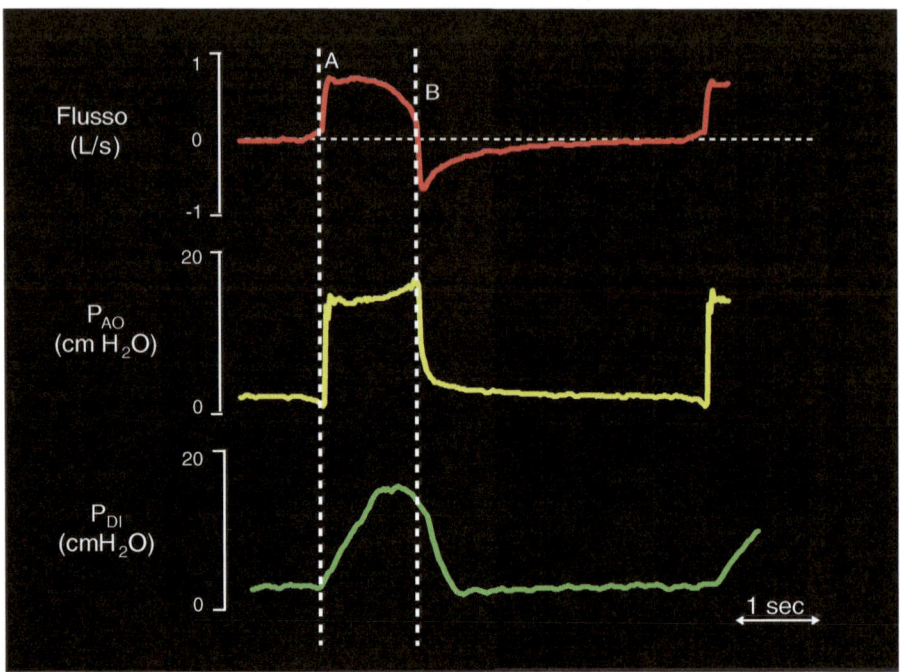

Fig. 7.2 Flow (*red trace*), airway opening pressure (P_{AO}- *yellow trace*) and transdiaphragmatic pressure (P_{DI}- *green trace*) during PSV. The dotted white line A indicates the inspiratory trigger phase. The dotted white line B indicates the expiratory trigger phase

2. Pressurization: during this phase, the ventilator maintains the preset level of positive pressure at the airway opening.
3. Recognition of the end of the inspiratory phase and start of the expiratory phase (expiratory trigger).

Generally, during PSV, the breaths are flow triggered but the pressure trigger mode can be used too.

With the pressure trigger, the ventilator starts to deliver the assistance when the patient's spontaneous respiratory effort generates a negative pressure inside the ventilator circuit. Instead, if the flow trigger is used, the assistance starts when the patient subtracts a predefined portion of a continuous gas flow ("bias" flow) that circulates in the circuit at end expiration. Any delay in the delivery of the assistance is named "inspiratory trigger delay". The amount of delay is greatly influenced by the technical features of the single ventilator but depends also on several clinical parameters, mainly patient's breathing pattern and the presence of dynamic hyperinflation [13].

The positive pressure applied by the ventilator to assist the spontaneous inspiratory effort is constant throughout the whole pressurization phase. During this phase, the ventilator maintains the preset level of positive pressure at the airway opening by replacing (virtually in real time) moment by moment the volume delivered to the patient. In most ventilators it is possible to adjust the pressurization rate (the time needed to reach the pressure support level, i.e. the slope of pressurization). In the common practice, the pressurization slope is set at 0.1–0.2 s. A peak and a subsequent approximately exponential decay characterize the inspiratory flow profile. The peak flow is greatly influenced by the slope of pressurization and by the early inspiratory effort. The subsequent flow rate decay depends on the interplay between the inspiratory efforts, the mechanical properties of the respiratory system and the amount of volume delivered to the patient. Ideally, until the inspiratory effort is active, after the inspiratory flow peak there will be a sustained, slowly decaying flow. When the inspiratory effort comes to an end, the inspiratory flow sharply decreases. The expiratory trigger is generally activated when the inspiratory flow decays below a given threshold, suggesting that the patient is no longer active in generating the inspiratory effort. Usually the expiratory trigger threshold is not fixed but is a percentage of the previous flow peak. For example, if the threshold is 30% of the inspiratory flow peak rate, the cycle will occur at 0.3 L/min if the peak flow is 1 L/min. In most ventilators, the expiratory trigger threshold is adjustable from 70 to 10% of the flow peak.

Figure 7.1 shows a typical ventilator screen during PSV. We can see pressure (PAO) and flow curves. The yellow arrows indicate the inspiratory trigger activation. The red dotted line represents the pressure support level. Note that the inspiratory time changes breath by breath (red arrows). The flow peak is also variable as indicated by red dotted cycles. The blue arrows indicate the expiratory trigger activation.

Figure 7.2 illustrates an ideal PSV breath. The diaphragmatic electrical activity (EAdi) trace (green line) is also visible. In this ideal situation, the diaphragm contraction activates the inspiratory trigger and the pressurization phase starts (PAO-yellow trace). Letter A indicates the flow peak. At the end of diaphragmatic contraction, the flow reduces and, at last, it decays to the expiratory trigger threshold.

In clinical practice, the level of support is titrated to obtain a VT between 5 and 8 ml/predicted body weight (PBW) and a RR between 15 and 30 breaths/min [9, 14]. That's why, according to physiological studies, a VT higher than 8 ml/PBW and a RR lower than 15 bpm are generally signs of over-assistance while, on the contrary, a VT lower than 5 ml/PBW and a RR higher than 30 bpm are signs of under-assistance [15].

Several physiological studies demonstrated the PSV ability, as compared with controlled mechanical ventilation, to reduce the adverse effects of prolonged sedation and ventilator-induced diaphragm dysfunction [5, 7, 9, 15]. Despite these positive reports, however, poor patient-ventilator interactions frequently occur during PSV. To understand why this occurs, it is convenient to introduce the "neuro-ventilatory coupling" concept [10] (Fig. 7.3). In healthy subjects, small changes in the respiratory effort determine high variations of flow and VT, and the physiological effort is about the 20–30% of the maximum inspiratory capacity (green line, Fig. 7.3) [16]. Whenever the neuro-ventilatory coupling is impaired, the slope and the variability of the neural output/VT or neural output/inspiratory flow relationship

Fig. 7.3 Neuro-ventilatory coupling. Neuro-ventilatory coupling relationship in healty subjects (*green line*), pathological subjects (*red line*), pathological subjects during PSV (*blue line*). The red point figures out the only one point in which physiological neuro-ventilatory coupling, during PSV, is preserved

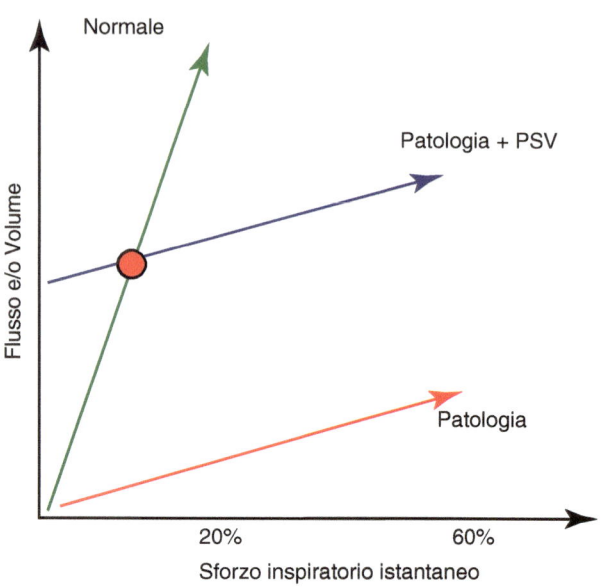

decrease (red line, Fig. 7.3). Considering a patient with an impaired neuro-ventilatory coupling ventilated in PSV, the slope of the neuro-ventilatory coupling remains a pathological one, but the inspiratory assistance provides a bust that translates each point of the line toward a higher VT and inspiratory flow. Accordingly there will be only one point (red point, Fig. 7.3), where the neuro-ventilatory coupling is "normal". This may explain why the over-assistance phenomenon frequently occurs during PSV. Over-assistance may reduce assisted mechanical ventilation advantages and side effects, generally associated with controlled mechanical ventilation, may prevail.

Over-assistance may frequently occur during PSV. Since the level of assistance is fixed and doesn't change with the patient's spontaneous effort, if the patient effort is weak and ceases very early, the ventilator inflates the passive patient up to the expiratory trigger threshold. Accordingly, the combination of high levels of PSV, weak and short inspiratory effort and low expiratory trigger threshold easily generates over-assistance during PSV. If the patient just triggers the ventilator and immediately ceases the inspiratory effort, the assistance delivery will be independent by the patient effort, and VT depends entirely on the level of assistance and the mechanical properties of the respiratory system. During over-assistance, the inspiratory mechanical time (Ti_{mech}) is longer than the neural inspiratory time (Ti_{neur}).

In most cases, as said above, when a patient is over-assisted, the VT is higher than 8–10 ml/Kg predicted body weight (PBW), and/or the RR is lower than 15 breaths/min. However, recent studies point out that, interestingly, over-assistance may occur even if RR and VT are in the suggested clinical range. Figure 7.5, adapted from ref. [17], shows the VT, RR and diaphragmatic WOB trend in 12 patients ventilated in PSV for 48 h [17]. Note that the diaphragmatic WOB was constantly under its physiological range throughout the period despite the PSV settings were in line with the clinical best practice, i.e. the PSV level was titrated to obtain a VT between 5 and 8 ml/PBW and RR between 15 and 30 breaths/min. Our group recently recorded the diaphragmatic electrical activity (EAdi) during prolonged PSV (12 h), in 17 patients (unpublished data). The EAdi represents the neural ventilator output and is strictly related with diaphragmatic WOB; we predefined four EAdi categories:

- NO EAdi: EAdi absent (the patient starts the breath with the accessory muscles and is subsequently over-assisted by the ventilator)
- LOW EAdi: EAdi under 5 µV
- NORMAL or MEDIUM: EAdi in the normal range of 5–15 µV
- HIGH: EAdi above 15 µV

The results are shown in Fig. 7.4. The NO EAdi condition occurred the 20.9% of the total recorded patients' breaths. The LOW EAdi condition occurred in the 52.8% of the total breaths and, finally the NORMAL and the HIGH EAdi conditions occurred in the 20.7 and the 5.6%, respectively.

Figure 7.5 illustrates PAO, flow and EAdi traces in one representative patient. Note that the EAdi decreased during the 12 h, whereas the flow and the PAO curves didn't change significantly.

Over-assistance is one of the most important causes of patient-ventilator asynchrony [18]. Several clinical trials have demonstrated that a high incidence of patient-ventilator asynchronies is correlated with a longer ICU length of stay and mechanical ventilation duration, a higher incidence of tracheostomy and, at last, a higher mortality [19–21].

Figure 7.6 shows the relationship between mechanical respiratory rate (RR_{mech}) and spontaneous "neural" respiratory rate (RR_{neur}) in 20 patients ventilated in PSV for 8 h (unpublished data). In a group of patients, that were mainly patients with moderate-severe COPD, the figure shows a severe discrepancy between RR_{mech} and RR_{neural}. Figure 7.7 shows the flow, the volume, the PAO and the oesophageal pressure (Pes) traces in one representative patient ventilated in PSV for 8 h. Each panel represents 30 s taken at the beginning of each hour of the study. In this patient,

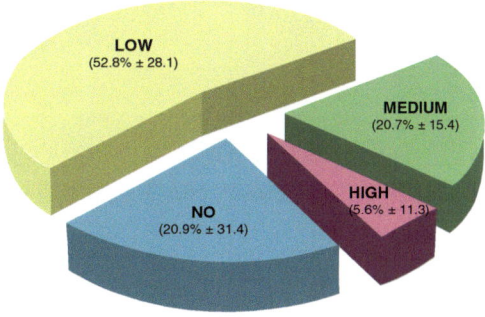

Fig. 7.4 Percentage of Eadi cathegories in 17 patients during prolonged PSV (12 hours). Please note the prevalence of NO-EAdi and LOW-Eadi conditions

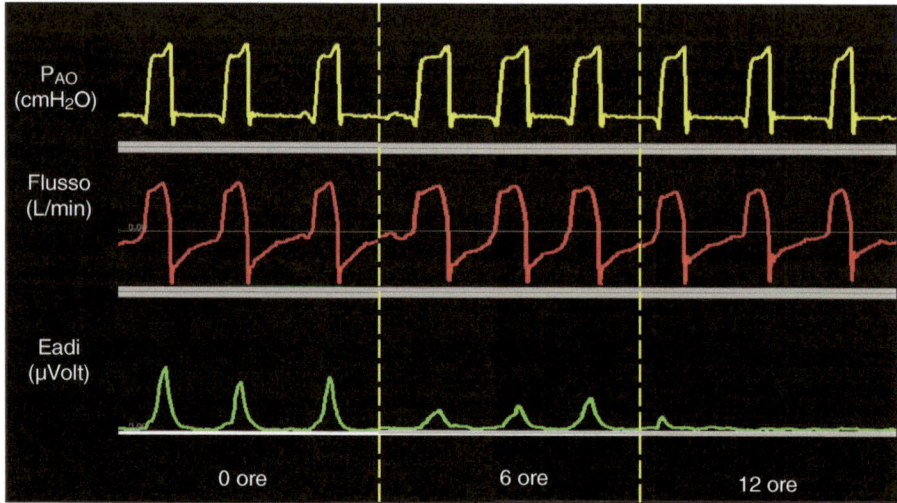

Fig. 7.5 P_{AO} (*yellow trace*), Flow (*red trace*) and Eadi (*green trace*) in one representative patient during the 12 hours of PSV. Eadi significantly decreased throughout the hours whether P_{AO} and flow traces remained unchanged

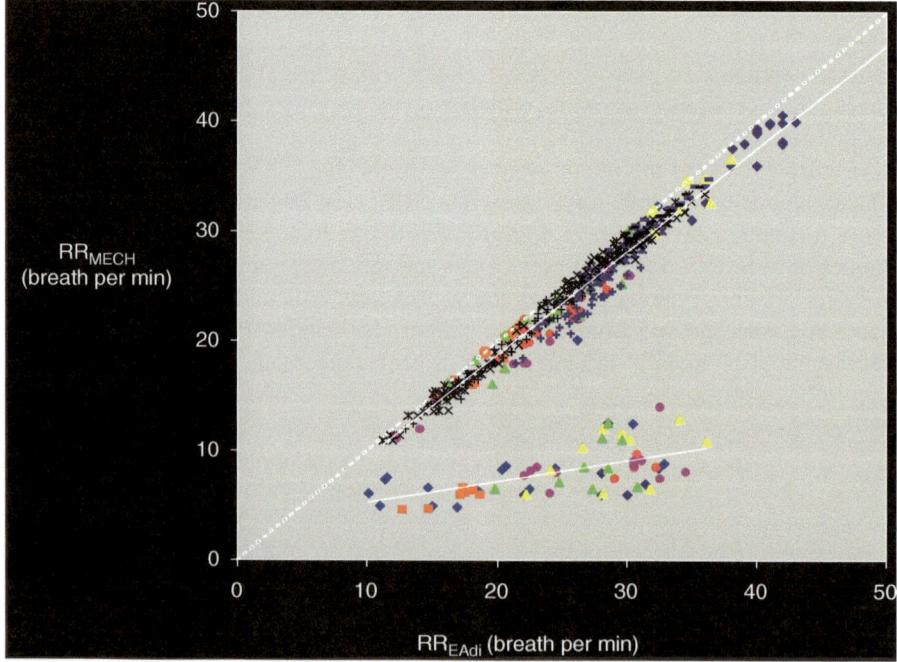

Fig. 7.6 Relationship between mechanical respiratory rate (RR_{mech}) and spontaneous "neural" respiratory rate (RR_{neural}) in 20 patients ventilated in PSV mode for 8 hours. The figure illustrates the discrepancy between RR_{mech} and RR_{neural} in some of the studied patients

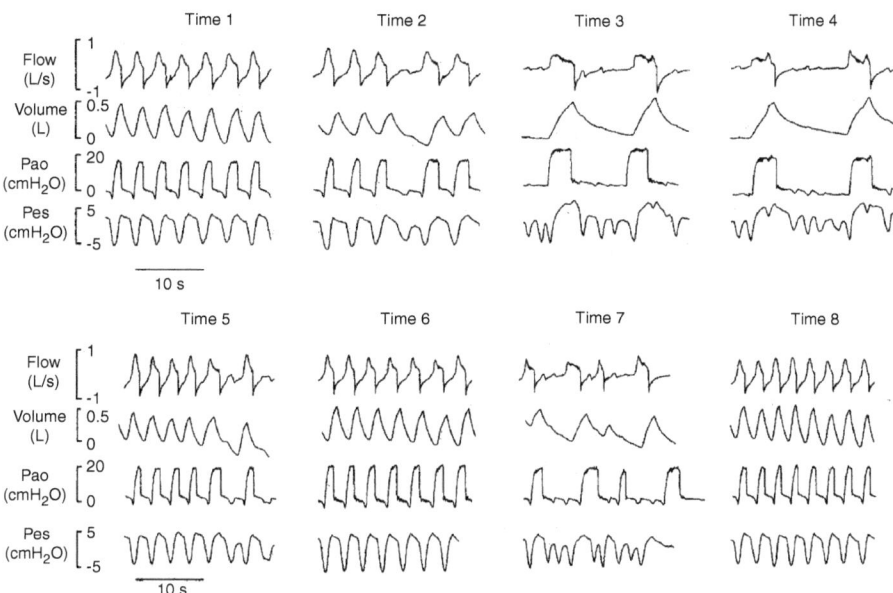

Fig. 7.7 Flow, volume, P_{AO} and esophageal pressure (P_{es}) in one representative patient during the 8 hours of PSV. We can see the changes in terms of patient-ventilator interactions throughout the study. Please note the high percentage of asynchronies at 3, 4, and 7 hours

patient-ventilator interactions remarkably varied throughout the study period. Asynchronies were evident at 3, 4 and 7 h.

Prolonging mechanical insufflation into neural expiration has been shown to worsen dynamic hyperinflation and cause ineffective inspiratory efforts. This may happen principally in COPD patients who need a higher respiratory effort to overcome the intrinsic PEEP ($PEEP_i$) [22].

A mean to improve the patient-ventilator interactions during PSV is to titrate the slope of pressurization, the level of assistance and the expiratory trigger threshold in order to optimize patient-ventilator interactions, assure the optimal diaphragmatic workload and minimize the asynchronies [20]. Generally speaking, the peak inspiratory flow increases with the slope of pressurization and vice versa, and, thus, the higher is the peak inspiratory flow the higher will be the mechanical inspiratory time (because the expiratory trigger threshold is a percentage of the peak inspiratory flow). On the other hand, the expiratory trigger threshold has a deep influence on the inspiratory time (the lower the threshold, the higher the mechanical inspiratory time). Titrating the assistance level could serve to circumvent over- and under-assistance. However, the PSV critically depends from the single clinicians' expertise, and one could consider it more an art than a science. The fact that during PSV the over-assistance may occur even if RR and VT are in the "optimal" range (see above) makes it difficult to trust solely on the flow and PAO traces to titrate the PSV level, the slope of pressurization and the expiratory trigger threshold. Experts are concordant in suggesting bedside monitoring of respiratory muscle activity to easily detect asynchronies and to avoid over- or under-assistance, but on the other hand, reliable indexes of diaphragmatic and intercostal muscle activity to be used at the bedside are scanty. The recent introduction in clinical practice of the EAdi monitoring (see below) and of diaphragmatic electromyography could represent a turning point to monitor diaphragm activity bedside on a breath-by-breath basis [23, 24].

7.3.1 EAdi and NAVA

During NAVA, the ventilator assistance is proportional to the patient's spontaneous diaphragmatic activity (EAdi). The diaphragmatic electromyography strictly correlated with phrenic nerve discharge [12, 25] and hence to the neuro-ventilatory drive. From a technical point of view, the EAdi is measured through an array of eight electrodes mounted within a nasogastric tube (NAVA catheter) (Fig. 7.8). The EAdi signal is obtained from the crural portion of the diaphragm, amplified and filtered from cardiac artefacts and other electrical contaminations.

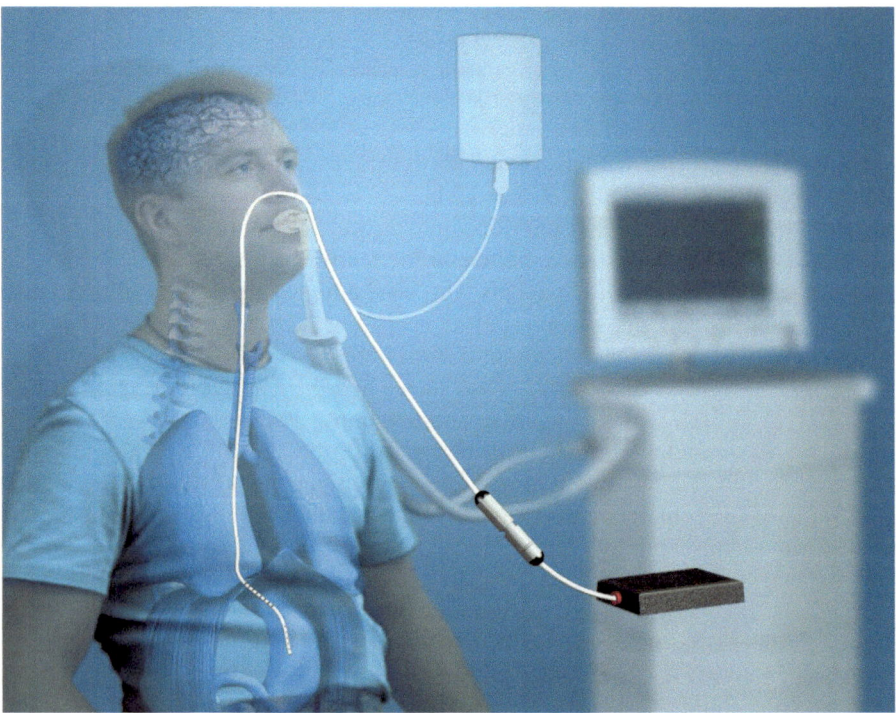

Fig. 7.8 Eadi signal acquisition during NAVA. Eadi is measured through a naso-gastric tube equipped with 8 electrodes (NAVA catheter) and is processed and visualized on the ventilator screen

Besides monitoring the neuro-ventilatory drive, the EAdi signal can be used to evaluate the diaphragmatic efficiency in terms of neuromechanical and neuro-ventilatory efficiency (NME and NVE, respectively) [23, 26]. The NME is calculated as the ratio between the negative pressure developed by the diaphragm and the EAdi peak during an end-expiratory occlusion and is expressed in $cmH_2O/\mu V$. The neuro-ventilatory efficiency, expressed in $ml/\mu V$, is calculated as the ratio between VT and the correspondent EAdi peak. Figure 7.9 shows how to calculate these two parameters. Bellani and co-workers validated a technique to continuously calculate the diaphragmatic WOB from NME and the EAdi signal [27]. Recently Liu and coll [26] demonstrated that the NME and NVE evaluation was useful to predict extubation readiness.

In the neurally adjusted ventilator assist mode (NAVA), the EAdi signal is used to drive the ventilator's assistance [25]. Briefly, during NAVA the EAdi triggers on and cycles off the ventilator, and, most important, the assistance delivery is proportional to EAdi according to the following formula:

$$PAO\left(cmH_2O\right) = NAVA\ level \times EAdi\left(\mu V\right).$$

The NAVA level must be set by the clinician. As an example, if the NAVA level is 1, the ventilator applies a positive pressure of 1 cmH_2O for each μV (Fig. 7.10).

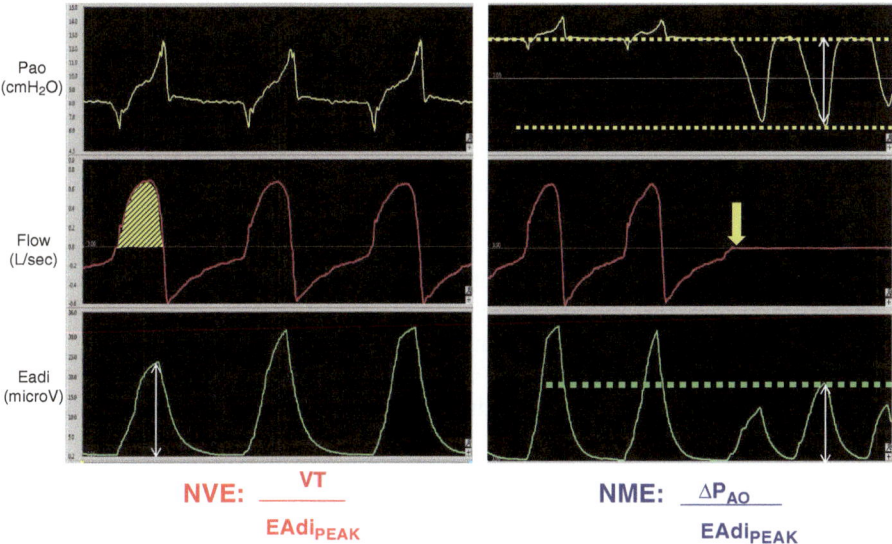

$$NVE: \frac{VT}{EAdi_{PEAK}} \qquad NME: \frac{\Delta P_{AO}}{EAdi_{PEAK}}$$

Fig. 7.9 Neuro-ventilatory efficiency (*NVE, panel on the left*) and neuro-mechanical efficiency (*NME, panel on the right*) calculation. The NVE is the ratio between tidal volume (*VT, yellow area under the flow trace, red trace*) and the Eadi peak (*white arrow under the green trace*). The NME is the ratio between negative pressure during an end-expiratory occlusion (*yellow trace*) and Eadi peak (*green trace*). During the expriratory occlusion the flow is zero (*red trace*)

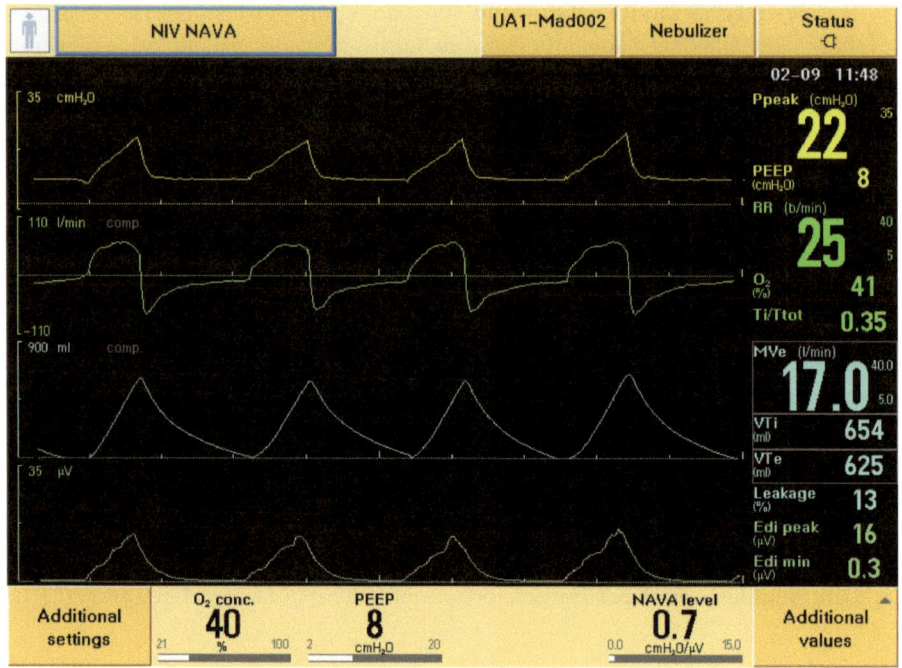

Fig. 7.10 Ventilator screen during NAVA. NAVA level, PEEP and O_2 concentration must be set by the clinician

Several physiological studies have shown the NAVA ability, as compared with PSV, to improve neuro-ventilatory coupling and patient-ventilator synchrony [12, 18]. Di Mussi and co-workers [17] compared NAVA vs PSV during a prolonged ventilation period (48 h) to test the impact of the two techniques on NVE and NME. Both NME and NVE significantly improved in patients randomized to NAVA whereas both were not affected by PSV. During the 48 h, the diaphragmatic WOB was constantly in the physiological range during NAVA and almost constantly under the physiological range during PSV, suggesting over-assistance. Patient-ventilator asynchronies were significantly less during NAVA than during PSV [17]. However in 20–30% of the patients included in the study, NAVA failed because of EAdi signal instability or difficult reading. Further studies are needed to evaluate the real percentage of NAVA failures in the clinical scenario.

7.3.2 Proportional Assist Ventilation (PAV)

PAV was first described in 1992 by Magdy Younes [10]. During PAV, the positive pressure applied to each breath is proportional to the spontaneous patient's inspiratory airflow, which is used as a surrogate of respiratory muscles effort [28]. The clinician can adjust the PAV gain, i.e. the percentage of total WOB to be performed from the ventilator.

To understand PAV one must preliminarily consider that, according to the "equation of motion" applied to mechanical ventilation, WOB is the result of (a) a resistive component to overcome airway resistance (R), proportional to the airway flow (resistive WOB = flow × R); (b) an elastic component that is needed to overcome the respiratory system elastance (E), proportional to the delivered gas volume (elastic WOB = volume × E); and a component needed to overcome positive intrinsic end-expiratory pressure (PEEPi). Provided that the ventilator software knows R, E and PEEPi, based on the "equation of motion" it can calculate the instantaneous patient's spontaneous inspiratory effort by measuring the spontaneous inspiratory flow and volume. Based on the instantaneous patient's WOB determination, the ventilator in the PAV mode applies positive pressure in proportion to the spontaneous WOB. Figure 7.11 shows the principles of the PAV algorithm. The ventilator is represented as a freely mobile piston inserted in a cylinder. The patient respiratory system is represented by a single alveolus (the airway resistances are represented by two orange triangles and the respiratory system elastance is represented by a single light blue triangle). The patient effort is represented by a yellow triangle. When the patient starts its spontaneous effort, the piston moves toward the patient: the velocity of the movement represents the instantaneous inspiratory flow, and the piston displacement represents the instantaneous inspired volume. The ventilator software is therefore able to calculate the instantaneous patient's WOB in terms of the elastic and resistive pressure generated by the respiratory muscles. The PAV assistance is applied by a motor that supports a predefined portion of the instantaneous piston movement toward the patient.

In the first PAV version, the clinician had to measure E, R and PEEPi to feed the ventilator algorithm. Considering the difficulties related to the assessment of respiratory mechanic in actively breathing patients, the quality of E and R estimation was strictly related to the clinicians' expertise. This was a major concern of the technique, since the quality of the quality of assistance was strictly dependent on the accuracy of E and R measurements. If E and R were underestimated, patients were

Fig. 7.11 Principles of PAV + algorythm. Freely mobile piston in the cilinder = ventilator; alveolous = patient's respiratory system; orange triangles = airway resistance; light blue triangle = respiratory system elastance; yellow triangle = patient's respiratory effort

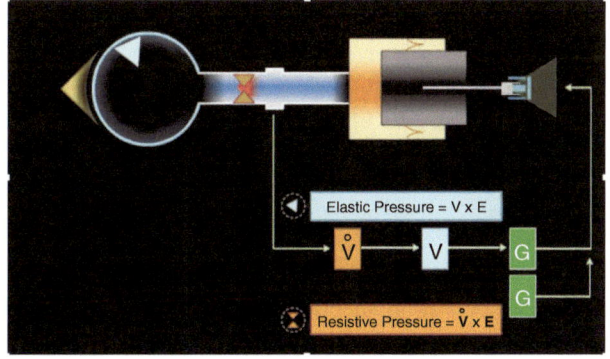

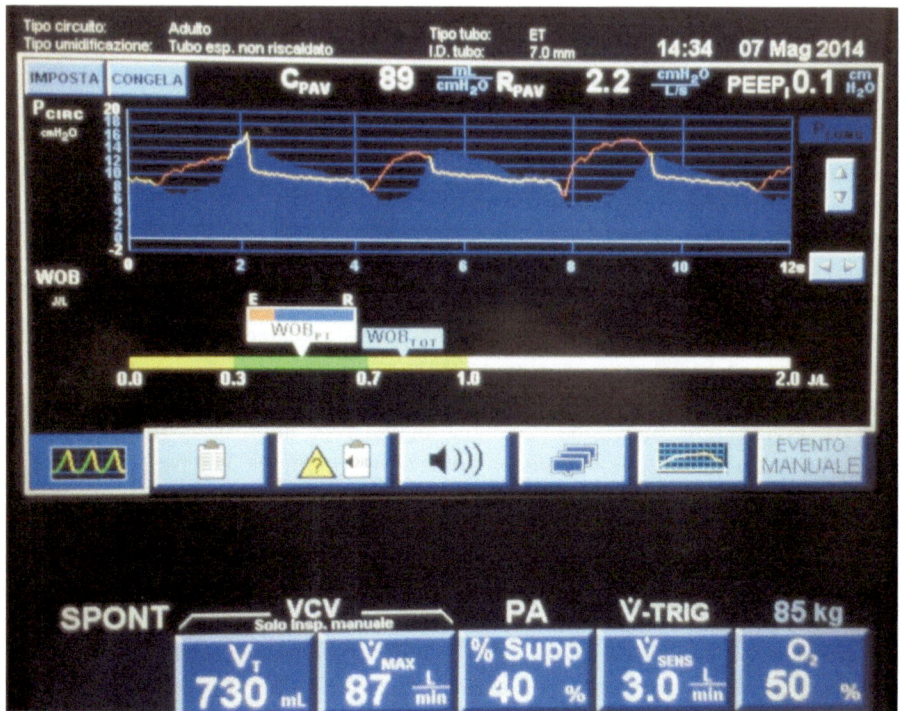

Fig. 7.12 Ventilator screen during PAV+ . Yellow dotted circles = respiratory mechanics values; Red circle = total work of breathing (WOB$_{total}$ = WOB$_{patient}$ + WOB$_{ventilator}$). Optimal WOB should be in the green part of the scale

over-assisted whereas, on other side, if E and R were overestimated, patients were under-assisted. In the last and definitive PAV version, the PAV plus (PAV +), E, R and PEEPi are automatically calculated by the ventilator through an end-inspiratory occlusion of 200 ms automatically performed every 10–15 breaths [29–31].

During PAV +, the ventilator screen continuously shows the WOB performed by the patient and by the ventilator, respectively. Accordingly, it is possible for the clinician to adjust the PAV + gain to keep the patient's spontaneous WOB in a physiological range. Figure 7.12 illustrates the ventilator screen during PAV +. The yellow dotted circles indicate the respiratory mechanics values. The red circle evidences the total WOB. The total WOB is composed by the WOB performed by the patient and the WOB performed by the ventilator (WOB$_{total}$ = WOB$_{patient}$ + WOB$_{ventilator}$). The patient's WOB is divided in the elastic and resistive components. The optimal WOB should be in the green part of the scale.

Figure 7.13 illustrates the impact of PAV + on the slope of the neuro-ventilatory coupling relationship [31]. In the lower panel, the depressed neuro-ventilatory coupling of a spontaneously breathing patient is compared with the physiological neuro-ventilatory coupling (blue-dotted line). In the middle panel, PAV + with a gain of 30% improves the physiological coupling improving its slope from 1.5 to 8. Finally, in the higher panel, a PAV gain of 80% further improves the slope [27].

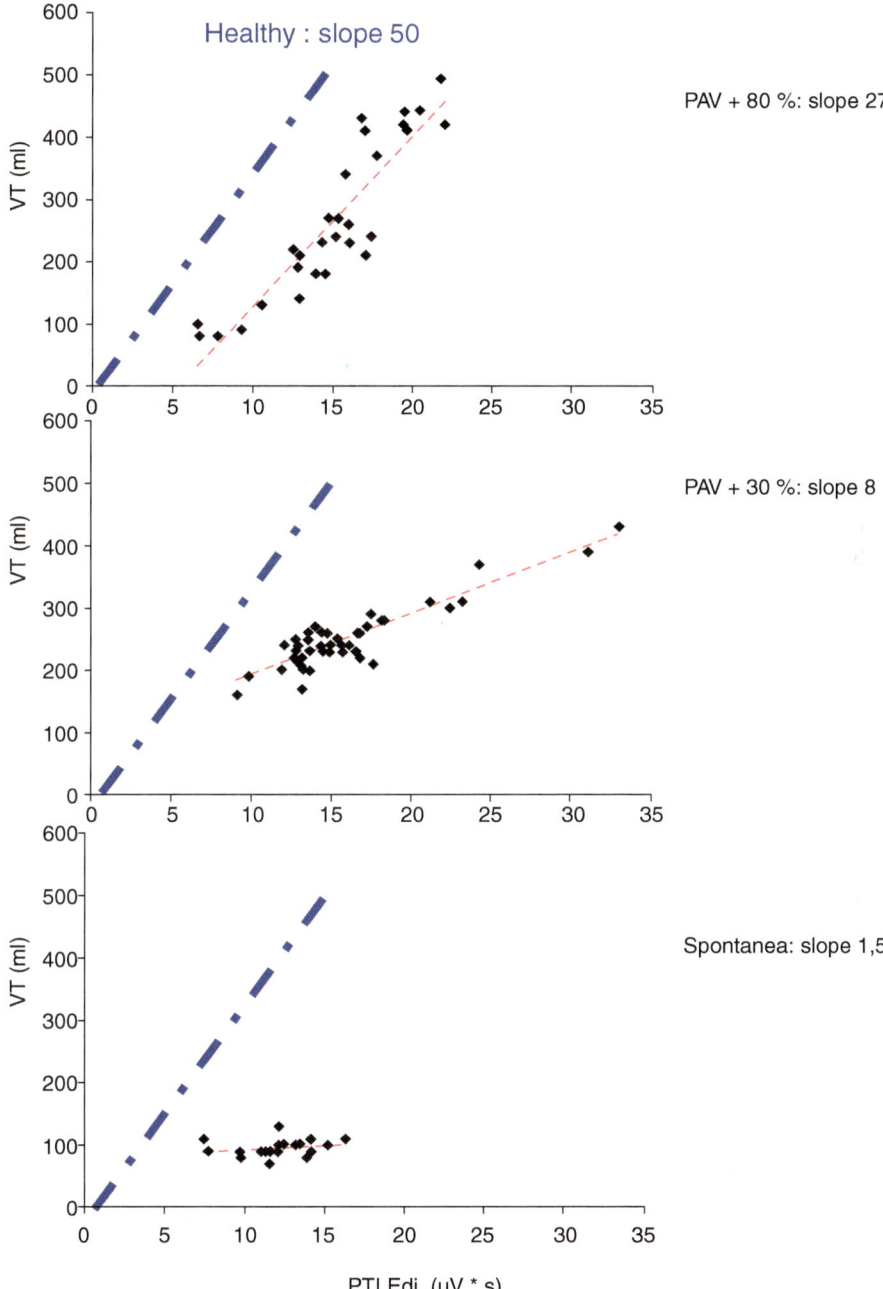

Fig. 7.13 Lower panel = physiological neuro-ventilatory coupling (blue dotted line) vs depressed neuroventilatory coupling in a spontaneously breathing patient (*red dotted line*). Middle panel= physiological neuro ventilatory coupling (*blue dotted line*) vs neuro-ventilatory coupling during PAV+ with the 30% of assistance (*red dotted line*). Upper panel: physiological neuro-ventilatory coupling (*blue dotted line*) vs neuro-ventilatory coupling during PAV+ with the 80% of assistance. The slope of the neuro-ventilatory coupling relationship increases at the same time as the % of assistance

From 1992 on, several physiological studies have clearly shown that, as compared with PSV, during PAV+ the breathing pattern is more variable (and hence more physiological), the number of patient-ventilator asynchronies, especially missed efforts, is decreased and the discrepancy between mechanical and neural inspiratory times significantly decreases [29, 32, 33]. PAV+ has been shown to unload respiratory muscles and prevent patient-ventilator asynchronies even in patients with severe chronic obstructive pulmonary disease (COPD) [34].

7.4 Indications and Contraindications to Assisted Ventilation

Assisted ventilation should be applied to patients able to trigger the ventilator and to subsequently sustain a spontaneous inspiratory effort [1, 8, 35]. The prerequisite for any assisted technique should be the integrity of the neuro-ventilatory drive. In critically ill patients, sedative drugs are often used. For this reason, in order to be confident that an excess of sedation could not excessively depress the neuro-ventilatory drive, it's important to quantify the sedation level. Considering that the level of sedation is strictly related to the quality and the concentration of sedative drugs [36–38], breathing pattern parameters and patient-ventilator interactions should be thoughtfully monitored in sedated patients. For example, with the Richmond agitation and sedation scale [39], only patients with a score between 0 (patient calm, alert, with open eyes that responds to simple orders) and −2 (patient with the eyes closed but briefly awakens—eye opening/eye contact—to voice) are suitable for assisted ventilation [36].

On the other hand, an excessively high respiratory drive during assisted ventilation may cause dynamic hyperinflation and haemodynamic derangement because of the increase of intrathoracic pressure and favour ventilation-induced lung injury (VILI) [40, 41]. In some instances the high respiratory drive results from the discrepancy between high respiratory load and the ability of the respiratory muscle to handle it. In these cases an attempt to decrease the inspiratory workload with assisted ventilation is warranted. However in some instances (ARDS, sepsis, fever, metabolic acidosis, some neurological conditions) the increased respiratory drive is independent from the mechanical load. In these instances assisted ventilation is not indicated. Several studies have shown the worsening of lung injury caused by assisted ventilation in patients with ARDS and an inappropriately high respiratory drive [42]. In these cases, sedation and eventually paralysis associated with controlled mechanical ventilation is the best choice, waiting for the normalization of the respiratory drive.

References

1. Tobin MJ, Jubran A, Laghi F. Patient-ventilator interaction. Am J Respir Crit Care Med. 2001;163(5):1059–63.
2. Petrof BJ, Hussain SN. Ventilator-induced diaphragmatic dysfunction: what have we learned? Curr Opin Crit Care. 2016;22(1):67–72.

3. Levine S, Nguyen T, Taylor N, Friscia ME, Budak MT, Rothenberg P, Zhu J, Sachdeva R, Sonnad S, Kaiser LR, et al. Rapid disuse atrophy of diaphragm fibers in mechanically ventilated humans. N Engl J Med. 2008;358(13):1327–35.
4. Heunks LM, van der Hoeven JG. Clinical review: the ABC of weaning failure—a structured approach. Crit Care. 2010;14(6):245.
5. Putensen C, Muders T, Varelmann D, Wrigge H. The impact of spontaneous breathing during mechanical ventilation. Curr Opin Crit Care. 2006;12(1):13–8.
6. Shekerdemian L, Bohn D. Cardiovascular effects of mechanical ventilation. Arch Dis Child. 1999;80(5):475–80.
7. Putensen C, Hering R, Wrigge H. Controlled versus assisted mechanical ventilation. Curr Opin Crit Care. 2002;8(1):51–7.
8. Tobin MJ. Advances in mechanical ventilation. N Engl J Med. 2001;344(26):1986–96.
9. Brochard L, Pluskwa F, Lemaire F. Improved efficacy of spontaneous breathing with inspiratory pressure support. Am Rev Respir Dis. 1987;136(2):411–5.
10. Younes M. Proportional assist ventilation, a new approach to ventilatory support theory. Am Rev Respir Dis. 1992;145(1):114–20.
11. Younes M, Puddy A, Roberts D, Light RB, Quesada A, Taylor K, Oppenheimer L, Cramp H. Proportional assist ventilation. Results of an initial clinical trial. Am Rev Respir Dis. 1992;145(1):121–9.
12. Terzi N, Piquilloud L, Roze H, Mercat A, Lofaso F, Delisle S, Jolliet P, Sottiaux T, Tassaux D, Roesler J, et al. Clinical review: update on neurally adjusted ventilatory assist—report of a round-table conference. Crit Care. 2012;16(3):225.
13. Piquilloud L, Vignaux L, Bialais E, Roeseler J, Sottiaux T, Laterre PF, Jolliet P, Tassaux D. Neurally adjusted ventilatory assist improves patient-ventilator interaction. Intensive Care Med. 2011;37(2):263–71.
14. Brochard L. Pressure support level before extubation. Chest. 1994;106(6):1932.
15. Berger KI, Sorkin IB, Norman RG, Rapoport DM, Goldring RM. Mechanism of relief of tachypnea during pressure support ventilation. Chest. 1996;109(5):1320–7.
16. Mead J. The control of respiratory frequency. Ann N Y Acad Sci. 1963;109:724–9.
17. Di Mussi R, Spadaro S, Mirabella L, Volta CA, Serio G, Staffieri F, Dambrosio M, Cinnella G, Bruno F, Grasso S. Impact of prolonged assisted ventilation on diaphragmatic efficiency: NAVA versus PSV. Crit Care. 2016;20(1):1.
18. Yonis H, Crognier L, Conil JM, Serres I, Rouget A, Virtos M, Cougot P, Minville V, Fourcade O, Georges B. Patient-ventilator synchrony in Neurally Adjusted Ventilatory Assist (NAVA) and Pressure Support Ventilation (PSV): a prospective observational study. BMC Anesthesiol. 2015;15:117.
19. Thille AW, Rodriguez P, Cabello B, Lellouche F, Brochard L. Patient-ventilator asynchrony during assisted mechanical ventilation. Intensive Care Med. 2006;32(10):1515–22.
20. Thille AW, Cabello B, Galia F, Lyazidi A, Brochard L. Reduction of patient-ventilator asynchrony by reducing tidal volume during pressure-support ventilation. Intensive Care Med. 2008;34(8):1477–86.
21. Blanch L, Villagra A, Sales B, Montanya J, Lucangelo U, Lujan M, Garcia-Esquirol O, Chacon E, Estruga A, Oliva JC, et al. Asynchronies during mechanical ventilation are associated with mortality. Intensive Care Med. 2015;41(4):633–41.
22. Ranieri VM, Grasso S, Fiore T, Giuliani R. Auto-positive end-expiratory pressure and dynamic hyperinflation. Clin Chest Med. 1996;17(3):379–94.
23. Doorduin J, van Hees HW, van der Hoeven JG, Heunks LM. Monitoring of the respiratory muscles in the critically ill. Am J Respir Crit Care Med. 2013;187(1):20–7.
24. Dres M, Rittayamai N, Brochard L. Monitoring patient-ventilator asynchrony. Curr Opin Crit Care. 2016;22(3):246–53.
25. Sinderby C, Navalesi P, Beck J, Skrobik Y, Comtois N, Friberg S, Gottfried SB, Lindstrom L. Neural control of mechanical ventilation in respiratory failure. Nat Med. 1999;5(12):1433–6.
26. Liu L, Liu H, Yang Y, Huang Y, Liu S, Beck J, Slutsky AS, Sinderby C, Qiu H. Neuroventilatory efficiency and extubation readiness in critically ill patients. Crit Care. 2012;16(4):R143.

27. Bellani G, Mauri T, Coppadoro A, Grasselli G, Patroniti N, Spadaro S, Sala V, Foti G, Pesenti A. Estimation of patient's inspiratory effort from the electrical activity of the diaphragm. Crit Care Med. 2013;41(6):1483–91.
28. Grasso S, Marco Ranieri V. Proportional assist ventilation. Semin Respir Crit Care Med. 2000;21(3):161–6.
29. Younes M, Brochard L, Grasso S, Kun J, Mancebo J, Ranieri M, Richard JC, Younes H. A method for monitoring and improving patient: ventilator interaction. Intensive Care Med. 2007;33(8):1337–46.
30. Younes M, Webster K, Kun J, Roberts D, Masiowski B. A method for measuring passive elastance during proportional assist ventilation. Am J Respir Crit Care Med. 2001;164(1):50–60.
31. Younes M, Kun J, Masiowski B, Webster K, Roberts D. A method for noninvasive determination of inspiratory resistance during proportional assist ventilation. Am J Respir Crit Care Med. 2001;163(4):829–39.
32. Giannouli E, Webster K, Roberts D, Younes M. Response of ventilator-dependent patients to different levels of pressure support and proportional assist. Am J Respir Crit Care Med. 1999;159(6):1716–25.
33. Meza S, Giannouli E, Younes M. Control of breathing during sleep assessed by proportional assist ventilation. J Appl Physiol. 1998;84(1):3–12.
34. Ranieri VM, Grasso S, Mascia L, Martino S, Fiore T, Brienza A, Giuliani R. Effects of proportional assist ventilation on inspiratory muscle effort in patients with chronic obstructive pulmonary disease and acute respiratory failure. Anesthesiology. 1997;86(1):79–91.
35. Tobin MJ, Mador MJ, Guenther SM, Lodato RF, Sackner MA. Variability of resting respiratory drive and timing in healthy subjects. J Appl Physiol (1985). 1988;65(1):309–17.
36. Vaschetto R, Cammarota G, Colombo D, Longhini F, Grossi F, Giovanniello A, Della Corte F, Navalesi P. Effects of propofol on patient-ventilator synchrony and interaction during pressure support ventilation and neurally adjusted ventilatory assist. Crit Care Med. 2014;42(1):74–82.
37. Ruokonen E, Parviainen I, Jakob SM, Nunes S, Kaukonen M, Shepherd ST, Sarapohja T, Bratty JR, Takala J. Dexmedetomidine versus propofol/midazolam for long-term sedation during mechanical ventilation. Intensive Care Med. 2009;35(2):282–90.
38. Jakob SM, Ruokonen E, Grounds RM, Sarapohja T, Garratt C, Pocock SJ, Bratty JR, Takala J. Dexmedetomidine vs midazolam or propofol for sedation during prolonged mechanical ventilation: two randomized controlled trials. JAMA. 2012;307(11):1151–60.
39. Sessler CN, Gosnell MS, Grap MJ, Brophy GM, O'Neal PV, Keane KA, Tesoro EP, Elswick RK. The Richmond agitation-sedation scale: validity and reliability in adult intensive care unit patients. Am J Respir Crit Care Med. 2002;166(10):1338–44.
40. Slutsky AS. Ventilator-induced lung injury: from barotrauma to biotrauma. Respir Care. 2005;50(5):646–59.
41. Slutsky AS, Ranieri VM. Ventilator-induced lung injury. N Engl J Med. 2013;369(22):2126–36.
42. Yoshida T, Uchiyama A, Matsuura N, Mashimo T, Fujino Y. Spontaneous breathing during lung-protective ventilation in an experimental acute lung injury model: high transpulmonary pressure associated with strong spontaneous breathing effort may worsen lung injury. Crit Care Med. 2012;40(5):1578–85.

Acute-on-Chronic Liver Failure: A New and Important Entity in the ICU

Gianni Biancofiore

Traditionally two types of liver failure were recognized: acute liver failure (ALF), characterized by a rapid deterioration of the liver function in the absence of a preexisting liver disease, and the progression with a slow deterioration over time of preexisting end-stage liver disease leading to an acute hepatic insult [1]. Recently, a new clinical form of liver failure has been described: Acute-on-chronic liver failure (ACLF). This new entity is characterized by acute complications of compensated or even decompensated cirrhosis with a high rate of organ failure and a high short-term mortality rate. ACLF is now an increasingly recognized entity in both the hepatology and critical care literature and poses several challenges to clinicians. In fact, the liver's position at the apex of multiple synthetic, detoxifying, metabolic, immunological, and hormonal processes predisposes patients with ACLF to a number of complications. The present review aims at summarizing the most updated knowledge about this particularly severe syndrome.

8.1 Definition of ACLF

Until 2013, there was no shared, established, evidence-based definition of ACLF, and the only published definitions were based on expert opinion. Moreover, the used definitions of ACLF differed between Eastern and Western countries. In Asia, the following liver-centered definition has been suggested: an acute hepatic insult manifesting as jaundice (serum bilirubin level > 5 mg/dL) and coagulopathy (international normalized ratio [INR] >1.5) complicated within 4 weeks by ascites

G. Biancofiore
Transplant Anesthesia and Critical Care Department, Azienda Ospedaliera
Universitaria Pisana, Pisana, Italy

Anesthesiolgy and Critical Care, University School of Medicine, Pisa, Italy
e-mail: g.biancofiore@med.unipi.it

© Springer International Publishing AG 2018
D. Chiumello (ed.), *Practical Trends in Anesthesia and Intensive Care 2017*,
http://doi.org/10.1007/978-3-319-61325-3_8

and/or encephalopathy in a patient with previously diagnosed or undiagnosed chronic liver disease [2]. In Europe and the USA, a different definition of ACLF was used identifying ACLF as an acute deterioration of liver function in patients with cirrhosis which usually is associated with a precipitating event and results in the failure of one or more organs and high short-term mortality rates [3]. Finally, the sequential organ failure assessment (SOFA) score was also used to diagnose organ failures in patients with cirrhosis admitted to the intensive care unit [4].

Since diagnostic criteria of ACLF were based in both definitions on personal expert opinions rather than on objective data, in 2009, a group of European investigators decided to create the Chronic Liver Failure (CLIF) Consortium with the objective of stimulating research on complications of cirrhosis. The Consortium was endorsed by the European Association for the Study of the Liver (EASL) resulting in the EASL-CLIF Consortium. One of the first decisions by the Steering Committee of the Consortium was to perform a multicenter, prospective, observational study in patients with an acute decompensation of cirrhosis. This study was named *CLIF Acute-on-Chronic Liver Failure in Cirrhosis (CANONIC) study* and aimed at assessing the prevalence, diagnostic criteria, precipitating events, natural course, and prognosis of ACLF. The CANONIC study prospectively enrolled 1343 patients with cirrhosis hospitalized in 29 liver units from 8 European countries between February and September 2011. Enrolled patients were hospitalized for at least 1 day and had an acute development of large ascites, hepatic encephalopathy, gastrointestinal hemorrhage, bacterial infections, or any combination of these [5]. For the diagnosis of organ failures, investigators used a modified SOFA scale, called the CLIF-SOFA scale, which had been designed specifically by the Writing Committee of the CANONIC study before the onset of this study. The CLIF-SOFA scale assesses the function of six organ systems (liver, kidneys, brain, coagulation, circulation, and lungs) but also takes into consideration some specificities of cirrhosis. Each organ system receives a subscore ranging from zero (normal) to four (most abnormal). A total CLIF-SOFA score ranging from 0 to 24 can thus be calculated. Notably, all variables included in the CLIF-SOFA are easy to obtain in every hospital.

In the CANONIC study, three types of risk factors obtained from the CLIF-SOFA score at enrollment were found to be related to high 28-day mortality rate: (1) the presence of two organ failures or more, (2) the presence of one organ failure when the organ that failed was the kidney, and (3) the coexistence of a single "non-kidney" organ failure with kidney dysfunction (i.e., serum creatinine level ranging from 1.5 to 1.9 mg/dL) and/or mild to moderate hepatic encephalopathy [5].

Based on the findings from the CANONIC study, four stages of ACLF can be nowadays recognized:

A. *No ACLF*. This group comprises three subgroups: (1) patients with no organ failure, (2) patients with a single "non-kidney" organ failure (i.e., single failure of the liver, coagulation, circulation, or respiration) who had a serum creatinine level > 1.5 mg/dL and no hepatic encephalopathy, and (3) patients with single cerebral failure who had a serum creatinine level > 1.5 mg/dL.

B. *ACLF grade 1*. This group includes three subgroups: (1) patients with single kidney failure; (2) patients with single failure of the liver, coagulation, circulation, or respiration who had a serum creatinine level ranging from 1.5 to 1.9 mg/dL and/or mild to moderate hepatic encephalopathy; and (3) patients with single cerebral failure who had a serum creatinine level ranging from 1.5 to 1.9 mg/dL.
C. *ACLF grade 2*. This group includes patients with two organ failures.
D. *ACLF grade 3*. This group includes patients with three organ failures or more.

These results show that ACLF is a new clinical entity that is distinct from decompensated cirrhosis.

8.2   Prevalence, Risk Factors, and Prognosis of ACLF (According to the CANONIC Study)

The prevalence of ACLF in the CANONIC Study was 30% (20% at admission and 10% during hospitalization), and the overall 28-day and 90-day mortality rates were 33% and 51%, respectively. Mortality rates in patients without ACLF were low (28-day, 1.9%; 90-day, 10%). The prevalence and 28-day and 90-day mortality rates associated with the different grades of ACLF were 15.8%, 22%, and 41%, respectively, in ACLF-1; 10.9%, 32%, and 55% in ACLF-2; and 4.4%, 73%, and 78% in ACLF-3 [5].

Patients with ACLF were significantly younger than those without ACLF, and the main etiologies were alcoholism (60%), hepatitis C (13%), and alcoholism plus hepatitis C (10%). In only 5% of patients, the main etiology was cirrhosis associated with hepatitis B virus (HBV) infection. The commonest organ failure in patients with ACLF was renal failure (56%) with liver coagulation and cerebral, circulatory, and respiratory failures (44%, 28%, 24%, 17%, and 9%, respectively) also very frequent. The prevalence of circulatory and respiratory failure was significant only in patients with ACLF-3. Most importantly, patients with ACLF showed systemic inflammation (high count of C-reactive protein and leukocyte concentration) which was independent on the presence or absence of recognized bacterial infections. Patients with no history of decompensated cirrhosis developed a more severe form of ACLF than patients with previous episodes of decompensation (28-day mortality of 42% vs. 29%).

The most common precipitating events were bacterial infections and active alcoholism. In patients with ACLF the prevalence of alcoholic cirrhosis (60%) was higher than the prevalence of active alcoholism, indicating that alcoholic hepatitis accounts for only part of cases of ACLF associated with alcoholic cirrhosis. There was a small proportion of other precipitating events. As a trigger, gastrointestinal hemorrhage was less frequent in patients with ACLF than in patients without ACLF, suggesting that hemorrhage, if not associated to other complications (i.e., active drinking and/or bacterial infections), is not related to ACLF development. Finally, a significant proportion of patients developing ACLF did so in the absence of any identifiable trigger. Mortality was independent of the presence and type of precipitating events, indicating that although triggers are important in the development of ACLF, mortality depends on other factors, such as the clinical course and number of organ failure [5, 6].

Regarding the prognostic relevance of ACLF, some findings have been reported as significant in determining patient outcomes [5]:

A. Among patients who are admitted for an acute decompensation and subsequently die, multiorgan failure (i.e., ACLF grade 3) is present in all patients before death.
B. The interval between the diagnosis of ACLF and death is 12.0 ± 7.5 days for ACLS grade 1, 11.0 ± 8.0 days for ACLS grade 2, and 8.0 ± 6.1 days for ACLS grade 3. Therefore, the greater the number of organ failures at diagnosis the shorter the time to death.
C. ACLF is not a temporally fixed syndrome. For example, 50% of patients with ACLF grade 1 at diagnosis improve and survive whereas one-third progress to ACLF grade 3 and die. A majority of patients with ACLF grade 3 at diagnosis acquire new organ failures and die. However, 16% of patients with ACLF grade 3 at diagnosis progress to a no ACLF status.
D. The finding that patients without any organ failure on admission have a 28-day mortality rate of approximately 5% and not 0% is explained by the fact that some of these patients develop in-hospital ACLF, which progresses to ACLF grade 3 and death. Conversely, patients who do not have ACLF on admission and remain free of this syndrome during the following 28 days have a very low short-term mortality rate (1.9%).

Another very important finding from the CANONIC study needs to be outlined: the fact that the presence or absence or the type of precipitating event is not related to the severity of ACLF and the short-term mortality rate [5]. Therefore, precipitating events are important in the occurrence of the syndrome but once it develops the prognosis depends on the number of organ failures. This observation indicates that the severity of ACLF probably depends more on the individual response to the precipitating event [6]. Finally, in almost half of patients enrolled in the CANONIC study with ACLF, the syndrome develops in the absence of a prior history of decompensation or has developed within a few weeks after the first episode of decompensation. This finding outlines that ACLF is not a terminal event in a long-lasting history of decompensated cirrhosis.

8.3 ACLS is Caused by a Derangement of the Inflammatory Pathway

The CANONIC study results clearly show that white cell count and plasma C-reactive protein (CRP) levels are higher in patients with ACLF than in those without indicating higher degree of systemic inflammation in the former patients [5]. Furthermore, the higher white cell count or CRP levels the higher the number of failing organs. All in all, these findings suggest that organ failures may result from an excessive inflammatory response, for which the term *immunopathology* was proposed [7]. Although the precise mechanisms involved in ACLF have yet to be clarified, the immune system seems to play a predominant role in the setting of cirrhosis. The homeostatic role of the liver in the systemic immune response is already well known, [8, 9] and the definition of "cirrhosis-associated immune dysfunction" which includes the main syndromic abnormalities of immune function, immunodeficiency and systemic inflammation, well depicts the key role of the immune system in this setting [10]. The immune dysfunction in cirrhosis is a dynamic condition which leads to oscillation from predominantly pro-inflammatory to predominantly immunodeficient situations, is multifactorial, and reflects a complex interaction between many systems predisposing these patients to infections [10]. It is thought that this susceptibility is not due to an only sole responsible factor but rather to the concomitant presence of various facilitating mechanisms such as portal hypertension with portosystemic shunting (thus impairing detoxification and reticuloendothelial system phagocytic activity), increased gut permeability and bacterial overgrowth (all of them increases the risk of bacteremia and the occurrence of endotoxemia), albumin and lipoprotein dysfunction, or aberrant toll-like receptor expression in hepatic Kupffer cells [1]. Moreover, comparing septic patients to ACLF patients, Wasmuth et al. formulated the concept of "sepsis- like immune paralysis" based on a profoundly decreased production of TNF-α and low monocyte HLA-DR expression in both groups. They also postulated that this cellular immune impairment could contribute to increased mortality [11]. Endotoxins have also been proposed to play a role in mediating the full activation of neutrophils, which paradoxically would render them unable to act against the insult. The role that cytokines play in ACLF remains a key point in the pathogenesis of the inflammatory response. Elevated serum levels of many cytokines including TNF-α, sTNF-αR1, sTNF-αR2, interleukin (IL)-2, IL-2R, IL-4, IL-6, IL-8, IL-10, and interferon-α has been described. In particular IL-6 and TNF-α had been proposed to have a dual action, producing hepatocyte death and also enhancing hepatocyte proliferation through a complex interplay with Kupffer cells and hepatocytes [1]. This entire cascade eventually leads to hepatocyte death and liver dysfunction. It has also been outlined that hepatocytes apoptosis rather than necrosis can be the predominant mode of cell death in ACLF, as high levels of some apoptosis markers occurs in ACLF patients [12].

8.4 Clinical Features of ACLF

8.4.1 Infections

Although the CANONIC study showed that the trigger of ACLF is not related to an infection in the 70% of cases, the presence of innate immune dysfunction in this class of patients can be inferred from susceptibility to infections: 30–50% of cirrhotic patients presented bacterial infections upon their admission or during hospitalization. The most common bacterial infections were spontaneous bacterial peritonitis (25%), urinary tract infections (20%), pneumonia (15%), and spontaneous bacteremia (12%). In a study of 184 cirrhotic patients from King's College

Hospital, 67 (36%) developed bloodstream infection (BSI) a median of 8 days after admission; BSI was independently associated with higher ICU mortality [13]. This may support the hypothesis that following the initial cytokine storm responsible for acute decompensation and multiorgan dysfunction, these patients enter a later phase of monocyte immunoparalysis (compensatory anti-inflammatory response), which further alters their susceptibility to sepsis and predisposes them to a higher rate of second infection and increased mortality [14, 15]. Finally, it is important to outline that data from a large multicenter study suggested that cirrhotic patients with septic shock, including those on mechanical ventilation or receiving renal replacement therapy, have benefited from the progress in septic shock and organ failures management obtained in recent years in the general population indicating that it is justified to admit ACLF patients to ICU [16].

8.4.2   Kidney Injury

Acute kidney injury (AKI) in critically ill cirrhotic patients is common and often multifactorial.

Renal complications of ACLF can be due to low flow state, infections, nephrotoxic drugs, and chronic diseases such as hypertension and diabetes which can predispose patients to chronic renal failure. However, the characteristic renal complication of end-stage liver diseases is the hepatorenal syndrome (HRS) which is characterized by splanchnic arterial vasodilatation leading to renal vasoconstriction in the setting of a low flow state due to decreased systemic vascular resistance [17, 18]. Although the incidence of HRS is unknown, especially in relation to other causes of renal failure, it is estimated to be 40% over a 5-year period in patients with cirrhosis and ascites [19]. There are two different forms of HRS, type 1 and type 2. Although HRS is associated with a very poor prognosis, overall the natural progression of the disease differs significantly based on the type, with type 1 experiencing a median survival of 2 weeks and type 2 exhibiting median survivals of 3–6 months. Diagnosis of HRS involves the demonstration of low glomerular filtration rate in the absence of shock, infection, fluid losses, and nephrotoxic agents, with no improvement after discontinuation of diuretics and administration of 1.5 L fluid and proteinuria of less than 500 mg/dL, with no ultrasonographic evidence of obstruction or intrinsic parenchymal disease [17, 18]. Recently, a consensus conference proposed that cirrhosis-associated AKI should be defined by an increase in serum creatinine by more than 50% from the stable baseline value in less than 6 months or by 0.3 mg/dl (27 mmol/l) in less than 48 h [20].

8.4.3   Cardiovascular Derangements

Hemodynamic changes observed in patients with end-stage liver disease are characterized by humoral and nervous dysregulation secondary to autonomic nervous system activation and include increased cardiac output, peripheral vasodilatation, decreased systemic vascular resistance (SVR), and decreased oxygen extraction. Circulatory failure in cirrhotic patients with ACLF is distributive in nature and characterized by a greater decrease in arterial pressure associated with signs of impaired tissue perfusion. Marked splanchnic vasodilatation results in a state of effective hypovolemia with water and sodium retention [19, 21]. Although mechanisms for this autonomic nervous system activation are still poorly understood, it has been associated with higher mortality. In addition to hemodynamic changes, a decline in cardiac function termed cirrhotic cardiomyopathy has also been described [21]. This is characterized by a combination of diastolic and systolic dysfunction. Cirrhotic cardiomyopathy can be associated with a prolonged QT interval and can lead to an increased risk of ventricular arrhythmias/sudden cardiac death.

8.4.4   Neurological Derangements

The most common manifestation is a confusional syndrome superimposed on varying degrees of cognitive impairment that can even evolve to coma [22]. Precipitating factors, such as infection or electrolyte abnormalities, may enhance the disturbances attributable to liver failure or exert a direct effect on the brain. Important contributing factors are the systemic inflammatory response, circulatory dysfunction, and failure of other organs [6]. The activation of inflammatory mediators, such as cytokines, may enhance the effects of neurotoxins such as ammonia. Neuroinflammation increases blood-brain barrier permeability and, by generation of nitric oxide and prostanoids, causes astrocyte swelling. Other cerebrovascular abnormalities include disturbances of neurotransmission, injury to astrocytes, energy impairment, brain edema, loss of autoregulation, and brain atrophy. In cirrhosis, cerebral edema is an uncommon finding; however, cases of increased intracranial pressure have been identified [22, 23]. Patients with ACLF are also more vulnerable to central pontine myelinolysis which has been reported even with relatively modest elevations in sodium in this population. However, the most common cause of changes in mental status is hepatic encephalopathy, a disease process thought to be caused by astrocyte swelling and cerebral edema due to the synergistic effects of excess ammonia and inflammation, although the precise underlying molecular mechanisms are unclear. Hepatic encephalopathy is rarely solely due to worsening liver function, rather a precipitating cause almost always is responsible and determining this precipitant is key to management [19].

8.4.5   Respiratory Derangements

Pulmonary vascular issues affecting patients with ACLF can be divided into two distinct abnormalities: hepatopulmonary syndrome (HPS) and portopulmonary hypertension (PPH). Hepatopulmonary syndrome is characterized by intrapulmonary vasodilation leading to a ventilation/perfusion mismatch with resultant hypoxemia that can be found in up to 40% of patients with end-stage liver disease.

Diagnosis is based on its identification identify either through pulse oximetry or on arterial blood gas and the demonstration of an intrapulmonary shunt (which can usually be demonstrated with contrast echocardiography) if there is a normal chest x-ray and pulmonary function tests [24]. Portopulmonary hypertension is the presence of pulmonary arterial hypertension due to increased pulmonary vascular resistance and pulmonary vasoconstriction leading to right heart failure in the setting of advanced liver disease. The disease is largely believed to be underdiagnosed as a cause of dyspnea and decreased exercise capacity. Doppler echocardiography is a highly sensitive tool for detecting portopulmonary hypertension, using a right heart catheterization for confirmation and definitive diagnosis. The diagnosis is made if mean pulmonary arterial pressure is >25 mm Hg or left ventricular end-diastolic pressure <15 mm Hg in the setting of liver disease or portal hypertension. In general, the presence of portopulmonary hypertension is a poor prognostic sign [24, 25]. Moreover, pulmonary function can also be compromised by direct mechanical effects of hydrothorax and abdominal ascites on diaphragmatic movement. Hydrothorax is defined as a significant pleural effusion, usually >500 mL in a patient with end-stage liver disease, exclusive of primary cardiac or pulmonary disease. A pleural effusion is observed in approximately 5% of patients with ACLF. Various mechanisms have been proposed such as decreased osmotic pressure, leakage of plasma from azygous venous system, and lymph leakage from the thoracic duct, although the prevailing thought is direct transport into pleural space through diaphragmatic defects [19]. Finally, the presence of an exaggerated inflammatory response, coupled with a relative immunocompromised state likely can predispose patients to acute lung injury. The risk of aspiration pneumonia is also high because of altered consciousness, swallowing dysfunction, gastric stasis, increased intra-abdominal pressure due to ascites, and ileus resulting from infection and electrolyte abnormalities [22].

8.4.6   Coagulation Derangements

Coagulopathy in patients with critical liver dysfunction is complex and can quickly decompensate to bleeding as well as to thrombosis [26]. Both are associated with worse outcome. Standard tests of coagulation can be altered as a consequence of impaired synthesis of coagulation factors and increased consumption. However, routine plasmatic coagulation tests such as PT and INR are not able to discriminate between hypo- and hypercoagulability and are not able to predict the risk of bleeding in patients with liver dysfunction. Therefore, prophylactic transfusion of FFP and platelets due to an increased INR should be avoided in this patient population, and hemostatic interventions should only be performed in case of clinically relevant bleeding. In contrast, thrombin generation assays in the presence and absence of thrombomodulin indicate that patients with severe liver dysfunction are rather hypercoagulable with the inherent risk of thrombosis [26]. Altogether, modified thrombin generation assays can be useful for determination of coagulation function in patients with liver dysfunction, but have the major drawback of not being available as routine laboratory tests. Spontaneous bleeding is rare in ACLS patients. However, bleeding associated with trauma or acute variceal hemorrhage may be more dramatic as a consequence of both attendant coagulopathy and enhanced fibrinolysis. A relative decrease in hepatic-derived anticoagulant factors serves to offset the decrease in procoagulant factors in the patient with cirrhosis who has compensated disease. Alternative techniques for assessing coagulation such as thromboelastography may be helpful in identifying this balance and for guiding blood product replacement [22].

8.4.7   Adrenal Insufficiency

Adrenal insufficiency is reported in 51–68% of patients with cirrhosis, particularly in more severe patients. The impaired adrenal response may reflect either or both primary and secondary adrenal insufficiency with inadequate pituitary response and low adrenocorticotropic hormone levels. Other proposed hypotheses to explain this phenomenon are: decreased cholesterol levels, overstimulation of the hypothalamus-pituitary-adrenal axis by cytokines and endotoxemia. Adrenal dysfunction is frequently reported in patients with chronic liver diseases (compensated or decompensated), and it is associated with increased mortality compared to patients without it [22, 27].

8.5   Management

8.5.1   General Considerations

At present, there is no treatment specific for ACLF. Current treatment consists of supportive measures and therefore it should rely on enhanced care in intensive care units (ICUs) where the management of patients with multiorgan failure is protocolised and patients can be closely monitored. The aim of the general management should be focused on early recognition of any condition or precipitating factor which can cause ACLF or on avoiding exposure to those factors known to trigger multiple organ failure. Although not proven, it is thought that the greatest impact on patient's outcome will be achieved by preventing or slowing a further progression of ACLF. Patients with ACLF present some unique features that may differentiate them from the non-cirrhotic patients and thus, a multidisciplinary approach is essential [1, 19, 22, 27].

8.5.2   Liver Transplantation

Available evidence about liver transplantation (LT) for patients with ACLF is scarce even though this represents the only definitive therapeutic option for the vast majority of patients with ACLF [28, 29]. Nonetheless, a number of factors, including advanced age, active alcoholism, uncontrolled infections, concomitant diseases, and the presence of associated organ failures, make patients with ACLF often unsuitable to undergo LT [1]. As ACLF is associated with high short-term mortality up to 50–90% and may evolve rapidly into a fatal clinical situation, the timeframe for evaluating patients and assessing them for LT is short. Moreover, evidences regarding the long-term outcome of patients transplanted for ACLF are very limited. Some studies showed similar survival rates of patients with ACLF to patients with chronic liver disease who underwent transplantation for other indications [30, 31]. When interpreting these data sets, differences between western and eastern transplant centers must be taken into consideration. Moreover, published studies are retrospective and have a limited sample size. Most importantly, only one study used intention-to-treat analysis and showed that some potential candidates are not even listed for transplantation and out of those listed mortality is of 50% [30]. Overall, only one-third of potential candidates reach liver transplantation according to this report. There is therefore a clear need for effective therapeutic methods that can "bridge" patients with ACLF to liver transplantation. A study reported outcomes in 183 critically ill patients with ACLF denied listing for LT. It was noted a substantially higher mortality in these patients compared with those who were listed for LT. Several variables were independently associated with mortality in this study. Some of these predictors, such as APACHE II scores, sepsis, and respiratory failure requiring mechanical ventilation are already known to predict mortality in other groups of patients with liver disease. Conversely, the presence of gastrointestinal bleeding is an independent predictor of decreased mortality [32]. Indeed, further studies are still necessary to determine timing of liver transplantation, optimal selection, and whether ACLF patients should be prioritized on a high urgency list.

8.5.3   Infections

Because overt signs of infection may be absent, a high index of suspicion is necessary for diagnosis. When the suspicion for infection is high, early initiation of antibiotics is mandatory. A study by the Cooperative Antimicrobial Therapy for Septic Shock research showed, in a group of 635 critically ill cirrhotic patients with septic shock, a hospital mortality of 76%. The median time to appropriate antimicrobial therapy was 7.3 (3.2–18.3) hours with each hour delay associated with significantly increased mortality (adj-odds ratio per hour 1.1) [33]. Sepsis in ACLF can be managed according to Surviving Sepsis Campaign guidelines [34]. Strict adherence to hand hygiene and "bundles" of care (e.g., ventilator and central line) are required to prevent hospital-acquired infections. For prolonged ICU stays, weekly swabs for resistant organisms should be obtained. Testing for Clostridium difficile infection should also be routinely performed and repeated in critically ill patients with diarrhea. For patients who have active C. difficile infections and are critically ill, a prompt specific treatment should be started. ACLF patients has previously been thought to be especially susceptible to specific sepsis-related complications to include hypoglycemia, adrenal insufficiency, defective arginine-vasopressin secretion, and compartment syndrome [35]. Although early goal-directed therapy (EGDT) with specific hemodynamic targets is a well-defined approach for general ICU patients, no study has assessed it or the optimal endpoints for resuscitation in cirrhotic patients [27]. Finally, while relative adrenal insufficiency has been identified in patients with septic end-stage liver disease, there are no further guidelines other than standard recommendations supporting the administration of hydrocortisone in cases of shock refractory to fluid and vasopressors [34].

8.5.4   Kidney Injury

AKI in critically ill cirrhotic patients is common and often multifactorial. In the setting of cirrhosis, serum creatinine (SCr) tends to overestimate renal function due to decreased creatine production by the liver, protein calorie malnutrition, muscle wasting, reduced physical activity, and enlarged volume of distribution in the setting of fluid overload. In addition, in the setting of AKI, Scr can lag by several hours to days despite a decrease in glomerular filtration rate especially in the setting of fluid overload [36]. Therefore, it is recommended that Scr values be interpreted with caution in ACLF patients due to overestimation of values. As for HRS, the cornerstone of management remains albumin (1 g/kg initially followed by 20–40 g/day) and vasopressor therapy to mitigate splanchnic and systemic vasodilatation. Terlipressin, a vasopressin analogue, has been shown to reverse Type 1 HRS in 50% of patients without a difference in mortality [37, 38]. Recommended doses currently are 1–2 mg/q4–6 h i.v. bolus for a minimum of 72 h. Other small studies have shown norepinephrine to be equally as effective as terlipressin in Type I HRS [27]. Renal replacement therapies are not a treatment for HRS/cirrhosis induced AKI but is often initiated as a bridge to either liver transplant or definitive decision. Nephrotoxic medications such as nonsteroidal anti-inflammatory drugs, intravascular volume depletion, and avoidance of large-volume paracentesis without albumin replacement should be avoided [14, 19].

8.5.5   Cardiovascular Issues

Management of cirrhotic cardiomyopathy is directed toward left ventricular failure with beta-blockade, angiotensin-converting enzyme inhibitor/angiotensin receptor blockers, and diuretics as tolerated, although the evidence to support this therapy is not specific to heart failure due to end-stage liver disease [19]. Although there are no clinical studies validating management strategies, afterload reduction is anecdotally not well tolerated if the patient is peripherally vasodilated. Usually, the disease process is subclinical and only becomes apparent during times of physiologic stress. Potential ICU events that can exacerbate cirrhotic cardiomyopathy include shunting of portal flow to systemic circulation after transjugular intrahepatic portosystemic shunt (TIPS) and bacterial infections/endotoxemia leading to a high output hypotensive state. Patients may be hypotensive despite presence of a hyperdynamic state and being unresponsive to volume challenge. Ventricular compliance is decreased and can be assessed by manipulation of intravascular volume. That is, the change in central venous pressure (CVP) after fluid challenge is more instructive than a single measurement of the CVP and, when properly applied, passive leg raise may be used to assess volume responsiveness [19, 22, 36]. Increased intra-abdominal pressure due to ascites may result in increased CVP without improving cardiac preload. Minimally invasive methods of assessing hemodynamic parameters such as stroke volume variation and pulse pressure variation have gained popularity in the ICU, however in patients who are spontaneously breathing, these methods have limited utility. Moreover, such monitors have failed to demonstrate acceptable accuracy in cirrhotic patients undergoing liver transplantation, which further questions their role in the ICU [39]. Echocardiography provides a much more robust assessment of ventricular function and response to volume infusion. Echocardiography is noninvasive and may be relatively inexpensive. Because pulmonary hypertension is associated with cirrhosis, pulmonary artery catheterization is required to measure pulmonary artery and pulmonary artery occlusion pressures [22, 36]. With regard to the hemodynamic goals, the optimal mean arterial pressure blood lactate or venous oxygen saturation are unknown. In septic shock, in the absence of liver disease, there appears to be no advantage to inducing hypertension. However, HRS responds to increasing perfusion pressure by administration of terlipressin. Circulating intravascular volume should be restored recognizing the difficulties in assessing volume. Vasopressors such as norepinephrine are titrated to achieve a mean arterial pressure of 65–70 mm Hg. Vasopressin (or terlipressin) is norepinephrine-sparing in sepsis and appears to have a similar effect in patients with cirrhosis [19, 36].

8.5.6 Neurological Issues

The mainstay of treatment of hepatic encephalopathy is use of lactulose and nonabsorbable antibiotics. Lactulose is a nonabsorbable disaccharide that is metabolized by colonic bacterial flora into lactic acid, creating an acidic environment in the gut which aids the conversion of ammonia (NH_3) to ionic ammonium (NH4+), which is then passed via fecal excretion. There remains academic debate concerning the routine use of lactulose for the treatment of acute hepatic encephalopathy, as several trials have failed to demonstrate a significant effect on mortality over placebo or antibiotics [19, 22, 36]. The optimal dose of lactulose is not well established; however, titration to two to three semiformed stools per day is recommended [22]. Avoidance of profuse diarrhea and its associated electrolyte abnormalities is essential. When advanced encephalopathy or mechanical ventilation precludes oral administration, administration should be via enteric tube or retention enema. Rifaximin is a poorly absorbed rifamycin-based antibiotic with broad activity against ammonia-producing aerobic and anaerobic enteric flora. Due to low systemic absorption, rifaximin is well tolerated, with a similar occurrence of adverse effects compared to placebo [19]. The combination of lactulose plus rifaximin was shown to be more effective than lactulose alone in the prevention and treatment of overt hepatic encephalopathy [40]. Avoidance of sedative agents is a mainstay of treatment. In patients who demonstrate signs of cerebral edema or increased ICP, the administration of mannitol is mandatory, and invasive ICP monitoring may be considered [19]. Endotracheal intubation for airway control is mandatory in patients with a Glasgow coma scale score of 8 and/or in the presence of active upper gastrointestinal bleeding [22].

8.5.7 Respiratory Issues

The only definitive treatment for HPS is liver transplantation, which will result in complete resolution in 80% of the cases. Other forms of medical therapy such as somatostatin, indomethacin, methylene blue, and plasma exchange have been used but remain invalidated [19]. Transjugular intrahepatic portosystemic shunt as treatment for HPS can allow for reversal of intrapulmonary vasodilatation and redistribution of pulmonary blood flow via increase in cardiac output. However, its efficacy is only described at the case report level and is therefore not the first-line therapy. With regard to PPH, the diagnosis has specific transplant implications, as orthotopic liver transplant is classified as high risk if mean pulmonary artery pressure is between 35 mm Hg and 50 mm Hg and contraindicated if mean pulmonary artery pressure is >50 mm Hg due to high mortality from acute right heart failure [41, 42]. Medical treatment is generally indicated as a bridge to transplant and is based on the continuous infusion of a prostacyclin such as epoprostenol for mean pulmonary artery pressures >25 mm Hg. Although effective, continuous epoprostenol infusions may be burdensome due to complex dosing and cost [19, 22]. There are reports describing the use of sildenafil. Pulmonary function can also be compromised by direct mechanical effects of hydrothorax and abdominal ascites on diaphragmatic movement. Workup includes chest x-ray, pleural fluid analysis, and echocardiography. Management largely involves thoracentesis, sodium restriction, and diuretics. Symptomatic and refractory hydrothorax can be managed with TIPS cost [19, 22].

8.5.8 Coagulation

Routine correction of coagulation abnormalities in the absence of active bleeding is not indicated as it may be associated with significant complications including transfusion-associated lung injury, transfusion-associated circulatory overload, and transfusion reactions. When correction of bleeding abnormalities is required in the presence of active bleeding, prothrombin time, complete blood count, and activated partial thromboplastin time can be used but with the knowledge that they do not provide an adequate assessment of hemostasis in cirrhosis to guide therapy and thromboelastography should be considered [36]. Correction of coagulation abnormalities prior to placement of central venous or arterial catheters, paracentesis, thoracentesis, or bronchoscopy and endoscopy without biopsy is not required. Vitamin K, given at 2 mg intravenously daily for 3–5 days, should be administered to eliminate vitamin K deficiency as a source of coagulopathy [22, 36]. Massive acute hemorrhage should be managed with transfusion of red blood cells and fresh frozen plasma given in a 1:1 or 2:1 ratio with transfusion of platelets and fibrinogen concentrates to address consumption. Fibrinolysis is common and is readily assessed by thromboelastography. Treatment of fibrinolysis with tranexamic acid is indicated when bleeding persists, despite correction of thrombocytopenia and clotting factors in the absence of disseminated coagulopathy [22, 36].

8.5.9 Referral to a Liver Transplant Center

The determination of transplant candidacy is complex. All patients admitted to the ICU with complications of cirrhosis deserve a consultation with a transplant center in order to assess candidacy for liver transplantation. "Perceived" contraindication to transplant should never preclude this consultation.

8.5.10 Liver Support Devices

When medical treatments fails, artificial liver support can be considered as a bridge therapy to liver transplantation or while the precipitating event is reversed. Liver support devices are intended to support liver function until such time as native liver function recovers or liver transplantation is feasible. Two types of devices can be distinguished: acellular devices such as albumin dialysis and plasma exchange [mainly molecular adsorbents recirculating system (MARS), and Prometheus devices], and cell-based devices, which incorporate cells from human, animal sources, or immortalized cells. The overall efficacy of liver support devices have, at this time, failed to reach a level sufficient strength of evidence. Recently, two European multicenter randomized control trials have evaluated the impact of MARS and Prometheus. The RELIEF trial concluded that despite biochemical improvement, there was no significant difference in 28-day survival between patients treated with MARS vs. standard medical therapy [43]. Similarly, the HELIOS trial compared Prometheus to standard medical therapy. This study showed no significant survival differences at day 28 or at day 90 [44]. Both of these studies were biased due to confounding by indication. Cirrhotic patients who were and were not liver transplant candidates were included in enrollment representing groups with very different prognoses. Future trials evaluating indications (liver transplant candidates only), timing of treatment and cost effectiveness are still needed to clarify the role for these therapies.

Conclusions

ACLF is a devastating syndrome. It is based not only on the presence of organ failure and high mortality rate but also on younger age, alcoholic etiology of cirrhosis, higher prevalence of some triggers (particularly bacterial infections and active alcoholism), and a higher level of systemic inflammation which make

ACLF a clinically, pathophysiologically, and prognostically distinct entity. ACLF is a new entity also because it cannot be entirely explained by severe sepsis or severe alcoholic hepatitis as a large proportion of cases remains of unknown origin. Rather, ACLF should be considered as a whole that includes subcategories such as severe sepsis, severe alcoholic hepatitis, and other categories that require a more precise definition. Hopefully, new research in end-stage liver disease will allow the determination of modifiable factors that predispose to ACLF in order to personalize their management based on clinical and genetic factors.

References

1. Blasco-Algora S, Masegosa-Ataz J, Gutiérrez-García ML, Alonso-López S, Fernández-Rodríguez CM. Acute-on-chronic liver failure: pathogenesis, prognostic factors and management. World J Gastroenterol. 2015;21:12125–40.
2. Sarin SK, Kumar A, Almeida JA, et al. Acute-on-chronic liver failure: consensus recommendations of the Asian Pacific Association for the Study of the liver (APASL). Hepatol Int. 2009;3:269–82.
3. Jalan R, Gines P, Olson JC, et al. Acute-on-chronic liver failure. J Hepatol. 2012;57:1336–48.
4. Levesque E, Hoti E, Azoulay D, et al. Prospective evaluation of the prognostic scores for cirrhotic patients admitted to an intensive care unit. J Hepatol. 2012;56:95–102.
5. Moreau R, Jalan R, Gines P, et al. Acute-on-chronic liver failure is a distinct syndrome that develops in patients with acute decompensation of cirrhosis. Gastroenterology. 2013;144:1426–37.
6. Arroyo V, Moreau R, Jalan R, Ginès P, On behalf of the investigators of the EASL-CLIF consortium CANONIC study. Acute-on-chronic liver failure: a new syndrome that will re-classify cirrhosis. J Hepatol. 2015;62:S131–43.
7. Medzhitov R, Schneider DS, Soares MP. Disease tolerance as a defense strategy. Science. 2012;335:936–41.
8. Racanelli V, Rehermann B. The liver as an immunological organ. Hepatology. 2006;43:S54–62.
9. Jenne CN, Kubes P. Immune surveillance by the liver. Nat Immunol. 2013;14:996–1006. 41-43
10. Albillos A, Lario M, Álvarez-Mon M. Cirrhosis-associated immune dysfunction: distinctive features and clinical relevance. J Hepatol. 2014;61:1385–96.
11. Wasmuth HE, Kunz D, Yagmur E, Timmer-Stranghöner A, Vidacek D, Siewert E, Bach J, Geier A, Purucker EA, Gressner AM, Matern S, Lammert F. Patients with acute on chronic liver failure display "sepsis-like" immune paralysis. J Hepatol. 2005;42:195–201.
12. Adebayo D, Morabito V, Andreola F, Pieri G, Luong TV, Dhillon A, Mookerjee R, Jalan R. Mechanism of cell death in acute-on-chronic liver failure: a clinico-pathologic-biomarker study. Liver Int. 2015;35:2564–74.
13. Karvellas CJ, Pink F, McPhail M, et al. Bacteremia, acute physiology and chronic health evaluation II and modified end stage liver disease are independent predictors of mortality in critically ill nontransplanted patients with acute on chronic liver failure. Crit Care Med. 2009;38:121–6.
14. Berry PA, Antoniades CG, Carey I, et al. Severity of the compensatory anti-inflammatory response determined by monocyte HLA-DR expression may assist outcome prediction in cirrhosis. Intensive Care Med. 2011;37:453–60.
15. Bajaj JS, O'Leary JG, Reddy KR, on behalf of NACSELD, et al. Second infections independently increase mortality in hospitalized patients with cirrhosis: the north American consortium for the study of end-stage liver disease (NACSELD) experience. Hepatology. 2012;56:2328–35.
16. Galbois A, Aegerter P, Martel-Samb P. Improved prognosis of septic shock in patients with cirrhosis: a multicenter study. Crit Care Med. 2014;42:16666–1675.

17. Møller S, Krag A, Bendtsen F. Kidney injury in cirrhosis: pathophysiological and therapeutic aspects of hepatorenal syndromes. Liver Int. 2014;34:1153–63.

18. Dundar HZ, Yılmazlar T. Management of hepatorenal syndrome. World J Nephrol. 2015;4:277–86.

19. DellaVolpe J, Garavaglia JM, Huang DT. Management of complications of end-stage liver disease in the intensive care unit. J Int Care Med. 2016;31:94–103.

20. Wong F, O'Leary JG, Reddy KR, et al. New consensus definition of acute kidney injury accurately predicts 30-day mortality in patients with cirrhosis and infection. Gastroenterology. 2013;145:1280–8.

21. Ruiz-del-Árbol L, Serradilla R. Cirrhotic cardiomyopathy. World J Gastroenterol. 2015;21:11502–21.

22. Olson JC, Wendon JA, Kramer DJ, et al. Intensive care of the patient with cirrhosis. Hepatology. 2011;54:1864–72.

23. Liu A, Perumpail RB, Kumari R, et al. Advances in cirrhosis: optimizing the management of hepatic encephalopathy. World J Hepatol. 2015;7:2871–9.

24. Raevens S, Geerts A, Van Steenkiste C, Verhelst X, Van Vlierberghe H, Colle I. Hepatopulmonary syndrome and portopulmonary hypertension: recent knowledge in pathogenesis and overview of clinical assessment. Liver Int. 2015;35:1646–60.

25. Ramsay M. Portopulmonary hypertension and right heart failure in patients with cirrhosis. Curr Opin Anaesthesiol. 2010;23:145–50.

26. Schadena E, Saner FH, Goerlinger K. Coagulation pattern in critical liver dysfunction. Curr Opin Crit Care. 2013;19:142–8.

27. Karvellas CJ, Bagshaw SM. Advances in management and prognostication in critically ill cirrhotic patients. Curr Opin Crit Care. 2014;20:210–7.

28. Chan AC, Fan ST. Criteria for liver transplantation in ACLF and outcome. Hepatol Int. 2015;9:355–9.

29. Reddy MS, Rajalingam R, Rela M. Liver transplantation in acute-on-chronic liver failure: lessons learnt from acute liver failure setting. Hepatol Int. 2015;9:508–13.

30. Finkenstedt A, Nachbaur K, Zoller H, et al. Acute-on-chronic liver failure: excellent outcomes after liver transplantation but high mortality on the wait list. Liver Transpl. 2013;19:879–86.

31. Bahirwani R, Shaked O, Bewtra M, et al. Acute-on-chronic liver failure before liver transplantation: impact on posttransplant outcomes. Transplantation. 2011;92:952–7.

32. Kress JP, Rubin A, Pohlman A, Hall JB. Outcomes of critically ill patients denied consideration for liver transplantation. Am J Respir Crit Care Med. 2000;162:418–23.

33. Arabi YM, Dara SI, Memish Z, et al. Antimicrobial therapeutic determinants of outcomes from septic shock among patients with cirrhosis. Hepatology. 2012;56:2305–15.

34. Rhodes A, Evans LE, Alhazzani W, Levy MM, Antonelli M, et al. Surviving sepsis campaign: international guidelines for management of sepsis and septic shock: 2016. Intensive Care Med. 2017;43:304–77.

35. Gustot T, Durand F, Lebrec D, et al. Severe sepsis in cirrhosis. Hepatology. 2009;50:2022–33.

36. Nadim MK, Durand F, Kellum JA, et al. Management of the critically ill patient with cirrhosis: a multidisciplinary perspective. J Hepatol. 2016;64:717–35.

37. Sanyal AJ, Boyer T, Garcia-Tsao G, et al. A randomized, prospective, doubleblind,placebo-controlled trial of terlipressin for type 1 hepatorenal syndrome. Gastroenterology. 2008;134:1360–8.

38. Martin-Llahi M, Pepin MN, Guevara M, et al. Terlipressin and albumin vs albumin in patients with cirrhosis and hepatorenal syndrome: a randomized study. Gastroenterology. 2008;134:1352–9.

39. Biancofiore G, Critchley LA, Lee A, et al. Evaluation of a new software version of the FloTrac/Vigileo (version 3.02) and a comparison with previous data in cirrhotic patients undergoing liver transplant surgery. Anesth Analg. 2011;113:515–22.

40. Sharma BC, Sharma P, Lunia MK, et al. A randomized, double-blind, controlled trial comparing rifaximin plus lactulose with lactulose alone in treatment of overt hepatic encephalopathy. Am J Gastroenterol. 2013;108:1458–63.

41. Krowka MJ, Plevak DJ, Findlay JY, et al. Pulmonary hemodynamics and perioperative cardiopulmonary-related mortality in patients with portopulmonary hypertension undergoing liver transplantation. Liver Transpl. 2000;6:443–50.
42. Krowka MJ, Mandell MS, Ramsay MA, et al. Hepatopulmonary syndrome and portopulmonary hypertension: a report of the multicenter liver transplant database. Liver Transpl. 2004;10:174–82.
43. Bañares R, Nevens F, Larsen FS, Jalan R, Albillos A, Dollinger M, Saliba F, et al. Extracorporeal albumin dialysis with the molecular adsorbent recirculating system in acute-on-chronic liver failure: the RELIEF trial. Hepatology. 2013;57(3):1153–62.
44. Kribben A, Gerken G, Haag S, Herget-Rosenthal S, Treichel U, Betz C, et al. Effects of fractionated plasma separation and adsorption on survival in patients with acute-on-chronic liver failure. Gastroenterology. 2012;142:782–9.

Lara Pisani, Giuliano Lo Bianco, Marinella Pugliesi, Jacopo Tramarin, and Cesare Gregoretti

9.1 Introduction

In the last decades, NIV has expanded greatly in several populations of patients with acute respiratory failure (ARF). As a result of emerging evidence, NIV has been shown to reduce the necessity of invasive ventilation and associated complications [1]. NIV is now considered the first-choice ventilator treatment for a large number of patients with ARF such as exacerbations of COPD along with a success percentage of 80–85% [2–5], acute cardiogenic pulmonary edema, pulmonary infiltrates in immuno-compromised patients, and weaning from mechanical ventilation in COPD patients [1]. NIV success is strongly dependent on the patient's degree of tolerance and collaboration during ventilation [3]. One of the most frequent causes of premature interruption of the NIV is mask intolerance due to pain, discomfort, or claustrophobia [6]. Relative contraindications to NIV are delirium and agitation [2]. Judicious sedation may play a crucial role in improving patient's tolerance in selected cases at risk of endotracheal intubation due to NIV failure. Although the use of sedative drugs can reduce the risk of NIV failure, the possibility and suitability of sedating a patient during NIV remain a debated issue [7–10]. This chapter will focus on a practical overview of sedation and analgesia during NIV.

L. Pisani
Department of Specialistic, Diagnostic and Experimental Medicine (DIMES),
Respiratory and Critical Care, Sant'Orsola Malpighi Hospital, Alma Mater Studiorum,
University of Bologna, Via Massarenti 9, Bologna 40126, Italy

G.L. Bianco • M. Pugliesi • J. Tramarin • C. Gregoretti (✉)
Department of Biopathology and Medical Biotechnology (DIBIMED),
Section of Anesthesia Analgesia Intensive Care and Emergency,
Policlinico Paolo Giaccone, University of Palermo, Palermo, Italy
e-mail: c.gregoretti@gmail.com

© Springer International Publishing AG 2018
D. Chiumello (ed.), *Practical Trends in Anesthesia and Intensive Care 2017*,
http://doi.org/10.1007/978-3-319-61325-3_9

9.2   Sedation and NIV in Clinical Practice

A survey published in 2007 [11] showed that in clinical practice, the use of sedatives varies according to the geographical location or by the type of hospital where the NIV is applied and by the specialist who prescribes it. This survey found that benzodiazepines were the most used drugs in North America, while opioids (morphine and fentanyl), although preferred in Europe, were only used in 29% of cases. In addition, sedation was usually administered as an intermittent intravenous bolus according to clinical experience rather than using standardized protocols.

Recently [12] a retrospective study evaluated the efficacy and safety of sedation in agitated patients treated with NIV after an episode of acute respiratory failure. Of 3506 patients 120 [81 patients with non-intubation code (DNI) and 39 non-DNI] were given sedatives to control agitation during NIV. Sedation was performed only intermittently in 72 (60%) patients, switched to continuously in 37 (31%), and provided only continuously in 11 (9%). The reasons for poor NIV tolerance were mask discomfort, pressure discomfort, or the combination of the two. Risperidone and haloperidol were the drugs of choice for the intermittent use; dexmedetomidine, midazolam, or propofol were chosen for continuous infusion. The Richmond Agitation-Sedation Scale (RASS) was used as an index of sedation level. Results suggest that sedation during NIV can be used to allow continuation of NIV in agitated patients with either a DNI or non-DNI status. Nevertheless 48% of patients in the study had diseases such as ARDS, severe pneumonia, and acute exacerbation of interstitial lung disease which have weak NIV recommendations.

Despite intolerance is commonly perceived as a reason for NIV failure that should respond to sedation and analgesia, recent studies suggest that they are not used very often for that indication. Muriel et al. found [13] that sedation and analgesia were used in only about 20% of patients using NIV, and they did not bring any benefit in terms of reduction of NIV failure. The level of evidence in favor of an extensive application of sedation during NIV is still limited, and further larger controlled trials are needed to clarify the indications of sedation during NIV.

9.3   Use of Sedation and Analgesia During NIV

Sedation and analgesia are commonly used in the ICU to improve quality of life in intubated and critically ill patients. Analgo-sedation increases tolerance to the endotracheal tube, reduces anxiety and reactions to painful stimuli, allows a better adaptation of the patient to the hospital environment, modulates patient respiratory effort and drive, and makes invasive procedures tolerable [14].

Additional goals of sedation include preserving day/night cycles, hemodynamic stability, conservation of diaphragmatic function, preservation of metabolic homeostasis, and attenuation of the stress/immune response.

In patients undergoing NIV, sedation should be administered by experienced staff using the minimum doses required to ensure a good control of agitation and to improve the patient-ventilator interaction, without inducing any respiratory drive depression. NIV is usually applied only in patients with a minimum spontaneous breathing capacity and able to trigger the ventilator and to protect the airway. The ideal sedative drug during NIV should have a rapid onset, a predictable duration of action, a constant half-life time, a no impact on the hemodynamic and respiratory drive, an organ-independent metabolism, a minimal drug interaction, and, finally, a low cost. However, no single sedative agent currently available fulfills the criteria for an ideal agent.

9.4   Analgesic Agents

Morphine and synthetic molecules such as fentanyl and remifentanil are used in analgo-sedation procedures. Opioids are able to overcome the blood-brain barrier, interacting with a variety of central and peripheral receptors. In particular, they have an agonist action on opioid μ and κ receptors, producing analgesic action. Instead, the interaction with other receptors contributes to adverse events such as respiratory depression and hypotension. In particular, hypotension depends on different factor combinations that include sympathicolysis, bradycardia, and vagal stimulus for histamine release. Other side effects are depression level of consciousness and intestinal hypomobility. All these aspects should be considered when opioids are administered during NIV. Opioids are risky in patients with obstructive sleep apnea syndrome (OSA) because they can cause pharyngeal collapse and inhibition of the rapid eye movement (REM) phase. Naloxone and naltrexone are able to displace the molecules of morphine and analogues from the receptors, thus interrupting their action. Naloxone has an extreme short onset of action; it is indeed the drug of choice for acute opioid intoxication.

9.4.1   Morphine

Morphine is a potent opioid analgesic characterized by hepatic metabolism and renal excretion with intermediate volume of distribution. Dose adjustment is recommended in patients with hepatic or renal impairment in order to avoid accumulation of morphine active metabolites which may cause prolonged effects. Morphine produces its major effects in the central nervous system (CNS), but action on peripheral receptors will also exert effects. CNS effects include analgesia, sedation, mood changes, respiratory depression, pruritus, nausea, and vomiting. Morphine has a rapid onset but requires continuous titration of dosage to avoid the risk of accumulation. Sleep apnea increases the risk of morphine-induced respiratory depression. The first study which analyzed analgo-sedation in patients undergoing NIV was published in 1999 [15]. In this pilot study morphine was used successfully in 9 of the 12 enrolled patients with ALI/ARDS who underwent a trial of NIV. Success rate defined as avoidance of intubation and no further assisted ventilation for 72 h was achieved on six of nine occasions (66%).

9.4.2 Remifentanil

Remifentanil is a short-acting opioid with μ receptor selectivity and a unique pharmacokinetic profile. This drug has an onset time of approximately 1 min and shows a rapid blood-brain equilibration time, and it has a reduced distribution volume [16].

Furthermore, no dose adjustment is necessary in patients with renal and hepatic impairment [17].

There are limited data regarding the use of remifentanil during noninvasive mechanical ventilation. In a prospective preliminary study, Constantin et al. [18] evaluated the efficacy and safety of the use of remifentanil in 13 patients (ten with acute hypoxemic respiratory failure and three with acute hypercapnic respiratory failure) at risk of failing noninvasive ventilatory treatment for discomfort and/or refusal to continue NIV.

Continuous infusion of remifentanil (mean remifentanil dose 0.1 ± 0.03 μg/kg/min) to obtain a conscious sedation (score 2–3 of the Ramsay scale) led to a decrease in respiratory rate and improvement of arterial blood gases after 1 h, avoiding intubation in 9 of 13 patients (69%).

Subsequently in a prospective uncontrolled trial [19], efficacy and safety of remifentanil was evaluated in 36 patients with persistent acute respiratory failure ($PaO_2/FiO_2 < 200$ after a first-line trial of NIV to avoid intubation) who refused to continue treatment because of intolerance to two different interfaces (helmet and total face mask). The initial dose of the drug was 0.025 μg/kg/min increased by 0.010 μg/kg/min every minute until score 2–3 of the Ramsay scale was reached; maximum dosage was set to 0.12 μg/kg/min. With this protocol 61% of patients continued NIV after the initiation of remifentanil infusion.

No patient showed hemodynamic changes or reduction in respiratory drive during the study period; 14 patients were intubated: 12 for the persisting discomfort and 2 for hemodynamic instability due to the presence of septic shock. In addition, analgo-sedation with remifentanil showed a decrease in respiratory rate and an improvement in blood gas values both in mask or helmet-ventilated patients.

Despite these promising results, the use of remifentanil-based sedation during NIV is still very limited. So far, there are no studies in literature which show a clear effect on the respiratory drive to the actual clinical practice drug dosage.

9.5 Sedative Drugs

9.5.1 Dexmedetomidine

Dexmedetomidine is a α2-adrenergic receptors agonist which inhibits the release of norepinephrine from sympathetic nerve endings [20].

Its sedative and analgesic profile is due to the activity on the α2-adrenoceptors located in the locus coeruleus. Unlike clonidine, dexmedetomidine has a shorter half-life and an eight times greater selectivity for α2-adrenoceptors.

Among all sedative drugs dexmedetomidine carries the lowest risk of depressing the respiratory centers [20].

Furthermore, dexmedetomidine works synergically with other sedatives, allowing lower doses to be used, finally decreasing its dose-dependent side effects.

Continuous intravenous infusion should start at a dose between 0.2 and 1.4 mg/kg/h, and no loading dose should be administered.

Dexmedetomidine has showed, through its central sympathetic action, bradycardia and hypotension, while hypertension due to vasoconstriction may be provoked at higher concentrations [21].

A Japanese pilot study reports the first application of dexmedetomidine as a sedative agent during NIV [22] where the authors evidenced, after an hour of infusion, an improvement in gas exchange and respiratory rate.

Senoglu et al. [23] tested the sedative profile and adverse events of dexmedetomidine against midazolam in an ICU population of patients undergoing NIV for acute respiratory failure secondary to COPD exacerbation. In both groups sedation was targeted to achieve either a score 2–3 RASS or a score 3/4 Riker sedation-agitation scale or a bispectral index level >85. No serious cardiovascular adverse events or NIV failures were documented. However, during the sedation induction period, heart rate and blood pressure were significantly lower in the group treated with dexmedetomidine (incidence of bradycardia: 18.2% vs. 0, $p = 0.016$).

In terms of respiratory frequency and gas exchanges, no significative differences were found between the two groups.

Comparable results are brought up by another randomized trial [24] which involved 62 patients with hypoxemic respiratory failure who rejected NIV treatment due to high discomfort and marked agitation. Authors established that dexmedetomidine and midazolam had both a similar safety profile. However, at the same level of sedation, dexmedetomidine showed to have a shorter half-life time, allowing patients to fully awaken more rapidly. In addition, healthcare-associated infections were reduced, apparently because with dexmedetomidine no blunting of the cough reflex was observed. Finally with the alpha-2 selective agonist, the length of stay in ICU was shorter.

However, a recently published work [25] concluded that in patients with acute respiratory failure, intravenous dexmedetomidine infusion starting soon after NIV initiation does not maintain adequate levels of sedation and does not improve NIV tolerance. The authors attested that in a population of subjects undergoing NIV treatment, of which only one-third showed at baseline signs of NIV intolerance, a routine and early dexmedetomidine infusion does not bring any advantage over an intermittent bolus of fentanyl and midazolam. In fact, there was no significant difference in the prevention of agitation and delirium, no reduction in NIV failure rate, or any improvement in patient/nursing staff comfort.

9.5.2   Propofol

Propofol is a highly lipophilic phenolic derivate; it is not soluble in water. Its intravenous formulation is an emulsion of soybean oil, egg lecithin, and glycerol.

Propofol which has no analgesic properties is known to produce hypnosis and a dose-dependent respiratory depression.

Propofol has a very rapid onset (about 90 s) and offset (20 min); its minimally active metabolites are excreted by the kidney.

No antagonist is available for this drug, and it shall not be used by any operator who is not able to manage the airways.

Important hemodynamic effects (hypotension due to a fall in peripheral vascular resistances and tachy- or bradycardia) may be caused by rapid propofol infusion.

Propofol may cause, if infused for a prolonged time at high doses (>4 mg/kg/h), propofol infusion syndrome (PRIS). This syndrome was reported in both adult and pediatric population and is characterized by a severe metabolic acidosis with renal failure and rhabdomyolysis [26, 27].

Clouzeau et al. [28] evaluated, in a population of ten patients with acute respiratory failure at risk of NIV failure due to poor tolerance, the safety of target-controlled infusion technique (TCI) propofol infusion for sedation. TCI is an infusion technique which allows, by means of an infusion pump with a build-in algorithm, to reach a specific desired plasma drug concentration. Furthermore, according to the patient's clinical response, rapid adjustments in the plasma concentration are allowed.

9.5.3 Benzodiazepine

Benzodiazepines are very common drugs used to achieve sedation in ICU. Midazolam and lorazepam are by far the two most common benzodiazepines used in ICU due to their pharmacology which allows administration by both intermittent boluses or by continuous infusion.

While only a low dose is requested to achieve anxiolysis, deeper sedation, amnesia, and muscle relaxation, anticonvulsive effects can be achieved with a higher dosage along with common side effects as respiratory and cardiovascular depression.

In fact, anxiety, epilepsy, or procedures that require sedation and amnesia are within the most common situations for benzodiazepine use. These drugs act on the central nervous system binding to a specific site on the inhibitory gamma-aminobutyric acid (GABA) receptor, facilitating GABA effects.

Caution must be taken since benzodiazepines, like opioids, may accumulate after repeated doses [14, 29]. Furthermore, cardiovascular and respiratory depressions are more likely to be caused if the two drugs are administered at the same time. In addition, a longer hospital length of stay and a higher incidence of delirium are more associated with prolonged sedation with benzodiazepines [14].

Recent guidelines, in order to reduce the duration of invasive mechanical ventilation, ICU stay, and the incidence of delirium, suggest the application of different sedation protocols involving drugs like propofol and dexmedetomidine as alternatives to benzodiazepines [14].

Conclusions

Although the use of analgo-sedation in patients intolerant to NIV may have a strong rationale, the real benefit in the clinical practice is uncertain until the lack of large randomized controlled trials will endure. Recently a prospective, observational, multicenter, international study has been published to evaluate the effects of analgo-sedation in case NIV failing [13]. The study involved 322 ICUs in 30 countries including more than 840 patients who had received, after being admitted to intensive care, at least 2 h of NIV as an initial treatment. Muriel et al. have shown that analgo-sedation was used only in 19.6% of patients, confirming the data of the study published in 2007. In these patients the use of sedative drugs to improve patient comfort did not bring any benefit in terms of reduction of NIV failure defined as the need to intubate the patient.

Furthermore, using a rigorous statistical method, an increased risk of failure of NIV and an increase of mortality have been proven within patients undergoing treatment with sedatives and analgesics simultaneously.

In conclusion, although analgo-sedation is not required in patients receiving NIV, it could be used in specific clinical setting only after a first non-pharmacological approach has been carried out to improve the patient's interaction/adaptation to ventilation.

Furthermore, the use of analgo-sedation cannot ignore the consideration of other aspects such as the level of experience of the medical and nursing staff, the use of clinical systems for determining/monitoring the level of pain, distress, and depth of sedation, as well as adequate pharmacovigilance.

References

1. Walkey AJ, Wiener RS. Use of noninvasive ventilation in patients with acute respiratory failure, 2000-2009: a population based study. Ann Am Thorac Soc. 2013;10:10–7.
2. Nava S, Hill N. Non-invasive ventilation in acute respiratory failure. Lancet. 2009;374:250–9.
3. Demoule A, Girou E, Richard JC, Taille S, Brochard L. Benefits and risks of success or failure of noninvasive ventilation. Intensive Care Med. 2006;32(11):1756–65.
4. Frat JP, Thille AW, Mercat A, Girault C, Ragot S, Perbet S, Prat G, Boulain T, Morawiec E, Cottereau A, Devaquet J, Nseir S, Razazi K, Mira JP, Argaud L, Chakarian JC, Ricard JD, Wittebole X, Chevalier S, Herbland A, Fartoukh M, Constantin JM, Tonnelier JM, Pierrot M, Mathonnet A, Béduneau G, Delétage-Métreau C, Richard JC, Brochard L, Robert R, FLORALI Study Group, REVA Network. High-flow oxygen through nasal cannula in acute hypoxemic respiratory failure. N Engl J Med. 2015;372(23):2185–96.
5. Plant PK, Owen JL, Elliott MW. A multicentre randomised controlled trial of the early use of non-invasive ventilation in acute exacerbation of chronic obstructive pulmonary disease on general respiratory wards. Lancet. 2000;355:1931–5.
6. Carlucci A, Richard JC, Wysocki M, Lepage E, Brochard L, SRLF Collaborative Group on Mechanical Ventilation. Noninvasive versus conventional mechanical ventilation. An epidemiologic survey. Am J Respir Crit Care Med. 2001;163:874–80.
7. Hilbert G, Clouzeau B, Nam Bui H, Vargas F. Sedation during non-invasive ventilation. Minerva Anestesiol. 2012;78:842–6.
8. Scala R. Sedation during non-invasive ventilation to treat acute respiratory failure. Shortness of Breath. 2013;2:35–43.

9. Hilbert G, Navalesi P, Girault C. Is sedation safe and beneficial in patients receiving NIV? Yes. Intensive Care Med. 2015;41:1688–91.
10. Conti G, Hill NS, Nava S. Is sedation safe and beneficial in patients receiving NIV? No. Intensive Care Med. 2015;41:1692–5.
11. Devlin JW, Nava S, Fong JJ, Bahhady I, Hill NS. Survey of sedation practices during noninvasive positive-pressure ventilation to treat acute respiratory failure. Crit Care Med. 2007;35:2298–302.
12. Matsumoto T, Tomii K, Tachikawa R, Otsuka K, Nagata K, Otsuka K, Nakagawa A, Mishima M, Chin K. Role of sedation for agitated patients undergoing noninvasive ventilation: clinical practice in a tertiary referral hospital. BMC Pulm Med. 2015;13:15–71.
13. Muriel A, Peñuelas O, Frutos-Vivar F, Arroliga AC, Abraira V, Thille AW, Brochard L, Nin N, Davies AR, Amin P, Du B, Raymondos K, Rios F, Violi DA, Maggiore SM, Soares MA, González M, Abroug F, Bülow HH, Hurtado J, Kuiper MA, Moreno RP, Zeggwagh AA, Villagómez AJ, Jibaja M, Soto L, D'Empaire G, Matamis D, Koh Y, Anzueto A, Ferguson ND, Esteban A. Impact of sedation and analgesia during noninvasive positive pressure ventilation on outcome: a marginal structural model causal analysis. Intensive Care Med. 2015;41:1586–600.
14. Barr J, Fraser GL, Puntillo K, et al. Clinical practice guidelines for the management of pain, agitation, and delirium in adult patients in the intensive care unit. Crit Care Med. 2013;41:263–306.
15. Rocker GM, Mackenzie MG, Williams B, Logan PM. Non invasive positive pressure ventilation: successful outcome in patients with acute lung injury/ARDS. Chest. 1999;115:173–7.
16. Kuhlen R, Putensen C. Remifentanil for analgesia based sedation in the intensive care unit. Crit Care. 2004;8:13–4.
17. Hoke JF, Shlugman D, Dershwitz M, Michałowski P, Malthouse-Dufore S, Connors PM, et al. Pharmaco-kinetics and pharmacodynamics of remifentanil in persons with renal failure compared with healthy volunteers. Anesthesiology. 1997;87:533–41.
18. Constantin JM, Schneider E, Cayot-Constantin S, Guerin R, Bannier F, Futier E, Bazin JE. Remifentanil-based sedation to treat noninvasive ventilation failure: a preliminary study. Intensive Care Med. 2007;33:82–7.
19. Rocco M, Conti G, Alessandri E, et al. Rescue treatment for noninvasive ventilation failure due to interface intolerance with remifentanil analgosedation: a pilot study. Intensive CareMed. 2010;36:2060–5.
20. Paris A, Tonner PH. Dexmedetomidine in anaesthesia. Curr Opin Anaesthesiol. 2005;18:412–8.
21. Bekker A, Sturatis M, Bloom M, Moric M, Golfinos J, Parker E, et al. The effect of dexdemetomidine on perioperative hemodynamics in patients undergoing craniotomy. Anesth Analg. 2008;107:1340–7.
22. Akada S, Takeda S, Yoshida Y, Nakazato K, Mori M, Hongo T, Tanaka K, Sakamoto A. The efficacy of dexmedetomidine in patients with noninvasive ventilation: a preliminary study. Anesth Analg. 2008;107:167–70.
23. Senoglu N, Oksuz H, Dogan Z, Yildiz H, Demirkiran H, Ekerbicer H. Sedation during noninvasive mechanical ventilation with dexmedetomidine or midazolam: a randomized, double-blind, prospective study. Curr Ther Res Clin Exp. 2010;71:141–53.
24. Huang Z, Chen YS, Yang ZL, Liu JY. Dexmedetomidine versus midazolam for the sedation of patients with non-invasive ventilation failure. Intern Med. 2012;51:2299–305.
25. Devlin JW, Al-Qadheeb NS, Chi A, Roberts RJ, Qawi I, Garpestad E, Hill NS. Efficacy and safety of early dexmedetomidine during noninvasive ventilation for patients with acute respiratory failure: a randomized, double-blind, placebo-controlled pilot study. Chest. 2014;145:1204–12.
26. Bray RJ. Propofol infusion syndrome in children. Pediatr Anaesth. 1998;8:491–9.
27. Cremer OL, Moons KG, Bouman EA, et al. Long term propofol infusion and cardiac failure in adult head-injuerd patients. Lancet. 2001;357:606–7.
28. Clouzeau B, Bui HN, Vargas F, Grenouillet-Delacre M, Guilhon E, Gruson D, Hilbert G. Target controlled infusion of propofol for sedation in patients with non-invasive ventilation failure due to low tolerance: a preliminary study. Intensive Care Med. 2010;36:1675–80.
29. Devlin JW, Roberts RJ. Pharmacology of commonly used analgesics and sedatives in the ICU: benzodiazepines, propofol, and opioids. Anesthesiol Clin. 2011;29:567–85.

Critical Care Management of Subarachnoid Hemorrhage (SAH)

10

Luciana Mascia, Anna Teresa Mazzeo, and Simone Caccia

10.1 Introduction

Nontraumatic subarachnoid hemorrhage (SAH) represents about 3% of all strokes in the USA. Worldwide the incidence of SAH is 2–16/100,000 people, and it has not undergone changes in the last three decades. Females are more commonly affected than males (F:M = 1.24:1), as are some ethnic groups (African Americans and Hispanics) compared to white Americans [1, 2]. SAH incidence increases with age (onset ≥ 50 years), while the prevalence rate is 3.2% [3]. In about 80% of cases, the cause of SAH is the rupture of a cerebral aneurysm (annual rupture rate 0.95%) [4]; in 15% of SAH, there is no evidence of source of bleeding with neuroimaging studies; and finally the remaining 5% of cases is explained by other causes (arteriovenous malformations, vasculitis). SAH is responsible for significant morbidity and mortality. Mortality rates vary widely between different studies (8–67%), but most of these studies do not take into account prehospital mortality (about 10–15%) [5].

A significant reduction of SAH mortality rates has been observed worldwide (30-day mortality 32–42%) [6], attributable to the improvements in patient care (neurosurgical intensive care, endovascular therapy, microsurgical techniques) which have increased the survival in hospitalized patients. Despite the reduction in fatality rates, about 50% of survivors have significant permanent reduction in health-related quality of life (loss of working capacity, social independence, and personal/family relationships at a 5-year follow-up). This quality of life reduction

L. Mascia (✉)
Dipartimento di Scienze e Biotecnologie Medico Chirurgiche, Sapienza University of Rome, Policlinico Umberto I Hospital, 00161 Rome, Italy
e-mail: luciana.mascia@uniroma1.it

A.T. Mazzeo • S. Caccia
Dipartimento di Anestesiologia e Rianimazione, Università di Torino, Ospedale S. Giovanni Battista-Molinette, Torino, Italy

© Springer International Publishing AG 2018
D. Chiumello (ed.), *Practical Trends in Anesthesia and Intensive Care 2017*,
http://doi.org/10.1007/978-3-319-61325-3_10

has multifactorial causes such as impairment of physical functions, cognitive deficits (executive function and memory), mood disorders (anxiety, depression, and posttraumatic stress disorder), and personality disorders [7, 8].

Several risk factors have been identified, both nonmodifiable (age, female sex, previous aneurysmal SAH, familiarity) and modifiable (hypertension, cigarette smoking, alcohol abuse, sympathomimetic drugs use). Other risk factors are some genetic diseases (autosomal dominant polycystic kidney disease, Ehlers-Danlos syndrome type IV, Marfan syndrome, neurofibromatosis type I, fibromuscular dysplasia), cerebral aneurysms of the anterior circulation in patients <55 years, cerebral aneurysms of the posterior circulation in male patients, cerebral aneurysms >7 mm in diameter, and finally patients with significant legal or financial problems over the last 30 days. It is unknown whether there are factors playing a predominant role but, if present simultaneously, many of them can interact among themselves with a synergistic effect [9–14]. Antihypertensive treatment is recommended and may reduce the risk of SAH, as well as avoiding tobacco and alcohol use and eating a diet rich in vegetables [2].

10.2 Clinical Features

Most of cerebral aneurysms are not diagnosed during life, or their detection is incidental. Inflammation appears to play an important role in the pathogenesis and growth of intracranial aneurysms [2]. Clinically the aneurysm may present with headache, bitemporal hemianopsia and bilateral hyposthenia of the lower limbs (anterior communicating artery), unilateral third cranial nerve palsy (posterior communicating artery), facial or orbital pain, epistaxis, progressive visual loss and/or ophthalmoplegia (intracavernous internal carotid artery), and with symptoms of brain stem dysfunction (posterior circulation).

SAH is the most common clinical presentation of an aneurysm [6]. A severe, sudden headache (thunderclap headache, often described as the worst headache a patient has ever had) is the typical onset of SAH, and it occurs in about 80% of patients, accompanied by nausea, vomiting, photophobia, neck pain and stiffness, and loss of consciousness [15]. Physical examination should include evaluation of level of consciousness, fundus oculi, meningeal signs, and presence of focal neurological deficits. Focal neurological deficits (including cranial nerve palsies) are present in 10% of SAH patients and are associated with worse prognosis when caused by the presence of thick subarachnoid clots or intraparenchymal hemorrhage.

A transient increase in intracranial pressure (ICP) is responsible for nausea, vomiting, and syncope; coma and even brain death can occur in case of more severe and prolonged increase in ICP values. Terson syndrome (vitreous hemorrhage associated with SAH) occurs in up to 40% of SAH patients [16, 17]. A sudden increase in ICP may cause preretinal hemorrhages associated with more severe SAH and increased mortality.

Occasionally some patients may have atypical SAH presentation with seizures, acute encephalopathy, concomitant subdural hematoma, and traumatic brain injury, making diagnosis more difficult. Some patients (10–43% of cases) experience days or weeks before aneurysmal SAH the so-called "sentinel" headache caused by a small blood loss from the aneurysm [18, 19]. Unfortunately this event often represents only retrospective information since sentinel headache is temporary, and head CT is negative in 50% of cases.

10.3 Diagnosis

10.3.1 Head CT

The initial and more appropriate diagnostic test for patients with suspected SAH is a non-contrast head CT [15]. CT sensitivity was found to be 98–100% in detecting subarachnoid blood within 12 h from symptoms onset, compared to lumbar puncture. CT sensitivity is reduced to 93% at 24 h and to 50% at 7 days after the event [20, 21]. The typical appearance of blood extravasated in the basal subarachnoid cisterns is hyperdense. Other localizations include the sylvian scissure, the interhemispheric scissure, the interpeduncular fossa, and suprasellar, ambient, and quadrigeminal cisterns. CT can also highlight intracerebral hemorrhage, intraventricular hemorrhage, and hydrocephalus. In the first 2 days of SAH presentation, MRI is as sensitive as CT but is rarely performed into this context for logistical reasons [22, 23]. Several days after SAH onset, MRI with hemosiderin-sensitive sequences (gradient echo and susceptibility-weighted imaging) or with FLAIR sequences (fluid-attenuated inversion recovery) is more sensitive than CT.

10.3.2 Lumbar Puncture

Lumbar puncture is recommended in all patients with clinical suspicion of SAH and negative or uncertain head CT. Cerebrospinal fluid (CSF) should be collected in four consecutive samples, and red blood cell counts should be performed in the first and fourth sample [15, 24]. Elevated opening pressure, elevated number of erythrocytes not significantly reducing in the fourth sample compared to the first one, and especially CSF xanthochromia are all elements that direct toward SAH diagnosis. Xanthochromia demonstrates intraliquoral hemolysis, and it can be detected by visual inspection of the sample or through spectrophotometry. Xanthochromia develops in about 12 h from SAH onset, and spectrophotometry seems to be more sensitive than visual inspection, which remains anyway the most widely used method. There is no clinical study that has determined the false negative rate for xanthochromia in different time intervals after SAH onset [25].

10.3.3 Source of Bleeding

All patients with diagnostic head CT and diagnostic or uncertain lumbar puncture must undergo CT angiography (CTA) or digital subtraction angiography (DSA) [15, 24].

DSA is traditionally considered the "gold standard" diagnostic test to detect the source of bleeding in SAH (especially aneurysmal SAH) and to plan the most suitable treatment. In many centers, CTA is commonly performed as a first-line diagnostic test, given its increasing availability. CTA has a 90–97% sensitivity and a 93–100% specificity (variability depends on technical factors such as the use of 16 or 64 slices, slice thickness, data processing algorithms, and finally the reader's experience [26, 27]). CTA may be unreliable in detecting small (<4 mm) or distal aneurysms. Finally the choice between performing CTA or DSA depends on the availability of resources and institutional protocols. In SAH patients presenting with loss of consciousness DSA should be performed even if CTA is negative. Patients with negative DSA should repeat it between 7 and 14 days since SAH onset, and if still negative, they should undergo magnetic resonance angiography (MRA) to detect possible cerebral, brainstem, or spinal vascular malformations [28].

10.3.4 Misdiagnosis

SAH may be not diagnosed because typical findings are not well defined or for an atypical clinical scenario. Since it is a medical emergency, a misdiagnosis is associated with a significant increase in mortality and disability (up to four times) in those patients presenting with no neurological deficits. Misdiagnosis has decreased from 60% in the early 1980s to 15% in recent years [29, 30]. It must be stressed how important is having a high index of suspicion in front of each new-onset headache to make a correct differential diagnosis. A recent study found a series of clinical factors assuring a 100% sensitivity in detecting SAH in patients with >40 years, including neck pain or stiffness, loss of consciousness, symptoms onset during physical exercise, thunderclap headache, and neck flexion pain ("The Ottawa SAH Rule") [31].

10.3.5 Perimesencephalic SAH

Imaging studies fail to demonstrate the source of bleeding in approximately 15% of SAH patients. It is estimated that 38% of these patients have a non-aneurysmal perimesencephalic SAH [32]. Fifty-four percent of patients with non-aneurysmal perimesencephalic SAH are male and have a lower risk of complications with better outcome than aneurysmal SAH patients. A correct diagnosis is important given the catastrophic consequences of not identifying a ruptured cerebral aneurysm. Non-aneurysmal perimesencephalic SAH occurs with negative CTA or DSA but with a characteristic head CT scan [33]. The hemorrhage origin is localized anterior to the midbrain, with or without blood spreading to the front portion of ambient cistern or to the basal part of sylvian scissure. Interhemispheric scissure is not completely occupied by the hemorrhage, and there is no intraventricular blood.

10.4   Initial Assessment

Initial assessment and management of SAH patients with impaired consciousness must focus on stabilizing airway, breathing, and circulation [2, 15, 22–24]. Once stabilized, patients should undergo head CT and, if the patient is unable to protect airway, must be immediately intubated. The most common indications for endotracheal intubation include coma, hydrocephalus, seizures, and the need for sedation. We must also avoid extreme values of blood pressure that could trigger rebleeding; therefore, controlling hypertension is critical [34]. On the basis of randomized controlled clinical trials, it is recommended to maintain mean arterial pressure (MAP) <110 mmHg or systolic blood pressure < 160 mmHg until ruptured aneurysm treatment, avoiding hypotension not to compromise cerebral perfusion [35, 36]. Usually blood pressure control is achieved by treating patient's pain, otherwise administering labetalol IV (5–20 mg), hydralazine (5–20 mg), or continuous nicardipine infusion (5–15 mg/h). To treat patient's pain, short-acting opioids are used.

10.4.1 Severity Assessment

The severity of neurological impairment and the amount of subarachnoid bleeding at patient's admission are the strongest predictors of neurological complications and outcome [15, 23]. It is therefore essential to assess the patient, after stabilization, using a scoring system. There are several scoring systems available such as the Hunt and Hess classification or the WFNS (World Federation of Neurosurgical Surgeons) grading system. The prognostic advantage of the one or the other scale is uncertain and both have limitations [37]. The WFNS scale has the advantage to have identified as a prognostic factor focal neurological deficit only in a patient with preserved consciousness. The modified Fisher scale categorizes SAH imaging findings on head CT, and the amount of subarachnoid bleeding is a predictor of cerebral vasospasm, delayed cerebral ischemia (DCI), and overall patient outcomes [38–40]. Currently WFNS scale is used for clinical grading (the score is derived from Glasgow Coma Scale (GCS) and neurological examination), and modified Fisher scale is used for radiological grading (the score is obtained by evaluating the amount of blood on head CT) [41, 42]. Elevated WFNS and modified Fisher scores are associated with poorer clinical outcome and a higher rate of neurological complications.

10.4.2 Admission in High-Volume Centers

SAH patients should be admitted in high-volume center, hospitalized in neurosurgical intensive care unit, and assessed by a multidisciplinary team for a correct cerebral aneurysm management [2, 43]. It has been demonstrated that admission of

SAH patients in low-volume centers is associated with increased 30-day mortality compared to admission in high-volume centers. Furthermore, hospitalization in neurosurgical intensive care unit managed by neurointensivists is associated with a reduced in-hospital mortality [44].

10.5   Aneurysm Treatment

In the management of cerebral aneurysms, there are two effective treatments: surgical clipping and endovascular coiling. The goal is to completely obliterate the aneurysm and exclude it from circulation whenever possible. Clipping consists in excluding the aneurysm sac from circulation by positioning a vascular clip at the aneurysm neck with microsurgical technique. Coiling is an endovascular treatment and consists in bringing an endovascular microcatheter to the aneurysm sac and releasing through these very thin metallic coils until complete aneurysm occlusion. The choice between this two treatment options depends on several factors including patient age, aneurysm localization and morphology, and the relationship with adjacent vessels. Since deciding on the most appropriate treatment for each patient is complex, it is important that the assessment is performed by a multidisciplinary team consisting of cerebrovascular neurosurgeons, endovascular-trained physicians, and neurointensivists to reach a consensus on therapy [2, 15, 22, 23, 30, 43]. A prospective randomized controlled clinical trial—ISAT (International Subarachnoid Aneurysm Trial)—was performed to evaluate patients with treatable aneurysms and candidates for both endovascular coiling and surgical clipping [45, 46]. Patients assigned to the coiling group showed a significantly better outcome (in terms of disability-free survival at a 1-year follow-up, evaluated with modified Rankin scale) and a lower risk of epilepsy compared to the clipping group. On the other hand, the risk of rebleeding and only partial aneurysm occlusion was lower in the clipping group. Overall, endovascular coiling should be preferred compared to surgical clipping whenever possible. Many aneurysms are not equally eligible for clipping or coiling. Characteristics such as advanced age, poor clinical grading, underlying multiple systemic comorbidities, aneurysms of basilar artery tip and vertebrobasilar circulation, aneurysms of intracavernous internal carotid artery, and high surgical risk make endovascular coiling preferable. Other features such as giant, fusiform aneurysms, with an elevated neck/body ratio (>0.5), localized at arterial bifurcations and middle cerebral artery aneurysms or associated with large parenchymal hematomas make surgical clipping more suitable. In young patients, surgical clipping is preferable as it provides better protection against SAH recurrence. After every aneurysm repair surgery, it is recommended to perform an immediate cerebrovascular imaging examination to identify promptly any residues or recurrences of aneurysmal pathology requiring further treatment [2]. Regardless of the chosen treatment, aneurysms should be treated as early as possible to prevent rebleeding and to safely and effectively treat vasospasm [6].

10.6   Anesthetic Management

The general goals of anesthesiologic management include hemodynamic control to minimize the risk of aneurysm re-rupture and strategies to protect the brain from ischemic injury. Depending on SAH severity, patients will exhibit a different degree of cerebrovascular reactivity impairment and of cerebral autoregulation impairment, making brain perfusion strictly dependent on MAP value. Therefore the patient should not be exposed to hypotension, with associated risk of DCI, or hypertension, with risk of rebleeding [47, 48]. The goal is to maintain the transmural pressure gradient through the aneurysm wall and to maintain the cerebral perfusion pressure (CPP), given by the subtraction MAP-ICP. A sudden increase in blood pressure along with a rapid reduction in ICP can alter the gradient and increase the risk of aneurysm rupture. It is therefore important to avoid hypotension or hypertension during induction of anesthesia, intubation, surgical incision, and opening of dura. Prior to induction of anesthesia, a central venous access and also an arterial access with intra-arterial blood pressure monitoring must be obtained to be able to continuously calculate CPP and the transmural pressure gradient through the aneurysm wall [49]. Many pharmacological agents have been used for neuroprotective purpose during aneurysm surgery, but no one has shown a significant improvement in outcome.

10.6.1 Anesthesia

The maintenance of anesthesia can be handled with inhaled agents, used with a minimum alveolar concentration ≤ 1 (MAC), along with the use of analgesics such as fentanyl, sufentanil, or remifentanil, and with an appropriate neuromuscular blockade obtained with non-depolarizing agents. The cerebral vasodilator effect of modern inhaled agents such as desflurane, isoflurane, and sevoflurane, used at MAC ≤ 1, is not clinically relevant as it depends on dosage and solubility coefficient of the gas in the blood [50, 51]. Alternatively maintenance of anesthesia can be achieved by total intravenous anesthesia (TIVA), based on propofol use. This technique may be preferable in patients with elevated ICP, as it reduces cerebral blood flow (CBF) and ICP, and also in patients monitored with evoked potentials, thus avoiding interferences with inhaled agents [52, 53]. It has not been demonstrated any superiority of TIVA compared to inhaled agents, in terms of anesthetic efficacy and neurological healing, and it is possible to use the two techniques in combination [54–56].

10.6.2 Neurophysiological Monitoring

Somatosensory evoked potentials (SSEP) and brain stem auditory evoked potentials (BAEP) can be used to monitor cerebral function. SSEP are used during aneurysm surgery in the area of both anterior and posterior cerebral circulation. BAEP are used during surgical interventions in the area of vertebrobasilar circulation. Monitoring through evoked potentials serves to guide the surgical procedure (removing or repositioning a vascular clip) and hemodynamic management (arterial blood pressure). Unfortunately this type of monitoring is not specific, and there are no studies that document an improvement in outcome [49].

10.6.3 ICP

ICP monitoring is particularly useful in the management of blood pressure during induction of anesthesia and in the postoperative period, especially in the patient who remains unconscious after surgery [49]. Elevated ICP management involves simple therapeutic measures such as lifting the headboard of the patient bed and preventing jugular venous compression. It is important to maintain $PaCO_2$ level around 35 mmHg ensuring a proper depth of anesthesia. To further reduce ICP, intravenous mannitol or hypertonic saline can be administered. Intravenous mannitol 20% is infused during 10–15 min at a dosage of 0.5 g/kg. The hypertonic saline should be administered via central venous access in order to avoid the risk of thrombophlebitis. There are no definitive data on the superiority of the one or the other solution. When all these therapeutic measures fail to control ICP, hyperventilation can be used, but it should be suspended as soon as the indication is ended [57]. Elevated ICP is a common complication in the first week after severe SAH in intensive care patients and is associated with the severity of initial brain injury and with mortality [58].

10.6.4 Hypothermia

The role of hypothermia in patients with surgically treated intracranial aneurysm has been studied in the IHAST II trial, whose results have shown that inducing mild hypothermia (33 °C), despite being relatively safe, is not associated with an improvement in neurological outcome and mortality. Since IHAST II has some limitations, the role of hypothermia cannot be completely denied and should be further evaluated [59].

10.7　Critical Care Management

In the early stage, SAH is often associated with severe systemic and intracranial consequences rather than further brain damage [60–63]. More than 75% of SAH patients experience a systemic inflammatory response syndrome (SIRS), probably due to high levels of inflammatory cytokines, associated with permanent neurocognitive dysfunction. SAH patients have an increased risk of developing several neurological complications, including hydrocephalus, cerebral edema, delayed cerebral ischemia, rebleeding, seizures, and neuroendocrine disorders leading to alteration of sodium, water, and glucose homeostasis. SAH also triggers alterations mediated by the hypothalamus increasing the orthosympathetic and parasympathetic tone, responsible for cardiac and pulmonary complications. Increased levels of circulating catecholamines are thought to be the basis of several cardiac manifestations including ECG alterations, arrhythmias, contractility disorder (Takotsubo cardiomyopathy), troponinemia, and myocardial necrosis. A similar pathophysiologic mechanism is probably the basis of pulmonary complications such as neurogenic pulmonary edema. It is important to recognize and treat all these systemic complications since they are associated with an increased risk of delayed cerebral ischemia and poor neurological outcome after SAH.

10.8   Neurological Complications

10.8.1 Rebleeding

Rebleeding is a major disabling complication of SAH, which involves high rates of mortality and morbidity. Four to fifteen percent of SAH patients rebleed within the first 24 h, but the risk is more elevated within the first 6 h after symptoms onset. The risk of rebleeding decreases over the next 2 weeks. The main associated risk factors include elevated systolic blood pressure (>160 mmHg), poor neurological grading, intracerebral or intraventricular hematomas, posterior circulation ruptured aneurysms and aneurysms >10 mm in diameter [34]. The best therapeutic measure to reduce rebleeding risk is the early treatment of the aneurysm [43]. When there is delay in treatment (clipping or coiling), tranexamic acid or aminocaproic acid should be given to the patient within 72 h and if there are no contraindications. The use of antifibrinolytic agents is justified by the fact that early risk of rebleeding is a consequence of activated fibrinolysis and therefore reduced clot stability in the first 6 h. It is also very important in the prevention of rebleeding blood pressure control before aneurysm repair. Nicardipine seems to provide better blood pressure control over labetalol and sodium nitroprusside, although there are no demonstrated differences in clinical outcome [64]. Since systemic hypertension following SAH is mediated by V1a receptors of vasopressin, it has been supposed that treatment with inhibitors of these receptors could reduce hemorrhage severity and prevent rebleeding, improving outcome [65]. Patients with suspected rebleeding should be immediately evaluated, performing head CT and DSA, and the aneurysm should be treated immediately. As far as endovascular treatment is concerned, it should only involve coiling of ruptured aneurysm. Stenting of cerebral aneurysm in the context of SAH should be avoided as it is associated with more hemorrhagic complications and poor outcome [2].

10.8.2 Hydrocephalus

Acute symptomatic hydrocephalus occurs in about 20% of SAH patients, usually within the first days after symptoms onset [2, 15, 22]. Patient's presentation is with a reduced level of consciousness and other signs of increased ICP, such as impaired upward movement of the eyes and hypertension. It is recommended to perform a control head CT in any suspected symptomatic hydrocephalus patient, followed by external ventricular drainage (EVD) placement. In patients with SAH complicated by communicating hydrocephalus, a lumbar drainage may be positioned, in some cases, instead of EVD. About 60% of SAH patients treated with EVD are successfully weaned, while the remaining is treated with the placement of a permanent ventriculoperitoneal shunt. The weaning of the patient from EVD should begin immediately after the treatment of the aneurysm or <48 h from the EVD positioning if the patient is neurologically stable. A fast weaning protocol is preferable as it has been shown that a gradual weaning (>24 h) is not effective in reducing the need for ventricular shunt.

10.8.3 Seizures

Defining the exact incidence of seizures in SAH patients is difficult and controversial since many patients (20–26%) experience seizure-like episodes that are unlikely to be correctly assessed as they occur at symptoms onset [15, 45, 46]. Generally, patients with middle cerebral artery aneurysms, thick subarachnoid clots, rebleeding, cerebral infarction, history of hypertension, concomitant intraparenchymal hematomas, and poor clinical grading are at higher risk of seizures, while patients treated with endovascular coiling have lower seizure rates. The long-term risk of developing epilepsy is low. A nonconvulsive status epilepticus is a strong predictor of poor outcome. Administering prophylactic antiepileptic drugs in SAH patients was common practice, but treatment, especially with phenytoin, was associated with worse clinical outcome and elevated incidence of drug-related complications [2]. It is therefore recommended to avoid phenytoin and, if treatment is needed, short-term administration of the antiepileptic drug, for 3–7 days. Prophylactic therapy is reasonable in patients in the acute stage of SAH to prevent further brain injury or rebleeding. In SAH patients with poor grading subclinical seizures may occur even with high frequency, so in this context, continuous EEG monitoring is recommended [43].

10.8.4 Delayed Cerebral Ischemia

Delayed cerebral ischemia (DCI) is one of the most feared complications after SAH and is the event with the greatest impact on functional outcome [62, 63]. It occurs in about 30% of SAH patients, usually between days 4 and 14 after symptoms onset. It is defined as any sign of neurological deterioration (focal or global) which is presumed to be secondary to cerebral ischemia, persistent for more than 1 h, and not explained by another neurological or systemic condition. This fact implies that DCI is a diagnosis of exclusion; therefore, there must be no hydrocephalus, sedation, hypoxemia, seizures, electrolytic alterations, and renal or hepatic dysfunction. Factors involved in DCI pathogenesis are different, including cerebral vasospasm, microcirculatory constriction, microthrombosis, cortical spreading depression (CSD), delayed cell apoptosis, loss of blood-brain barrier integrity, cerebral edema, and loss of cerebral autoregulation [66, 67]. Most likely, the principal factor triggering all these processes is the release of oxyhemoglobin and other erythrocyte components through hemolysis, which activates a number of inflammatory and proapoptotic factors. CSD is a depolarizing wave spreading through cerebral gray matter at a speed of 2–5 mm/min, and it depresses spontaneous and evoked EEG activity. Cluster diffusion of these slow waves causes severe vasoconstriction, impaired cerebral electrolyte homeostasis, and recurrent tissue ischemia [68–70]. Microthrombosis is a consequence of coagulation cascade activation following initial hemorrhage.

Vasospasm of cerebral arteries occurs more frequently 7–10 days after aneurysm rupture, and it resolves spontaneously after 21 days. It affects both arterial and arteriolar circulation, and 50% of the angiographically detectable cases cause ischemic neurological symptoms. The risk of cerebral vasospasm increases on the basis of thickness, density, localization and persistence of subarachnoid blood, onset of neurological condition, transcranial Doppler (TCD) flow velocity, Lindegaard ratio (ratio between mean CBF velocity in middle cerebral artery and mean CBF velocity in extracranial internal carotid artery), and ratio between TCD flow velocity and CBF (spasm index) [71]. Also poor clinical grading, loss of consciousness at event onset, cigarette smoking, cocaine use, systemic inflammatory response syndrome (SIRS), hyperglycemia, and hydrocephalus are factors increasing the risk of DCI and poor neurological outcome [72]. Predicting which patients may develop DCI is very difficult but would have important consequences such as a reduction in the level of monitoring in SAH patients with low risk of DCI, thus avoiding potential adverse effects of aggressive management and reducing resource utilization. The best predictors for reducing the level of monitoring include older age (> 65 years), WFNS scale grades I–III, and a modified Fisher scale score < 3.

The best studied interventions to prevent DCI are calcium channel blockers use and monitoring of intravascular volume status. The use of nimodipine is recommended to reduce the risk of DCI and poor functional outcome [23, 62]. It is enterally administered at a dose of 60 mg every 4 h for a period of 21 days. Nimodipine provides neuroprotection without reducing angiographic vasospasm incidence. The most common adverse effects include constipation and hypotension, and the latter may be problematic since it can lead to hypoperfusion given by a CPP reduction. For this reason, during nimodipine administration, systolic blood pressure of the patient should not be altered.

SAH patients often face a hypovolemic status and negative water balance, which is associated with higher incidence of cerebral infarction and poor neurological outcome. In the past this fact led to the introduction of prophylactic hypervolemic therapy that has not demonstrated to improve CBF or to reduce cerebral vasospasm or DCI incidence. On the contrary, prophylactic hypervolemia increases the incidence of cardiopulmonary complications, so it should not be established, and it is recommended to maintain euvolemia after SAH [2, 43]. The methodology to ensure patient euvolemia is still being subject of controversy. There are several methods such as close monitoring of water balance, central venous pressure, stroke volume variation, and echocardiography. Generally, to ensure euvolemia, it is necessary to reintegrate fluid lost with diuresis and eventually administer fludrocortisone or hydrocortisone in patients with significant diuresis.

The possible neuroprotective role of statin therapy on cerebral hemodynamics has been investigated. However, a randomized multicenter trial (STASH) did not show any benefit in the use of simvastatin in SAH patients regarding both short-term and long-term outcomes. Therefore, although a safe treatment, statin is not indicated [73]. Also early treatment with magnesium sulfate did not show any benefit in terms of outcome and DCI development [74]. Treatment with albumin administered up to 1.25 g/kg/day for 7 days may be neuroprotective and is tolerated by patients [75]. It is also associated with a reduced incidence of TCD-detected vasospasm, DCI, and cerebral infarction at day 90 in a dose-dependent manner [76].

10.8.5 Diagnosis and Monitoring

Diagnosing DCI is not simple, but the combination of neurological examination with imaging studies can increase early diagnosis and management. SAH patients should be admitted to neurosurgical intensive care unit where they can be examined frequently, at least every 2 h. DCI should be suspected in case of developing focal neurological impairment or in case of a GCS 2-point reduction that lasts for more than 1 h and cannot be explained by another cause. In addition, all SAH patients should undergo head CT or MRI 24–48 h after aneurysm repair. Any new hypodensity found at CT imaging after this time window, not attributable to EVD insertion or intraparenchymal hematoma, should be considered cerebral infarction caused by DCI, regardless of clinical signs. Expert opinion recommends that SAH patients should routinely undergo further imaging studies and/or further physiological monitoring during the period at risk for developing DCI [2, 43]. Usually monitoring is multimodal and includes ICP, CPP, CBF, EEG, TCD, DSA, CTA, perfusion CT, and cerebral tissue oxygenation. Among all these methods, the more investigated one is TCD, which has sensitivity and specificity suitable to detect DCI secondary to cerebral vasospasm in major arteries, compared to DSA. The limits of this technique are the operator's experience and the patient's cranial acoustic window [77]. The TCD threshold values to diagnose vasospasm are as follows: mean CBF velocity < 120 cm/s excludes vasospasm; mean CBF velocity > 200 cm/s or Lindegaard ratio > 6 are diagnostic for vasospasm. In addition, mean CBF velocity increase of >50 cm/s within 24–48 h are associated with DCI.

DSA is the gold standard method to detect vasospasm in large arteries, but it is an invasive technique that puts the patient at risk of stroke by arterial dissection, embolism, and arterial rupture [78]. CTA has become widely available and could replace DSA for vasospasm screening with a high degree of specificity. Detecting an elevated mean transit time on perfusion CT (> 6.4 s; a recommended threshold for reduced cerebral perfusion) can be a predictive factor of DCI, additional to CTA, along with the visual qualitative interpretation of perfusion CT. Moreover, CTA and perfusion CT use can result not only in clinical benefit but also in economic advantage, in terms of cost-effectiveness [79].

Cerebral tissue oxygenation and CBF monitoring may add more information if used in a multimodal approach context, always taking into account the limitations of the different methods. Continuous EEG monitoring allows to monitor wide cerebral regions and to detect in a non-invasive way any epileptiform event. It is particularly useful in patients with poor grading where neurological examination is very limited. There is some variability regarding timing and frequency of the use of different neuromonitoring techniques [62]. Generally SAH patients are stratified in low risk (old age, WFNS 1–2, Fisher < 3), high risk (WFNS 1–3, Fisher 3), and high risk with poor neurological grading (sedated patient, WFNS 3–5, Fisher 4). All patients with aneurysmal SAH should be monitored with TCD (daily) and should undergo head CT (and even CTA/perfusion CT or DSA) on admission, on days 3–5, and on days 7–10 for reduced cerebral perfusion screening and vasospasm screening. High-risk patients with poor neurological grading deserve further neuromonitoring (EEG, cerebral tissue oxygenation, CBF).

10.8.6 Invasive Monitoring

The possibility to directly or indirectly monitor cerebral physiology and metabolism can help diagnosing cerebral vasospasm, adding important information about its course and effectiveness of treatment. In particular, techniques such as microdialysis and cerebral tissue oxygenation monitoring, which can detect neurometabolic and cerebral oxygenation alterations, can contribute to early diagnosis of DCI, thus improving outcome [80]. In SAH patients vasospasm affects energetic metabolism, leading to neurological deterioration. It may be useful to monitor cerebral metabolism through microdialysis, since it could correlate with clinical condition of the patient, and it may early detect metabolic dysfunction [81]. *Cerebral microdialysis* is a neuromonitoring technique offering the possibility of continuous, almost real time, sampling of endogenous neurochemical molecules (neurotransmitters, metabolites) that can help understand the underlying pathophysiological cascades and detect DCI after SAH. It allows to monitor, through analytes fluctuations, the neurochemical events of brain extracellular space. Lactate, glucose, and pyruvate are parameters of energetic metabolism important to detect secondary cerebral damage following SAH. In addition, the level of glutamate in dialysate, excitatory amino acid which plays an important role in secondary cerebral damage, closely correlates with ischemic alterations and poor outcome. During ischemia, witnessing the transition to an anaerobic brain energy metabolism, we will have high lactate, reduced extracellular glucose which negatively affects the outcome, and reduced pyruvate due to lack of substrates. A lactate/pyruvate ratio > 40 correlates with a condition of regional cerebral ischemia. The increase of glutamate in extracellular fluid of SAH patients, as a result of secondary damage, correlates with unfavorable outcome [82]. Following SAH, ischemia raises extracellular glutamate concentration, causing neuronal damage. The accumulation of glutamate is due both to an increased release from neurons and to a reduced reuptake by the synaptic fissure, and this fact enhances the neurotoxic effect of ischemia. Possible early markers of DCI following SAH are glyceraldehyde-3-phosphate dehydrogenase (GAPDH) and HSP7C protein, the concentrations of which vary before symptomatic vasospasm onset. FGF2 levels show the tendency to be higher in SAH patients, and NO can be monitored in SAH patients undergoing surgery. Microdialysis monitoring is able to predict DCI and cerebral infarction with sensitivity and specificity between 75 and 90%, on average 11 h before clinical onset [83].

The role of endothelin-1 (ET-1) in the development of cerebral vasospasm following SAH was evaluated [84]. ET-1 levels in cerebrospinal fluid are increased under severe neurological damage conditions, irrespective of whether the cause is either vasospasm or primary hemorrhagic event, and they also correlate with neurological deterioration but are not predictive of DCI. The role of clazosentan, an endothelin receptor antagonist, has been investigated in the treatment of SAH patients. A first trial (CONSCIOUS-1) demonstrated a significant reduction in moderate and severe angiographic vasospasm in a dose-dependent manner [85]. Clazosentan was then studied in patients treated with clipping (CONSCIOUS-2) and coiling (CONSCIOUS-3), without demonstrating a significant beneficial effect on mortality and functional outcome [86, 87]. A meta-analysis also showed that the use of endothelin receptor antagonists does not improve functional outcome following SAH, increasing the risk of some complications (pulmonary edema, hypotension, and anemia) [88]. Recently, in experimental models of rat arteries, it has been demonstrated that CSF of SAH patients which developed vasospasm causes vasoconstriction, mediated by endothelin, in an endothelium-dependent manner. In addition, it has been observed that only antagonizing in a combined way of two different endothelin receptors, it is possible to inhibit vasoconstriction [89].

The outcome after SAH is therefore not only affected by the severity of primary damage but also by the cascade of secondary damage. Eighty-three percent of patients who develop an ICP increase following SAH show cerebral metabolic alterations that precede the ICP increase [90]. A thin catheter (0.5 mm in diameter) is inserted into cerebral parenchyma for cerebral tissue oxygenation monitoring [91]. This technique can help not only in the early diagnosis of DCI but also in evaluating the effect of treatments such as nimodipine and angioplasty and in avoiding ischemic events during and following aneurysm surgery. CPP < 70 mmHg is associated with metabolic alterations and cerebral tissue hypoxia by secondary damage, resulting in increased mortality and poor functional recovery following SAH [92].

10.8.7 Treatment

All SAH patients should be treated with nimodipine and maintenance of euvolemia. Low-risk patients, whose neurological examination remains unchanged and do not show signs of vasospasm and hypoperfusion on TCD and CTA/perfusion CT, can be transferred to units with lower intensity of care starting from day 5 after the event. High-risk patients with good neurological status and with unchanged neurological examination and imaging can be transferred starting from day 7 after the event. High-risk patients with poor neurological status, whose neurological examination remains unchanged and neuromonitoring values remain within the normal range, can be transferred starting from day 14 after SAH. When an increase in TCD mean CBF velocity or CTA/perfusion, CT alterations are observed; the intensity and frequency of neuromonitoring must be augmented.

The development of neurological deterioration suggestive of DCI determines the starting of rescue therapy. It is important to work on hemodynamics to improve cerebral perfusion. In case of cerebral autoregulation alteration, a MAP increase results in a parallel CBF increase. Initially the hemodynamic approach consisted in triple H therapy (hemodilution, hypervolemia, hypertension), but scientific literature demonstrated the only usefulness of hypertension with maintenance of euvolemia; thereafter, guidelines indicate induced hypertension as first-line treatment [2, 43]. IV fluid bolus is usually infused (1–2 l physiological saline 0.9%) and hypertension is induced with vasopressor drugs use (noradrenaline). The increase in blood pressure is achieved gradually with frequent neurological examination (every 10 mmHg of mean or systolic blood pressure increase, without exceeding 200 mmHg of systolic blood pressure) to determine the final target pressure. Inotropic agents use (dobutamine, milrinone) is reserved for patients with impaired cardiac function. If neurological deficit persists, then the patient must undergo head CT/CTA/perfusion CT or DSA and must be treated with endovascular therapy once cerebral vasospasm has been confirmed. On the basis of prospective and retrospective observational data, endovascular treatment with intra-arterial vasodilators (papaverine) and/or angioplasty is recommended. Induced hypertension should be maintained for at least 72 h or until stability is achieved, and then progressive slow weaning is started. Prophylactic angioplasty, in a patient with positive imaging but no neurological deterioration, is not recommended since it is associated with elevated complication rate. In many cases in high-risk patients with poor neurological grading, DCI diagnosis and treatment are driven by data found on neuromonitoring (alterations in TCD mean CBF velocity, cerebral tissue oxygenation, CBF suggestive of vasospasm indicate induced hypertension, and further investigation with imaging studies).

10.9 Medical Complications

10.9.1 Cardiopulmonary

Cardiopulmonary alterations are among the most common systemic SAH complications and may range from minor ECG abnormalities to severe dilated cardiomyopathy and acute respiratory distress syndrome (ARDS) [61]. ECG alterations and elevated cardiac enzymes (troponin T and I) are rather frequent after SAH; they are characteristic of what is called neurogenic stress cardiomyopathy (NSC) and, depending on severity, are significant factors for clinical outcome. ECG alterations include sinus tachycardia, peaked T waves, T wave inversion, ST-segment depression or ST-segment elevation, and QT prolongation. ECG alterations affect 25–75% of SAH patients, whereas arrhythmias are present in about 100% of cases. Troponin increase occurs in up to 30% of patients. Troponin I is a highly sensitive and specific myocardial dysfunction marker, and in SAH patients, it is predictive of increased risk of hypotension, pulmonary edema, left ventricular systolic dysfunction, and DCI. In SAH patients there is also an increase in plasma BNP. The exact pathogenesis of cardiac alterations is not fully understood but it could be explained by catecholamine-related myocardial damage. In fact, structural brain injury and sudden increase in ICP induce high tissue and plasma levels of catecholamine due to significant autonomic stimulation. Plasma noradrenaline is increased three times the baseline value within the first 48 h following SAH, and it remains elevated even after 1 week. Excessive myocardial noradrenaline concentration induces myocitary calcium overload and cell death resulting in cardiac dysfunction [93]. High levels of inflammatory cytokines present in patients CSF and serum contribute to NSC damage. Echocardiography can help distinguish patients with SAH-related widespread cardiac dysfunction from those with underlying cardiac ischemia, showing regional wall motility abnormalities in irroration areas of relative coronary vessels. Regional or global wall motion abnormalities occur in 8–13% of patients, usually within the first 2 days from the event, and their prevalence is reduced in the following 3–8 days. From a clinical point of view, SAH patients may develop a significant cardiac dysfunction that manifests itself as left ventricular heart failure with compromised cardiac output, hypotension, and pulmonary edema. These cardiovascular dysfunctions lead to severe hypoperfusion, reduced CPP or cerebral tissue oxygenation, increasing the catastrophic consequences on a cerebral tissue already suffering and vulnerable to DCI, and poor neurological outcome. The concept of stunned myocardium is valid for SAH patients presenting with hypoxemia and cardiogenic shock with pulmonary edema within a few hours from onset. Takotsubo cardiomyopathy (characterized by the typical balloon-like shape of ventricular apex, visible on echocardiogram) may occur in patients with poor neurological status, and it increases the risk of DCI. In more than 50% of NSC cases following SAH, it has been described a "preserved apex" pattern, characterized by basal and mid-ventricular left ventricular wall contraction abnormalities, without apex involvement (less innervated from an orthosympathetic point of view). Therefore, from a cardiac point of view, monitoring of SAH patients through the execution of serial cardiac enzymes, ECG and echocardiography can be beneficial especially in front of myocardial dysfunction signs. If there is also hemodynamic instability, it may be useful to monitor cardiac output, even if there are no outcome data demonstrating its effectiveness.

Neurogenic pulmonary edema seems to be explained by a significant orthosympathetic drive caused by neurological injury, and it is associated with reduced global and segmental left ventricular systolic function [94]. It reflects subarachnoid bleeding severity, and it is associated with poor outcome [95, 96]. Recommendations for treating pulmonary edema or ARDS in SAH patients consist in avoiding excessive fluid administration and rationally use diuretics to reach euvolemia. Standard treatment for heart failure is also indicated, considering the importance of maintaining CPP in the normal range [43]. Protective mechanical ventilation should be set, considering however to carefully monitor hypercapnia, which should be readily managed so as to avoid further ICP increase. Cardiopulmonary function should also be supported by the use of intra-aortic balloon pump if necessary, since these anomalies usually improve a few days after the onset.

10.9.2 Fever

Fever is the most common non-neurological SAH complication, and it occurs in up to 70% of patients during hospitalization [2, 43]. It occurs more frequently in patients with poor neurological status and high score on modified Fisher scale. During SAH, fever is associated with poor clinical outcome, and it is probably associated with a systemic inflammatory response syndrome (SIRS) rather than an infectious event. There is currently no evidence for a benefit in body temperature control of SAH patients. It is recommended to monitor body temperature frequently and to look for, and eventually treat, infectious processes. In addition, during the period at risk for DCI, temperature control must be carried out gradually, starting with standard antipyretic medications, then switching to the use of surface cooling devices, and finally intravascular temperature control, always avoiding the phenomenon of shivering.

10.9.3 Thromboembolism

Deep venous thrombosis (DVT) incidence following SAH varies between 2 and 20% according to the screening methodology used, and the risk is greater in patients with poor neurological status [43]. Given DVT elevated incidence and its potentially fatal consequences, prophylactic treatment should be administered, and intermittent pneumatic compression is recommended for all SAH patients. Unfractionated heparin use in prophylaxis is indicated following aneurysm repair, and it can be started after 24 h from the procedure.

10.9.4 Glycemic Alterations

Hyperglycemia is a common phenomenon following SAH. The real impact of this condition is not yet well defined, but hyperglycemia is associated with DCI development and poor clinical outcome. It is also indicated to prevent intraoperative hyperglycemia during aneurysm surgery. Hypoglycemia is associated with worse clinical outcome. Methods, timing, and aggressiveness of glycemic control have not been studied well in SAH patients. It is recommended to maintain blood glucose level between 80 and 200 mg/dl while awaiting further evidence [43].

10.9.5 Hyponatremia

Hyponatremia is the most common electrolyte disorder in SAH patients, it occurs in approximately 30% of patients, and it is associated with clinical and sonographic vasospasm onset, DCI development, and poor clinical outcome [2, 15, 43]. It may be secondary to cerebral salt-wasting syndrome (CSWS) or to syndrome of inappropriate antidiuretic hormone secretion (SIADH). CSWS is caused by an excessive secretion of natriuretic peptides, and it results in hyponatremia, with possible hypovolemia, by excessive natriuresis. The treatment of these syndromes, in patients without SAH, provides for CSWS fluid infusion, while for SIADH fluid restriction. Following SAH, the CSWS patient treated with aggressive fluid resuscitation has an improvement in risk for cerebral ischemia. In SAH patients who develop SIADH, since it is often difficult to calculate water balance of neurosurgical intensive care unit patients, and since hypovolemia is associated with poor clinical outcome, fluid restriction should be avoided. The goal of hyponatremia treatment during SAH is therefore restriction of free water per os, maintaining patient's euvolemia. Patients can be treated with continuous infusion of hypertonic saline (1.5–3%) that in patients with severe SAH seems to increase CBF, tissue oxygenation, and pH. In case of active diuresis preventing adequate water balance maintenance, fludrocortisone is administered. It is important to look for thyroid and adrenal dysfunction, especially in SAH patients needing treatment with vasopressors to maintain normal blood pressure.

10.9.6 Hemoglobin

In most SAH patients a reduction in hemoglobin level occurs during hospitalization, which may compromise cerebral oxygen distribution. It can be caused by several factors, including excessive blood sampling, blood loss from other causes, or systemic inflammation [43]. Anemia is associated with DCI and poor clinical outcome, but the optimal hemoglobin value in SAH patients has not been determined. Blood transfusions have not yet shown an improvement in clinical outcome but significantly increase cerebral oxygen distribution reducing oxygen extraction ratio. It is recommended to minimize blood sampling and blood losses and to maintain a hemoglobin value greater than 8–10 g/dl.

Conclusion

SAH is a neurological emergency associated with high morbidity and mortality. It is more common in females than males and in ethnic minorities compared to white Americans. When treating a SAH patient, the determining factors are prompt assessment and diagnosis, transfer to an appropriate center, rapid diagnosis and treatment of the source of bleeding, and overall management in neurosurgical intensive care unit consistent with the available guidelines. The main neurological complications of SAH include hydrocephalus, seizures, cerebral edema, DCI, and neuroendocrine disorders. Frequently patients manifest cardiopulmonary complications, which may be potentially fatal [97]. Following SAH patient discharge, it is reasonable to conduct a comprehensive assessment, including cognitive, behavioral, and psychosocial status [2].

References

1. Go AS, et al. Heart disease and stroke statistics--2014 update: a report from the American Heart Association. Circulation. 2014;129(3):e28–e292.
2. Connolly ES Jr, et al. Guidelines for the management of aneurysmal subarachnoid hemorrhage: a guideline for healthcare professionals from the American Heart Association/American Stroke Association. Stroke. 2012;43(6):1711–37.
3. Vlak MH, et al. Prevalence of unruptured intracranial aneurysms, with emphasis on sex, age, comorbidity, country, and time period: a systematic review and meta-analysis. Lancet Neurol. 2011;10(7):626–36.
4. Investigators UJ, et al. The natural course of unruptured cerebral aneurysms in a Japanese cohort. N Engl J Med. 2012;366(26):2474–82.
5. Lovelock CE, Rinkel GJ, Rothwell PM. Time trends in outcome of subarachnoid hemorrhage: population-based study and systematic review. Neurology. 2010;74(19):1494–501.
6. D'Souza S. Aneurysmal subarachnoid hemorrhage. J Neurosurg Anesthesiol. 2015;27(3): 222–40.
7. Tjahjadi M, et al. Health-related quality of life after spontaneous subarachnoid hemorrhage measured in a recent patient population. World Neurosurg. 2013;79(2):296–307.
8. Lo B, Macdonald RL. Health-related quality of life after aneurysmal subarachnoid hemorrhage: new data from a large series in Germany. World Neurosurg. 2013;79(2):243–4.
9. Broderick JP, et al. Greater rupture risk for familial as compared to sporadic unruptured intracranial aneurysms. Stroke. 2009;40(6):1952–7.
10. Lindner SH, Bor AS, Rinkel GJ. Differences in risk factors according to the site of intracranial aneurysms. J Neurol Neurosurg Psychiatry. 2010;81(1):116–8.
11. Etminan N, et al. The impact of hypertension and nicotine on the size of ruptured intracranial aneurysms. J Neurol Neurosurg Psychiatry. 2011;82(1):4–7.
12. Shiue I, et al. Life events and risk of subarachnoid hemorrhage: the Australasian cooperative research on subarachnoid hemorrhage study (ACROSS). Stroke. 2010;41(6):1304–6.
13. Andreasen TH, et al. Modifiable risk factors for aneurysmal subarachnoid hemorrhage. Stroke. 2013;44(12):3607–12.
14. Wiebers DO, et al. Unruptured intracranial aneurysms: natural history, clinical outcome, and risks of surgical and endovascular treatment. Lancet. 2003;362(9378):103–10.
15. Suarez JI, Tarr RW, Selman WR. Aneurysmal subarachnoid hemorrhage. N Engl J Med. 2006;354(4):387–96.
16. Hassan A, et al. Terson's syndrome. Neurocrit Care. 2011;15(3):554–8.
17. McCarron MO, Alberts MJ, McCarron P. A systematic review of Terson's syndrome: frequency and prognosis after subarachnoid haemorrhage. J Neurol Neurosurg Psychiatry. 2004;75(3):491–3.
18. Linn FH, et al. Prospective study of sentinel headache in aneurysmal subarachnoid haemorrhage. Lancet. 1994;344(8922):590–3.
19. Leblanc R. The minor leak preceding subarachnoid hemorrhage. J Neurosurg. 1987;66(1):35–9.
20. Sames TA, et al. Sensitivity of new-generation computed tomography in subarachnoid hemorrhage. Acad Emerg Med. 1996;3(1):16–20.
21. Boesiger BM, Shiber JR. Subarachnoid hemorrhage diagnosis by computed tomography and lumbar puncture: are fifth generation CT scanners better at identifying subarachnoid hemorrhage? J Emerg Med. 2005;29(1):23–7.
22. Raya AK, Diringer MN. Treatment of subarachnoid hemorrhage. Crit Care Clin. 2014;30(4): 719–33.

23. Rabinstein AA, Lanzino G, Wijdicks EF. Multidisciplinary management and emerging therapeutic strategies in aneurysmal subarachnoid haemorrhage. Lancet Neurol. 2010;9(5):504–19.
24. Edlow JA, Malek AM, Ogilvy CS. Aneurysmal subarachnoid hemorrhage: update for emergency physicians. J Emerg Med. 2008;34(3):237–51.
25. Perry JJ, et al. Should spectrophotometry be used to identify xanthochromia in the cerebrospinal fluid of alert patients suspected of having subarachnoid hemorrhage? Stroke. 2006;37(10):2467–72.
26. McKinney AM, et al. Detection of aneurysms by 64-section multidetector CT angiography in patients acutely suspected of having an intracranial aneurysm and comparison with digital subtraction and 3D rotational angiography. AJNR Am J Neuroradiol. 2008;29(3):594–602.
27. Donmez H, et al. Comparison of 16-row multislice CT angiography with conventional angiography for detection and evaluation of intracranial aneurysms. Eur J Radiol. 2011;80(2):455–61.
28. Dupont SA, et al. The use of clinical and routine imaging data to differentiate between aneurysmal and nonaneurysmal subarachnoid hemorrhage prior to angiography. Clinical article. J Neurosurg. 2010;113(4):790–4.
29. Kowalski RG, et al. Initial misdiagnosis and outcome after subarachnoid hemorrhage. JAMA. 2004;291(7):866–9.
30. van Gijn J, Kerr RS, Rinkel GJ. Subarachnoid haemorrhage. Lancet. 2007;369(9558):306–18.
31. Perry JJ, et al. Clinical decision rules to rule out subarachnoid hemorrhage for acute headache. JAMA. 2013;310(12):1248–55.
32. Kapadia A, et al. Nonaneurysmal perimesencephalic subarachnoid hemorrhage: diagnosis, pathophysiology, clinical characteristics, and long-term outcome. World Neurosurg. 2014;82(6):1131–43.
33. Rinkel GJ, et al. Nonaneurysmal perimesencephalic subarachnoid hemorrhage: CT and MR patterns that differ from aneurysmal rupture. AJNR Am J Neuroradiol. 1991;12(5):829–34.
34. Tang C, Zhang TS, Zhou LF. Risk factors for rebleeding of aneurysmal subarachnoid hemorrhage: a meta-analysis. PLoS One. 2014;9(6):E99536.
35. Anderson CS, et al. Rapid blood-pressure lowering in patients with acute intracerebral hemorrhage. N Engl J Med. 2013;368(25):2355–65.
36. Butcher KS, et al. The intracerebral hemorrhage acutely decreasing arterial pressure trial. Stroke. 2013;44(3):620–6.
37. Rosen DS, Macdonald RL. Subarachnoid hemorrhage grading scales: a systematic review. Neurocrit Care. 2005;2(2):110–8.
38. Fisher CM, Kistler JP, Davis JM. Relation of cerebral vasospasm to subarachnoid hemorrhage visualized by computerized tomographic scanning. Neurosurgery. 1980;6(1):1–9.
39. Frontera JA, et al. Prediction of symptomatic vasospasm after subarachnoid hemorrhage: the modified fisher scale. Neurosurgery. 2006;59(1):21–7. discussion 21-7
40. Nomura Y, et al. Retrospective analysis of predictors of cerebral vasospasm after ruptured cerebral aneurysm surgery: influence of the location of subarachnoid blood. J Anesth. 2010;24(1):1–6.
41. Report of world Federation of Neurological Surgeons Committee on a universal subarachnoid hemorrhage grading scale. J Neurosurg. 1988;68(6):985–6.
42. Claassen J, et al. Effect of cisternal and ventricular blood on risk of delayed cerebral ischemia after subarachnoid hemorrhage: the Fisher scale revisited. Stroke. 2001;32(9):2012–20.
43. Diringer MN, et al. Critical care management of patients following aneurysmal subarachnoid hemorrhage: recommendations from the Neurocritical care Society's multidisciplinary consensus conference. Neurocrit Care. 2011;15(2):211–40.
44. Suarez JI, et al. Length of stay and mortality in neurocritically ill patients: impact of a specialized neurocritical care team. Crit Care Med. 2004;32(11):2311–7.
45. Molyneux A, et al. International subarachnoid aneurysm trial (ISAT) of neurosurgical clipping versus endovascular coiling in 2143 patients with ruptured intracranial aneurysms: a randomised trial. Lancet. 2002;360(9342):1267–74.
46. Molyneux AJ, et al. International subarachnoid aneurysm trial (ISAT) of neurosurgical clipping versus endovascular coiling in 2143 patients with ruptured intracranial aneurysms: a ran-

domised comparison of effects on survival, dependency, seizures, rebleeding, subgroups, and aneurysm occlusion. Lancet. 2005;366(9488):809–17.

47. Jaeger M, et al. Continuous monitoring of cerebrovascular autoregulation after subarachnoid hemorrhage by brain tissue oxygen pressure reactivity and its relation to delayed cerebral infarction. Stroke. 2007;38(3):981–6.

48. Jaeger M, et al. Clinical significance of impaired cerebrovascular autoregulation after severe aneurysmal subarachnoid hemorrhage. Stroke. 2012;43(8):2097–101.

49. Priebe HJ. Aneurysmal subarachnoid haemorrhage and the anaesthetist. Br J Anaesth. 2007;99(1):102–18.

50. Sponheim S, et al. Effects of 0.5 and 1.0 MAC isoflurane, sevoflurane and desflurane on intracranial and cerebral perfusion pressures in children. Acta Anaesthesiol Scand. 2003;47(8):932–8.

51. Fraga M, et al. The effects of isoflurane and desflurane on intracranial pressure, cerebral perfusion pressure, and cerebral arteriovenous oxygen content difference in normocapnic patients with supratentorial brain tumors. Anesthesiology. 2003;98(5):1085–90.

52. Petersen KD, et al. Intracranial pressure and cerebral hemodynamic in patients with cerebral tumors: a randomized prospective study of patients subjected to craniotomy in propofol-fentanyl, isoflurane-fentanyl, or sevoflurane-fentanyl anesthesia. Anesthesiology. 2003;98(2):329–36.

53. Conti A, et al. Cerebral haemodynamic changes during propofol-remifentanil or sevoflurane anaesthesia: transcranial Doppler study under bispectral index monitoring. Br J Anaesth. 2006;97(3):333–9.

54. Lauta E, et al. Emergence times are similar with sevoflurane and total intravenous anesthesia: results of a multicenter RCT of patients scheduled for elective supratentorial craniotomy. J Neurosurg Anesthesiol. 2010;22(2):110–8.

55. Citerio G, et al. A multicentre, randomised, open-label, controlled trial evaluating equivalence of inhalational and intravenous anaesthesia during elective craniotomy. Eur J Anaesthesiol. 2012;29(8):371–9.

56. Magni G, et al. No difference in emergence time and early cognitive function between sevoflurane-fentanyl and propofol-remifentanil in patients undergoing craniotomy for supratentorial intracranial surgery. J Neurosurg Anesthesiol. 2005;17(3):134–8.

57. Stocchetti N, et al. Hyperventilation in head injury: a review. Chest. 2005;127(5):1812–27.

58. Zoerle T, et al. Intracranial pressure after subarachnoid hemorrhage. Crit Care Med. 2015;43(1): 168–76.

59. Todd MM, et al. Mild intraoperative hypothermia during surgery for intracranial aneurysm. N Engl J Med. 2005;352(2):135–45.

60. Macdonald RL, Diringer MN, Citerio G. Understanding the disease: aneurysmal subarachnoid hemorrhage. Intensive Care Med. 2014;40(12):1940–3.

61. Etminan N, Macdonald RL. Medical complications after aneurysmal subarachnoid hemorrhage: an emerging contributor to poor outcome. World Neurosurg. 2015;83(3):303–4.

62. Macdonald RL. Delayed neurological deterioration after subarachnoid haemorrhage. Nat Rev Neurol. 2014;10(1):44–58.

63. Vergouwen MD, Ilodigwe D, Macdonald RL. Cerebral infarction after subarachnoid hemorrhage contributes to poor outcome by vasospasm-dependent and -independent effects. Stroke. 2011;42(4):924–9.

64. Woloszyn AV, et al. Retrospective evaluation of nicardipine versus labetalol for blood pressure control in aneurysmal subarachnoid hemorrhage. Neurocrit Care. 2012;16(3):376–80.

65. Hockel K, et al. Vasopressin V(1a) receptors mediate posthemorrhagic systemic hypertension thereby determining rebleeding rate and outcome after experimental subarachnoid hemorrhage. Stroke. 2012;43(1):227–32.

66. Budohoski KP, et al. Impairment of cerebral autoregulation predicts delayed cerebral ischemia after subarachnoid hemorrhage: a prospective observational study. Stroke. 2012;43(12):3230–7.

67. Rowland MJ, et al. Delayed cerebral ischaemia after subarachnoid haemorrhage: looking beyond vasospasm. Br J Anaesth. 2012;109(3):315–29.

68. Woitzik J, et al. Delayed cerebral ischemia and spreading depolarization in absence of angiographic vasospasm after subarachnoid hemorrhage. J Cereb Blood Flow Metab. 2012;32(2):203–12.

69. Lauritzen M, et al. Clinical relevance of cortical spreading depression in neurological disorders: migraine, malignant stroke, subarachnoid and intracranial hemorrhage, and traumatic brain injury. J Cereb Blood Flow Metab. 2011;31(1):17–35.
70. Dreier JP, et al. Cortical spreading ischaemia is a novel process involved in ischaemic damage in patients with aneurysmal subarachnoid haemorrhage. Brain. 2009;132(Pt 7):1866–81.
71. Gonzalez NR, et al. Vasospasm probability index: a combination of transcranial Doppler velocities, cerebral blood flow, and clinical risk factors to predict cerebral vasospasm after aneurysmal subarachnoid hemorrhage. J Neurosurg. 2007;107(6):1101–12.
72. de Rooij NK, et al. Delayed cerebral ischemia after subarachnoid hemorrhage: a systematic review of clinical, laboratory, and radiological predictors. Stroke. 2013;44(1):43–54.
73. Kirkpatrick PJ, et al. Simvastatin in aneurysmal subarachnoid haemorrhage (STASH): a multicentre randomised phase 3 trial. Lancet Neurol. 2014;13(7):666–75.
74. Dorhout Mees SM, et al. Early magnesium treatment after aneurysmal subarachnoid hemorrhage: individual patient data meta-analysis. Stroke. 2015;46(11):3190–3.
75. Suarez JI, et al. The albumin in subarachnoid hemorrhage (ALISAH) multicenter pilot clinical trial: safety and neurologic outcomes. Stroke. 2012;43(3):683–90.
76. Suarez JI, et al. Effect of human albumin on TCD vasospasm, DCI, and cerebral infarction in subarachnoid hemorrhage: the ALISAH study. Acta Neurochir Suppl. 2015;120:287–90.
77. Suarez JI, et al. Symptomatic vasospasm diagnosis after subarachnoid hemorrhage: evaluation of transcranial Doppler ultrasound and cerebral angiography as related to compromised vascular distribution. Crit Care Med. 2002;30(6):1348–55.
78. Heiserman JE. MR angiography for the diagnosis of vasospasm after subarachnoid hemorrhage. Is it accurate? Is it safe? AJNR Am J Neuroradiol. 2000;21(9):1571–2.
79. Sanelli PC, et al. Cost-effectiveness of CT angiography and perfusion imaging for delayed cerebral ischemia and vasospasm in aneurysmal subarachnoid hemorrhage. AJNR Am J Neuroradiol. 2014;35(9):1714–20.
80. Kolias AG, Sen J, Belli A. Pathogenesis of cerebral vasospasm following aneurysmal subarachnoid hemorrhage: putative mechanisms and novel approaches. J Neurosci Res. 2009;87(1):1–11.
81. Noske DP, et al. Cerebral microdialysis and positron emission tomography after surgery for aneurysmal subarachnoid hemorrhage in grade I patients. Surg Neurol. 2005;64(2):109–15. discussion 115
82. Bullock R, et al. Factors affecting excitatory amino acid release following severe human head injury. J Neurosurg. 1998;89(4):507–18.
83. Skjoth-Rasmussen J, et al. Delayed neurological deficits detected by an ischemic pattern in the extracellular cerebral metabolites in patients with aneurysmal subarachnoid hemorrhage. J Neurosurg. 2004;100(1):8–15.
84. Mascia L, et al. Temporal relationship between endothelin-1 concentrations and cerebral vasospasm in patients with aneurysmal subarachnoid hemorrhage. Stroke. 2001;32(5):1185–90.
85. MacDonald RL, et al. Clazosentan to overcome neurological ischemia and infarction occurring after subarachnoid hemorrhage (CONSCIOUS-1): randomized, double-blind, placebo-controlled phase 2 dose-finding trial. Stroke. 2008;39(11):3015–21.
86. MacDonald RL, et al. Clazosentan, an endothelin receptor antagonist, in patients with aneurysmal subarachnoid haemorrhage undergoing surgical clipping: a randomised, double-blind, placebo-controlled phase 3 trial (CONSCIOUS-2). Lancet Neurol. 2011;10(7):618–25.
87. Macdonald RL, et al. Randomized trial of clazosentan in patients with aneurysmal subarachnoid hemorrhage undergoing endovascular coiling. Stroke. 2012;43(6):1463–9.
88. Vergouwen MD, Algra A, Rinkel GJ. Endothelin receptor antagonists for aneurysmal subarachnoid hemorrhage: a systematic review and meta-analysis update. Stroke. 2012;43(10):2671–6.
89. Assenzio B, et al. Cerebrospinal fluid from patients with subarachnoid haemorrhage and vasospasm enhances endothelin contraction in rat cerebral arteries. PLoS One. 2015;10(1):E0116456.
90. Nagel A, et al. Decompressive craniectomy in aneurysmal subarachnoid hemorrhage: relation to cerebral perfusion pressure and metabolism. Neurocrit Care. 2009;11(3):384–94.

91. Mazzeo AT, Bullock R. Monitoring brain tissue oxymetry: will it change management of critically ill neurologic patients? J Neurol Sci. 2007;261(1–2):1–9.
92. Schmidt JM, et al. Cerebral perfusion pressure thresholds for brain tissue hypoxia and metabolic crisis after poor-grade subarachnoid hemorrhage. Stroke. 2011;42(5):1351–6.
93. Mazzeo AT, et al. Brain-heart crosstalk: the many faces of stress-related cardiomyopathy syndromes in anaesthesia and intensive care. Br J Anaesth. 2014;112(5):803–15.
94. Mayer SA, et al. Cardiac injury associated with neurogenic pulmonary edema following subarachnoid hemorrhage. Neurology. 1994;44(5):815–20.
95. Muroi C, et al. Neurogenic pulmonary edema in patients with subarachnoid hemorrhage. J Neurosurg Anesthesiol. 2008;20(3):188–92.
96. Davison DL, Terek M, Chawla LS. Neurogenic pulmonary edema. Crit Care. 2012;16(2):212.
97. Suarez JI. Diagnosis and management of subarachnoid hemorrhage. Continuum (Minneap Minn). 2015;21(5):1263–87.

High-Flow Oxygen Therapy

11

Cristina Mietto and Davide Chiumello

11.1 Introduction

Oxygen (O_2) therapy is essential for treating hypoxemic patients. First records about oxygen therapy date back to the eighteenth century, but only during the First World War specific nasal cannula systems for oxygen supplementation were developed to treat gas-poisoned patients [1]. Since then oxygen delivery systems progressed to meet individual patient's need with higher gas flow and fraction of inspired oxygen (FiO_2). Ventilatory support may be required in patients with acute respiratory failure (ARF), going from continuous positive airway pressure (CPAP) and noninvasive ventilation (NIV) to endotracheal intubation and mechanical ventilation depending on patient's characteristics.

Low gas flow systems (i.e., the supplied gas flow is lower than patient's peak inspiratory flow (PIF); therefore, the oxygen flow mixes with room air and the actual FiO_2 will be lower than expected) are usually the first-line devices for oxygen supplementation in clinical practice and include:

- Low-flow nasal cannula: oxygen delivery is restricted to low flows and allows only minor increase in FiO_2. The maximal O_2 flow is 5–6 l/min, because higher gas flow rates cause excessive dryness of nasal mucosa despite the use of bubble humidifiers and are not tolerable for the patient.

C. Mietto (✉)
Department of Anesthesia and Critical Care, ASST Ovest Milanese Ospedale di Legnano, Legnano, Italy
e-mail: cristina.mietto@gmail.com

D. Chiumello
Department of Anesthesia and Critical Care, ASST Santi Paolo e Carlo, Università Degli Studi di Milano, Milano, Italy
e-mail: chiumello@libero.it

© Springer International Publishing AG 2018
D. Chiumello (ed.), *Practical Trends in Anesthesia and Intensive Care 2017*,
http://doi.org/10.1007/978-3-319-61325-3_11

Table 11.1 Consequences of dry and cold oxygen supplementation

Consequences of dry and cold oxygen supplementation
Injury to the airway mucosa
Bronchoconstriction and increase in airway resistance
Dryness of airway secretions
Mucociliary dysfunction
Increase in work of breathing

- Simple and non-rebreather mask: these devices deliver higher gas flows, usually up to 15 l/min, but anyway without control of the actual FiO_2 supplied to the patient and with similar problems of dryness of respiratory mucosa with bubble humidifiers. Moreover, face masks limit patient's interaction with the environment, causing difficulties in basic life activities (such as eating, speaking, drinking, etc.), effective communication with healthcare personnel, and claustrophobia.

Classical high-flow systems for oxygen therapy, the Venturi mask, apply the Bernoulli principle to ensure a fixed FiO_2. These devices work with a constant gas flow (O_2 is set usually between 4 and 8 l/min) that is squeezed through a narrow central space causing an increase in gas velocity and a decrease in static pressure. The consequence is that room air is drawn inside the device through peripheral openings by the subatmospheric pressure at the center of the device. Previous limitations about inadequate gas humidification and interference with patient's interaction are unchanged compared to low-flow face masks (Table 11.1). Moreover, a dilution effect of the delivered FiO_2 is always present in patients with high respiratory drive and work of breathing.

Following on from these limits in conventional oxygen therapy, the high-flow nasal cannula system (HFNC) was developed to supply controlled mixture of properly heated and humidified oxygen at high flow rates. First applied in neonatal and pediatric population with respiratory failure [2], HFNC treatment in adult patients is recently increasing [3]. HFNC system delivers a gas flow up to 20 l/min in children and 60 l/min in adult patients with a constant FiO_2 ranging from 21 to 100%. Main advantages of this technique are (1) the possibility to supply high gas flow rates that exceed patient's PIF, (2) the delivered gas is optimally heated and humidified with a constant FiO_2, and (3) the nasal cannula are more comfortable than face masks and allow better patient-environment interaction.

11.2 Setting the High-Flow Nasal Cannula System

Different HFNC devices are available on the market, each one with distinctive features but basic principles apply to all systems. Key components of any HFNC device are a set of nasal cannula, a gas delivery blender that allows control on gas flow and FiO_2, and an active humidifier.

Ideally, the system should allow titration of gas flow rates between 0 and 60 l/min in order to adapt to patient's need. Most common HFNC systems use two rotameters connected through a Y connection or a high-flow Venturi valve. The system must include a flowmeter and a gas analyzer on the inspiratory line, in order to monitor the actual flow and FiO_2 of the gas mixture provided to the patient.

Proper humidification is required for effectiveness and tolerability of the HFNC therapy. International guidelines (American Society for Testing and Materials, http://www.astm.org) recommend a minimum absolute humidity of 10 mg H_2O/l for gas flow that pass through the upper airways [4]. This value roughly corresponds to standard room air characteristics, that is, a relative humidity of 50% at 22 °C. The development of active humidifiers for HFNC systems is rather new, and these devices are analogous to those already in use for invasive mechanical ventilation. Indeed, the most efficient bubble humidifier is able to reach the required absolute humidity only for gas flow up to 15 l/min [5]. Active heated humidification systems deliver a relative humidity of nearly 100% for gas flow exceeding 40 l/min at 36.5 °C [5]. An additional useful feature is the presence of heated plastic circuits of larger diameter compared to standard low-flow nasal cannula. The larger dimension of the tubes allows for lower resistance to gas flow, while the heated wire circuit avoids condense formation at the interface between plastic and cold room air, reducing the risk of tube obstruction due to water accumulation inside the circuit.

Setting HFNC system is rather simple: First choose the nasal cannula size and circuit adequate for the patient. Nasal cannula must fit comfortably the nares, without excessive leaking or total obstruction. Active humidification must be on and working before starting the treatment, and gas flow temperature must be set between 34 and 37 °C. Gas flow must be started around 6 l/min and subsequently step-by-step increased to the target flow of 35–60 l/min during a few minutes time, in order to allow the patient to progressively adapt to the treatment.

11.3   Physiological Effects of HFNC System

Different physiological mechanisms have been suggested for the benefits and efficacy of HFNC oxygen therapy in pediatric and adult patients with acute respiratory failure (Table 11.2):

- Controlled FiO_2

Oxygen supplementation delivered through low-flow nasal cannula is an open system in which oxygen mixes with room air, and the maximum FiO_2 is not greater

Table 11.2 Mechanisms of action and benefits of HFNC

Mechanisms of action
Stable and controlled FiO_2
Washout of upper airway dead space
Reduction in airway resistance
Positive end-expiratory pressure (PEEP)
Alveolar recruitment
Superior patient's comfort
Advantage in clearance of bronchial secretions

than 30%. Moreover, the dilution effect is more extensive in case of respiratory distress – consequently, actual FiO_2 is lower in patients with dyspnea and tachypnea in which PIF is increased and varies from 30 to 120 l/min [6, 7]. HFNC systems deliver gas flow close to real patient's effort to breathe, up to 60 l/min, with excellent comfort and without injury to the upper airway mucosa. Real high FiO_2 (close to 100%) is guarantee even in hypoxemic patients with respiratory distress [8]. HFNC systems deliver FiO_2 higher than non-rebreather masks as well, as a consequence to minor room air admixture and washout of the upper airway dead space [7].

• Nasopharyngeal anatomical dead space washout

The nasopharynx is a complex anatomical space, and mouth-nasal breathing in patients with respiratory distress makes difficult a precise description of gas distribution during respiration. Numerous authors hypothesize that high gas flow rates during HFNC therapy promote the washout of the nasopharyngeal space from the expiratory air (containing CO_2) coming from the lungs. The resulting effect is double: first anatomical dead space is reduced with advantage in alveolar ventilation; moreover, the washed-out space acts as a reservoir of highly oxygenated air in the oropharynx [9]. Intratracheal insufflation techniques use different devices to obtain similar results, showing to be effective in reducing anatomical dead space with improved alveolar-to-minute ventilation ratio and clearance of CO_2 [10]. High-flow oxygen therapy, HFNC or intratracheal insufflation, compared to conventional oxygen therapy with low-flow devices showed to improve resistance to physical exercise and to reduce dyspnea symptoms in patients with chronic obstructive pulmonary disease (COPD) [11]. In another study, COPD patients showed improved oxygenation, respiratory mechanics, and resistance to exhaustion during physical exercise with HFNC oxygen supplementation [12].

• Reduction of airway inspiratory resistance

Nasopharyngeal space is essential to heat and humidify inspiratory room air. Optimal heating and humidification of inspiratory gas during HFNC therapy blunt the bronchoconstriction reflex caused by the administration of dry and cold gas. The consequence is the reduction in work of breathing [13]. Moreover, in predisposed patients, such as those with obstructive sleep apnea syndrome (OSAS), the soft tissue of the pharynx can collapse and obstruct during inspiration, leading to desaturation and CO_2 retention. High gas flow rates typical of HFNC may be equal or even superior to patient's inspiratory effort, thus to prevent upper airway collapse and reduce supraglottic resistance. HFNC promotes the development of a positive pressure in the nasopharyngeal space that contrasts tissue obstruction [9].

• Positive end-expiratory pressure (PEEP)

Graves and Tobin were the first authors to prove the development of airway positive pressure associated with HFNC treatment in adults [14]. The amount of positive pressure produced depends upon the supplied flow rate, anatomy of patient's airway, and individual respiratory system mechanical characteristics. Positive pressure linearly correlates with gas flow rate and system leakage [14]. Essential features for an effective HFNC support are good seal of nasal cannula, closure of patient's mouth, and gas flow higher, or at least equal, to PIF. Numerous studies measured actual delivered PEEP, but the results showed a wide interindividual variability. In healthy volunteers median PEEP was 7.4 cmH$_2$O (95% confidence interval (CI) 5.4–8.8 cmH$_2$O) with a gas flow of 60 l/min and close mouth [15]. Airway pressure was positive even during the inspiration phase of breathing, indicating adequate gas flow, with a median value of 1.6 cm H$_2$O (95%CI 0.8–2.9 cmH$_2$O) [15]. Post-cardiac surgery patients showed a mean positive pressure of 2.7 ± 1.04 cmH$_2$O with gas flow of 35 l/min and close mouth during the postoperative period [16]. Ritchie et al. assessed a positive correlation between gas flow rates and mean nasopharyngeal positive pressure, used as surrogate of airway pressure, in healthy volunteers: 3 cmH$_2$O with a flow of 30 l/min, 4 cmH$_2$O with 40 l/min, and 5 cmH$_2$O with 50 l/min [17]. Similarly, another study found that airway pressure increased at 0.69 cmH$_2$O for every increment of 10 l/min in gas flow when the subject breathes with his mouth close; the increase associated with airflow is lower (0.35 cmH$_2$O) when the mouth is open during respiration [18].

- Alveolar recruitment

Positive airway pressure causes improvement in gas exchange and respiratory system mechanics only if it is associated with alveolar recruitment of the lung parenchyma. Corley et al. used electrical impedance tomography (EIT) to study the association between PEEP and alveolar recruitment during HFNC therapy in post-cardiac surgery patients [19]. HFNC therapy significantly increased both PEEP (3.0 cmH$_2$O, 95%CI 2.4–3.7 cmH$_2$O) and end-expiratory lung volume (EELV) (25.6%, 95%CI 24.3–26.9%) compared to standard oxygen delivery systems. Moreover, the authors found an increase in minute ventilation associated with HFNC therapy (tidal volume increase 10.5%, 95%CI 6.1–18.3%). The eventual effect was an improvement in gas exchange and respiratory system mechanics, mirrored by a reduction in respiratory rate and dyspnea relief [19].

- Patient's comfort

Optimal humidification and heating of the supplied gas is essential to guarantee a tolerable and effective therapy during HFNC support. Such high gas flow rates would be otherwise harmful for the respiratory system mucosa and would cause an increase in airway resistance by eliciting the bronchoconstriction reflex through activation of nasal receptors [20]. Mechanically ventilated children showed a reduction of lung compliance after only 5 min of ventilation with cold and dry air [21]. Furthermore, patients in acute respiratory failure show increased bronchial secretions. Active heated humidifiers prevent dryness and promote the clearance of respiratory secretions, especially in patients with chronic respiratory comorbidities

Table 11.3 Contraindications
to HFNC support

Contraindications
Impaired consciousness
Impaired patency of airway
Facial injury
Cardiac arrest
Hemodynamic instability

(i.e., COPD, cystic fibrosis, bronchiectasis, etc.). Roca et al. found that patient's comfort is superior and dyspnea relief is greater with HFNC therapy than standard oxygen mask supports [22]. If properly set and delivered, HFNC therapy can be used for prolonged periods of time without complications or patient's refusal to treatment (Table 11.3) [23, 24].

11.4   Clinical Trials in Adult Population

HFNC systems are widely applied for treatment of newborns and children with acute respiratory distress, and literature strongly supports the efficacy in these populations [25]. Recently, increasing interest is shown about the implementation of HFNC therapy in adults with ARF. Evidences about HFNC treatment in adults are reported accordingly to different clinical scenario.

11.5   HFNC Therapy in Hypoxemic Respiratory Failure

Oxygen supplementation is the first-line therapy in hypoxemic patients, regardless of the cause of respiratory failure. Numerous studies compared the efficacy of HFNC therapy to other noninvasive techniques of respiratory support.

In a prospective sequential study, Roca et al. showed that 30 min of HFNC support increased oxygenation and reduced respiratory rate compared to standard oxygen mask in patients admitted to intensive care unit (ICU) for acute hypoxic respiratory failure (defined as $SpO_2 \leq 96\%$ with a $FiO_2 \geq 50\%$) [22]. All patients reported better comfort and dyspnea relief with HFNC therapy. Similar results were obtained in other two observational prospective trials in patients with ARF and respiratory distress [26, 27]. Rello et al. published their experience in hypoxemic patients with ARF caused by influenza A/H1N1 infection [28]. Nine patients improved with HFNC therapy, and all survived, while 11 patients required intubation and invasive mechanical ventilation with an ICU mortality of 27%. Factors associated with HFNC failure were requirement of inotropic/vasopressor therapy, SOFA score > 4, APACHE score > 12, failure of improvement in oxygenation, and/or tachypnea after 6 h of HFNC support.

In a multicenter randomized trial, Frat et al. compared the efficacy of HFNC and NIV as first respiratory support in patients with ARF and a PaO_2/FiO_2 ratio below 300 [29]. Three hundred and ten patients were enrolled, 94 were randomized to standard oxygen mask, 106 were treated with HFNC at a minimum flow rate of

50 l/min, and a third group of 110 patients underwent NIV through face mask (ventilatory setting: PEEP between 2 and 10 cmH$_2$O, pressure support tailored to obtain a tidal volume of 7–10 ml/kg$_{IBW}$); FiO$_2$ (and PEEP in the NIV group) was modified to maintain a SpO$_2$ equal or above 92%. The authors did not find any difference in rate of intubation among the different treatments (38% for HFNC, 47% for standard oxygen mask, and 50% for NIV patients). Otherwise, the HFNC group showed a statistically significant benefit in survival, 90 days of mortality hazard ratio was 2.01 (95%CI 1.01–3.99, $p = 0.046$) for standard oxygen mask and 2.50 (95%CI 1.31–4.78, $p = 0.006$) for NIV compared to HFNC support [29].

The use of HFNC in acute respiratory distress syndrome (ARDS) was specifically addressed by a single-center observational study [30]. Out of the total 45 ARDS patients treated with HFNC support during the study period, 26 subjects successfully improved, 1 patient required NIV, and 18 were eventually intubated and mechanically ventilated. Risk factors for HFNC failure were severe hypoxemia, hemodynamic shock with inotropic/vasopressor therapy, and high SAPS II score at ICU admission [30].

Recently, a meta-analysis of six RCTs comparing efficacy of HFNC and conventional oxygen therapy or NIV in hypoxic patients found that intubation rate was significantly lower with HFNC therapy than with conventional oxygen support (RR 0.60, 95%CI 0.38–0.94). No significant difference was found between HFNC therapy and NIV (RR 0.86, 95%CI 0.68–1.09) [31]. No difference in oxygenation was found between HFNC therapy and conventional oxygen mask; NIV achieved higher PaO$_2$/FiO$_2$ ratio, although with similar PaCO$_2$ levels to HFNC therapy. Mortality was not different: there were 52 (5.9%) deaths in the HFNC group, 30 (6.7%) in the conventional oxygen therapy group, and 50 (9.5%) in the NIV group [31].

In conclusion, HFNC is a useful noninvasive option in ARF patients who do not require intubation and invasive mechanical ventilation. Nevertheless, additional studies are necessary to establish possible benefits in the most severely hypoxemic patients.

11.6   Post-extubation HFNC Therapy

Patients often require oxygen therapy in the post-extubation period in order to correct residual hypoxemia. Reintubation is associated to increased morbidity and mortality; thus, optimal oxygenation is essential during this phase. Numerous studies focused on the use of HFNC support in this setting.

Tiruvoipati et al. performed a crossover and randomized study to evaluate the benefits of HFNC therapy compared to standard oxygen mask during the post-extubation period [32]. No differences in gas exchange were found in a cohort of 42 patients, although treatment comfort was superior with HFNC therapy. In a similar study, Rittaymai et al. looked for differences in clinical variables during the first 60 min after extubation [33]. HFNC support was associated with decreased dyspnea, tachypnea, and tachycardia [33]. Moreover, improvement of gas exchange associated to HFNC therapy was reported in 34 patients who received HFNC immediately after endotracheal tube removal and showed a subsequent increase in oxygenation after extubation (PaO_2/FiO_2 rose from 224 to 270, $p < 0.05$); in the other group (33 patients) treated with standard oxygen mask, an opposite trend occurred with a worst oxygenation in spontaneous breathing (PaO_2/FiO_2 decreased from 256 to 183, $p < 0.05$) [34]. Consequently, post-extubation oxygenation was significantly higher in the HFNC group ($p < 0.0001$). Patients who received HFNC support had lower reintubation rate (3% versus 18%, $p = 0.004$) and higher free-ventilation days [34]. Similarly, HFNC support proved to be superior to Venturi mask in patients with a PaO_2/FiO_2 ratio lower than 300 at extubation [35]. Maggiore et al. randomized 53 patients to HFNC therapy for 48 h post-extubation and showed a steady increased oxygenation at 24, 36, and 48 h compared to the group treated with Venturi mask. Respiratory rate and $PaCO_2$ were lower already after 3 h of HFNC support. Patient's comfort and mouth dryness were reduced with HFNC treatment; fewer desaturation and spontaneous removal of the device were recorded in the interventional group. Lastly, patients randomized to HFNC therapy had a lower extubation failure rate, requiring reintubation or NIV, although mortality was similar in the two groups [35]. A subsequent study focused on post-cardiac surgery obese patients ($BMI > 30$ kg/m^2) and enrolled 155 patients who were randomized to elective HFNC support immediately after extubation (81 patients) or standard of care with oxygen mask (75 patients) [36]. Authors did not find any significant difference regarding oxygenation, respiratory rate at 24 h, dyspnea relief, and presence of atelectasis at 1 and 5 post-extubation days. Reintubation rate did not differ either between the two groups (three patients were reintubated in the HFNC group compared to five patients in the standard mask group) [36]. Differences in the enrolled population, timing of enrollment and treatment after extubation, and control group protocols can account for the contrasting results [35, 36].

Previous studies compared HFNC to standard oxygen therapy through mask, but frequently patients who develop post-extubation respiratory failure are treated with NIV. In a recent Spanish multicenter study, 527 patients mechanically ventilated for longer than 12 h and with a low risk of reintubation were recruited to HFNC therapy or standard oxygen support immediately after extubation. Reintubation within 72 h post-extubation was lower in the HFNC group (4.9% in the HFNC group versus 12.2% in the conventional group, with an absolute difference of 7.2%, 95%CI 2.5–12.2% $p = 0.004$) [37]. HFNC therapy was independently and inversely associated with all-cause reintubation (OR 0.32, 95%CI 0.16–0.66), and the number needed to treat (NNT) to prevent reintubation was 14 (95%CI 8–40). There was no difference in ICU length of stay, but all patients comfortably tolerated HFNC treatment, and no adverse event was recorded [37]. In a previous study, the same group published the use of HFNC therapy in patients at high risk of extubation failure [38]. Patients were randomized to HFNC therapy (290 subjects) or NIV (314 patients) support for 24 h post-extubation. Reintubation occurred in 60 patients (19.1%) in the NIV group and 66 patients (22.8%) in the HFNC group (risk difference –3.7%, 95%CI–9.1%–∞). Median time to reintubation was not significantly different in the two groups: 26.5 h (interquartile range (IQR) 14–39 h) in the HFNC group versus 21.5 h (IQR 10–47 h) in the NIV group (absolute difference –5 hours; 95%CI–34–24 hours) [38]. Similarly, Stéphan et al. designed a large multicenter randomized study to evaluate the efficacy of HFNC support in post-cardiac surgery patients that developed hypoxemic respiratory failure after extubation or with multiple risk factors for post-extubation respiratory distress [39]. A total of 830 patients were enrolled, 414 subjects were randomized to continuous HFNC therapy (50 l/min, FiO_2 50%), and 416 patients received NIV (PEEP 4 cmH_2O, PS 8 cmH_2O, FiO_2 50%) through face mask for at least 4 consecutive hours per day. HFNC therapy showed to be not inferior to NIV in the treatment of post-extubation respiratory failure: treatment failure (87 case in HFNC versus 91 cases in the NIV group), reintubation rate (57 case in HFNC versus 58 cases in the NIV group), and mortality (6.8% in HFNC versus 5.5% in the NIV group, $p = 0.66$) were similar in the two groups [39]. Although studies found that delayed reintubation may be associated to higher mortality [40, 41], no difference in time to reintubation was between the two groups in the described studies.

Instead, HFNC therapy during the first postoperative day after abdominal surgery (procedures lasting longer than 2 h and no planned postoperative ICU admission) in patients at risk for respiratory failure did not improve oxygenation or requirement of any respiratory support during the first 7 days [42].

In conclusion, evidences suggest that HFNC therapy is a useful and well-tolerated option in patients that develop post-extubation hypoxemic respiratory failure, although reintubation should not be delayed if clinically required. A recent meta-analysis confirmed the previously reported results. HFNC therapy is associated with lower reintubation risk compared to conventional oxygen therapy (OR 0.47, 95%CI 0.27–0.84, $p = 0.01$), but not in the comparison with NIV (OR 0.73, 95%CI 0.47–1.13, $p = 0.16$). No significant difference was found in mortality rate or ICU length of stay [43].

11.7   HFNC Therapy in Special Population

HFNC support, being noninvasive and assuring good comfort for the patient, may play a central role in those circumstances in which invasive mechanical ventilation is contraindicated (palliative care) or burdened by very high mortality (immuno-compromised patients or affected by hematological malignancies):

- Palliative care

Peters et al. reviewed the clinical charts of all patients admitted to ICU in two American hospitals during the time period 2010–2011. The authors identified 50 patients with do-not-intubate (DNI) orders treated with HFNC support for respiratory distress, hypoxemia, and mild hypercapnia ($PaCO_2 > 65$ mmHg and pH < 7.28) [44]. HFNC was associated with a reduction in tachypnea (respiratory rate 31 versus 25 breaths/min, $p < 0.001$) and increase in oxygenation (SpO_2 89 versus 95%, $p < 0.001$). Nine patients (18%) required intensifying treatment with NIV, while 41 patients (82%) were maintained on HFNC support. Mean duration of HFNC support was 30 h; overall mortality was 60% without any difference between those who received NIV and HFNC therapy [44].

- Lung transplant patients

Roca et al. performed a retrospective analysis on the effects of HFNC therapy in patients admitted to ICU for acute respiratory failure after lung transplant [45]. The authors analyzed 35 patients for a total of 40 ARF events; 18 cases were initially treated with standard oxygen mask and had a relative risk for intubation of 1.50 (IC95% 1.05–2.21) in comparison to HFNC therapy. The prompt institution of HFNC support showed the ability to reduce intubation rate about 30%, with a NNT of 3 in avoiding intubation. Logistic regression showed an odd ratio of 0.43 (IC95% 0.002–0.88) for HFNC failure and subsequent intubation requirement. Shock and ARDS diagnosis were risk factors for HFNC failure and invasive mechanical ventilation [45].

- Oncologic patients

On a cohort of 1424 patients with hematological malignancies admitted to ICU during the period 2012–2014, Lee et al. found 45 patients with ARF that underwent HFNC as first-line treatment [46]. Fifteen patients recovered with HFNC, while in 30 cases intubation and mechanical ventilation was implemented after few hours of HFNC therapy. The only risk factor associated to respiratory deterioration was the diagnosis of bacterial pneumonia (73% patients with bacterial pneumonia deteriorated in HFNC support compared to 27% cases affected by ARF for any other causes, $p = 0.004$); HFNC failure and intubation were correlated with a steep increase in mortality (13% versus 87%) [46]. In a similar paper, Mokart et al. studied oncologic patients admitted to ICU with acute respiratory failure requiring oxygen mask support with a gas flow higher than 9 l/min [47]. Out of the overall 178 patients enrolled, 8 continued standard oxygen mask, 20 were treated with HFNC therapy, 74 were supported with NIV and standard oxygen mask, and lastly 76 patients required cycles of both NIV and HFNC. Primary outcome was 28-day mortality; secondary endpoints were 28-day ventilation-free days and long-term mortality. Compared to all the other groups, patients treated with both HFNC therapy and NIV showed lower mortality (37% versus 52%, $p = 0.045$), longer time to intubation (34 versus 16 h, $p = 0.01$), and a trend toward longer ventilation-free days (24 versus 8 days, $p = 0.06$). The authors developed a severity propensity score at ICU admission to identify a subgroup of severely ill patients (138 patients); study results were consistent with those found in the total population: mortality was lower for patients treated with HFNC and NIV cycles (36% versus 54%, $p = 0.027$), and all secondary endpoints were significantly improved in this group. Moreover, HFNC support was independently associated with survival benefits (65% versus 43%, $p = 0.008$), and no similar result was found for NIV treatment [47].

Conclusions

HFNC therapy showed numerous benefits compared to standard oxygen mask support. Constant and reliable FiO_2, nasopharyngeal anatomical dead space washout, upper airway resistance reduction, PEEP and subsequent alveolar recruitment, and better comfort for the patient are some of the hypothesized mechanisms to support HFNC use in ARF patients. Literature provided evidence about the usefulness of HFNC systems during the post-extubation period and ARF and in patients for whom intubation is contraindicated. Further studies are required to evaluate its role in the most severely hypoxemic patients.

References

1. Leigh JM. The evolution of oxygen therapy apparatus. Anaesthesia. 1974;29:462–85.
2. Hutchings FA, Hilliard TN, Davis PJ. Heated humidified high-flow nasal cannula therapy in children. Arch Dis Child. 2015;100:571–5.
3. Ricard J-D. High flow nasal oxygen in acute respiratory failure. Minerva Anestesiol. 2012;78:836–41.
4. O'Driscoll BR, Howard LS, Davison AG. BTS guideline for emergency oxygen use in adult patients. Thorax. 2008;63(Suppl 6):vi1–68.
5. Malinowski T, Lamberti J. Oxygen concentrations via nasal cannula at high flow rates. Respir Care. 2002;47:1039.
6. L'Her E, Deye N, Lellouche F, Taille S, Demoule A, Fraticelli A, et al. Physiologic effects of noninvasive ventilation during acute lung injury. Am J Respir Crit Care Med. 2005;172: 1112–8.
7. Wettstein RB, Peters JI, Shelledy DS. Pharyngeal oxygen concentration in normal subjects wearing high flow nasal cannula. Respir Care. 2004;49:1444.
8. Tiep B, Barnett M. High flow nasal vs high flow mask oxygen delivery: tracheal gas concentrations through a head extension airway model. Respir Care. 2002;47:1079.
9. Spence KL, Murphy D, Kilian C, McGonigle R, Kilani RA. High-flow nasal cannula as a device to provide continuous positive airway pressure in infants. J Perinatol. 2007;27:772–5.
10. Miller TL, Blackson TJ, Shaffer TH, Touch SM. Tracheal gas insufflation-augmented continuous positive airway pressure in a spontaneously breathing model of neonatal respiratory distress. Pediatr Pulmonol. 2004;38:386–95.
11. Dewan NA, Bell CW. Effect of low flow and high flow oxygen delivery on exercise tolerance and sensation of dyspnea. A study comparing the transtracheal catheter and nasal prongs. Chest. 1994;105:1061–5.
12. Chatila W, Nugent T, Vance G, Gaughan J, Criner GJ. The effects of high-flow vs low-flow oxygen on exercise in advanced obstructive airways disease. Chest. 2004;126:1108–15.
13. Itagaki T, Okuda N, Tsunano Y, Kohata H, Nakataki E, Onodera M, et al. Effect of high-flow nasal cannula on thoraco-abdominal synchrony in adult critically ill patients. Respir Care. 2014;59:70–4.
14. Groves N, Tobin A. High flow nasal oxygen generates positive airway pressure in adult volunteers. Aust Crit Care. 2007;20:126–31.
15. Miller MJ, DiFiore JM, Strohl KP, Martin RJ. Effects of nasal CPAP on supraglottic and total pulmonary resistance in preterm infants. J Appl Physiol (1985). 1990;68:141–6.
16. Parke R, McGuinness S, Eccleston M. Nasal high-flow therapy delivers low level positive airway pressure. Br J Anaesth. 2009;103:886–90.
17. Ritchie JE, Williams AB, Gerard C, Hockey H. Evaluation of a humidified nasal high-flow oxygen system, using oxygraphy, capnography and measurement of upper airway pressures. Anaesth Intensive Care. 2011;39:1103–10.
18. Parke RL, McGuinness SP. Pressures delivered by nasal high flow oxygen during all phases of the respiratory cycle. Respir Care. 2013;58:1621–4.
19. Corley A, Caruana LR, Barnett AG, Tronstad O, Fraser JF. Oxygen delivery through high-flow nasal cannulae increase end-expiratory lung volume and reduce respiratory rate in post-cardiac surgical patients. Br J Anaesth. 2011;107:998–1004.

20. Fontanari P, Burnet H, Zattara-Hartmann MC, Jammes Y. Changes in airway resistance induced by nasal inhalation of cold dry, dry, or moist air in normal individuals. J Appl Physiol (1985). 1996;81:1739–43.
21. Greenspan JS, Wolfson MR, Shaffer TH. Airway responsiveness to low inspired gas temperature in preterm neonates. J Pediatr. 1991;118:443–5.
22. Roca O, Riera J, Torres F, Masclans JR. High-flow oxygen therapy in acute respiratory failure. Respir Care. 2010;55:408–13.
23. Boyer A, Vargas F, Delacre M, Saint-Leger M, Clouzeau B, Hilbert G, et al. Prognostic impact of high-flow nasal cannula oxygen supply in an ICU patient with pulmonary fibrosis complicated by acute respiratory failure. Intensive Care Med. 2011;37:558–9.
24. Chikata Y, Izawa M, Okuda N, Itagaki T, Nakataki E, Onodera M, et al. Humidification performance of two high-flow nasal cannula devices: a bench study. Respir Care. 2014;59:1186–90.
25. Mayfield S, Jauncey-Cooke J, Hough JL, Schibler A, Gibbons K, Bogossian F. High-flow nasal cannula therapy for respiratory support in children. Cochrane Database Syst Rev. 2014;3:CD009850.
26. Sztrymf B, Messika J, Mayot T, Lenglet H, Dreyfuss D, Ricard J-D. Impact of high-flow nasal cannula oxygen therapy on intensive care unit patients with acute respiratory failure: a prospective observational study. J Crit Care. 2012;27:324.e9–13.
27. Sztrymf B, Messika J, Bertrand F, Hurel D, Leon R, Dreyfuss D, et al. Beneficial effects of humidified high flow nasal oxygen in critical care patients: a prospective pilot study. Intensive Care Med. 2011;37:1780–6.
28. Rello J, Perez M, Roca O, Poulakou G, Souto J, Laborda C, et al. High-flow nasal therapy in adults with severe acute respiratory infection: a cohort study in patients with 2009 influenza a/H1N1v. J Crit Care. 2012;27:434–9.
29. Frat J-P, Thille AW, Mercat A, Girault C, Ragot S, Perbet S, et al. High-flow oxygen through nasal cannula in acute hypoxemic respiratory failure. N Engl J Med. 2015;372:2185–96.
30. Messika J, Ben Ahmed K, Gaudry S, Miguel-Montanes R, Rafat C, Sztrymf B, et al. Use of high-flow nasal cannula oxygen therapy in subjects with ARDS: a 1-year observational study. Respir Care. 2015;60:162–9.
31. Ou X, Hua Y, Liu J, Gong C, Zhao W. Effect of high-flow nasal cannula oxygen therapy in adults with acute hypoxemic respiratory failure: a meta-analysis of randomized controlled trials. CMAJ. 2017;189:E260–7.
32. Tiruvoipati R, Lewis D, Haji K, Botha J. High-flow nasal oxygen vs high-flow face mask: a randomized crossover trial in extubated patients. J Crit Care. 2010;25:463–8.
33. Rittayamai N, Tscheikuna J, Rujiwit P. High-flow nasal cannula versus conventional oxygen therapy after endotracheal extubation: a randomized crossover physiologic study. Respir Care. 2014;59:485–90.
34. Brotfain E, Zlotnik A, Schwartz A, Frenkel A, Koyfman L, Gruenbaum SE, et al. Comparison of the effectiveness of high flow nasal oxygen cannula vs. standard non-rebreather oxygen face mask in post-extubation intensive care unit patients. Isr Med Assoc J. 2014;16:718–22.
35. Maggiore SM, Idone FA, Vaschetto R, Festa R, Cataldo A, Antonicelli F, et al. Nasal high-flow versus Venturi mask oxygen therapy after extubation. Effects on oxygenation, comfort, and clinical outcome. Am J Respir Crit Care Med. 2014;190:282–8.
36. Corley A, Bull T, Spooner AJ, Barnett AG, Fraser JF. Direct extubation onto high-flow nasal cannulae post-cardiac surgery versus standard treatment in patients with a BMI >/=30: a randomised controlled trial. Intensive Care Med. 2015;41:887–94.
37. Hernández G, Vaquero C, González P, Subira C, Frutos-Vivar F, Rialp G, et al. Effect of postextubation high-flow nasal cannula vs conventional oxygen therapy on reintubation in low-risk patients. A randomized clinical trial. JAMA. 2016;315:1354–61.
38. Hernández G, Vaquero C, Colinas L, Cuena R, González P, Canabal A, et al. Effect of postextubation high-flow nasal cannula vs noninvasive ventilation on reintubation and postextubation respiratory failure in high-risk patients. A randomized clinical trial. JAMA. 2016;316:1565–74.
39. Stephan F, Barrucand B, Petit P, Rezaiguia-Delclaux S, Medard A, Delannoy B, et al. High-flow nasal oxygen vs noninvasive positive airway pressure in hypoxemic patients after cardiothoracic surgery: a randomized clinical trial. JAMA. 2015;313:2331–9.

40. Esteban A, Frutos-Vivar F, Ferguson ND, Arabi Y, Apezteguía C, González M, et al. Noninvasive positive-pressure ventilation for respiratory failure after extubation. N Engl J Med. 2004;350:2452–60.
41. Kang BJ, Koh Y, Lim CM, Huh JW, Baek S, Han M, et al. Failure of high-flow nasal cannula therapy may delay intubation and increase mortality. Intensive Care Med. 2015;41:623–32.
42. Futier E, Paugam-Burtz C, Godet T, Khoy-Ear L, Rozencwajg S, Delay JM, et al. OPERA study investigators. Effect of early postextubation high-flow nasal cannula vs conventional oxygen therapy on hypoxaemia in patients after major abdominal surgery: a French multicentre randomised controlled trial (OPERA). Intensive Care Med. 2016;42:1888–98.
43. Ni YN, Luo J, Yu H, Liu D, Ni Z, Cheng J, et al. Can high-flow nasal cannula reduce the rate of endotracheal intubation in adult patients with acute respiratory failure compared with conventional oxygen therapy and noninvasive positive pressure ventilation? A systematic review and meta-analysis. Chest. 2017;151:764–75.
44. Peters SG, Holets SR, Gay PC. High-flow nasal cannula therapy in do-not-intubate patients with hypoxemic respiratory distress. Respir Care. 2013;58:597–600.
45. Roca O, de Acilu MG, Caralt B, Sacanell J, Masclans JR. Humidified high flow nasal cannula supportive therapy improves outcomes in lung transplant recipients readmitted to the intensive care unit because of acute respiratory failure. Transplantation. 2015;99:1092–8.
46. Lee HY, Rhee CK, Lee JW. Feasibility of high-flow nasal cannula oxygen therapy for acute respiratory failure in patients with hematologic malignancies: a retrospective single-center study. J Crit Care. 2015;30:773–7.
47. Mokart D, Geay C, Chow-Chine L, Brun J-P, Faucher M, Blache J-L, et al. High-flow oxygen therapy in cancer patients with acute respiratory failure. Intensive Care Med. 2015;41:2008–10.

Hypermetabolism in Critical Care: The Role of Metabolism Measurement and Its Nutritional Implications

12

Marco Dei Poli, Nicholas S.M. Bianchi Bosisio, and Valeria Musso

In recent years a key role has been assumed in all areas of critical care medicine by the accurate assessment of the patient's energy state. A definition of needs is crucial in responding adequately to the state of acute imbalance that almost all illnesses bring about. Nutrition in relation to the metabolism plays a key role in influencing prognosis and patient outcome. Criticality goes hand in hand with complex responses from the biochemical point of view. Knowing these and how exactly to define them is the topic of this brief chapter.

12.1 The Definition of "Hypermetabolism"

"Hypermetabolism" is a state of enhanced metabolic activity, characterised by an increase of the basal metabolic rate. Catabolic reaction rate is higher than anabolic one. These changes are the result of a systemic response to a damage or a trauma suffered by the organism under stress. As for the autonomic nervous system, the sympathetic component is intensely active, while the parasympathetic activity is reduced.

Some of the main clinical and biochemical features of hypermetabolic patients are:

1. Increase of energy expenditure and oxygen consumption
2. Stress-induced hyperglycaemia
3. Hyperlactatemia
4. Loss of muscle mass due to hypercatabolism of proteins
5. Negative nitrogen balance

M. Dei Poli (✉) • N.S.M. Bianchi Bosisio • V. Musso
General Intensive Care Unit, IRCCS Policlinico, San Donato, San Donato, MI, Italy
e-mail: marco.deipoli@grupposandonato.it

© Springer International Publishing AG 2018
D. Chiumello (ed.), *Practical Trends in Anesthesia and Intensive Care 2017*,
http://doi.org/10.1007/978-3-319-61325-3_12

12.2   Biochemistry of Hypermetabolism [3, 9, 14]

Gluconeogenesis (Focus On)
Gluconeogenesis is a metabolic pathway that leads to generation of glucose using non-glucidic substrates, such as pyruvate, lactate, glycerol, ethanol and gluco-genic amino acids. This process occurs when blood glucose level is low, and in humans it happens mainly in the liver. Most steps of gluconeogenesis are the reverse of those we find in glycolysis (except for three exergonic reactions). Gluconeogenesis begins in the mitochondria, where pyruvate is converted to oxa-loacetate and then to malate. Malate is then transported to cytoplasm, where it is oxidised to oxaloacetate and converted to phosphoenolpyruvate. Other reactions take place in the cytoplasm and they are the same as in reversed glycolysis.

Fructose1,6-bisphosphatase is the key enzyme in this process. This is con-trolled by allosteric regulation (by binding an effector molecule to allosteric site, the enzyme's active site will be able to catalyse reactions). Fructose1,6-bisphosphatase can bind positive allosteric modulators such as citrate, enhanc-ing its attraction to substrates, or negative effectors such as AMP (adenosine monophosphate) and fructose2,6-bisphosphate, reducing its affinity to reagents. The reaction catalysed by fructose1,6-bisphosphatase is the rate-limiting step of gluconeogenesis.

Stress response is characterised by a raise of energy expenditure: proteins are used as an energy source by the liver, where gluconeogenesis is highly active. Hepatocytes are able to produce glucose, using pyruvate as a substrate. The energy needed for this metabolic pathway is provided by beta oxidation and later by the citric acid cycle.

Acute-phase proteins: they are serum proteins whose levels rise (positive acute-phase proteins) or decrease (negative acute-phase proteins) when inflammation occurs. They are a useful marker to detect inflammation, and together with fever, leucocytosis and other symptoms such as tachycardia, hypertension, shivering, anorexia and malaise, they constitute the so-called acute-phase reaction.

Positive proteins: they are part of the innate immune system, but they serve several different functions. Some of them destroy or inhibit microbes (i.e. C-reactive protein, mannose-binding protein, complement factors, ferritin, ceruloplasmin, serum amyloid A and haptoglobin); others give negative feed-back to the inflammatory response, such as serpins (serine protease inhibitor). Coagulation factors and alpha-2-macroglobulin mainly stimulate coagulation, probably in order to trap pathogens and to limit the infection. Other products of the coagulation system can increase vascular permeability, acting as che-motactic agents for phagocytic cells.

Negative proteins: they include albumin, transferrin, transthyretin, retinol-binding protein, antithrombin and transcortin. When inflammation occurs, these proteins' synthesis decreases with the purpose of sparing amino acids to produce positive acute-phase proteins. Transferrin reduction is also due to an upregulation of its receptors, but this mechanism does not seem to change in relation with inflammation.

When a patient undergoes stress response, protein synthesis is reduced, and hepatocytes begin producing *acute-phase proteins*. There is an enhancement of plasma concentration of positive acute-phase proteins (e.g. C-reactive protein, ferritin, ceruloplasmin) and a decrease of negative acute-phase protein concentration, for example, serum albumin levels. *Protein hypercatabolism* attempts to respond to the increased energy needs. This leads to one of the main features of stress response: the loss of patient's lean body mass. An important difference between starvation and *stress reaction* is the *inflammatory response* (first local and then systemic) activated by the injury. Inflammation causes the release of cytokines, hormones and neuronal signalling molecules to the hypothalamus. These changes in the hormonal profile determine a strong *fight-or-flight*-like response. The so-called stress hormone (e.g. catecholamines, cortisol, glucagon) levels are increased, inducing various consequences on the organism. This response is a maladaptive process.

The systemic response to stress causes several biochemical changes, for example, the increase of oxygen consumption and body temperature and the alteration of metabolic profile to keep up with the high oxygen demand. Gluconeogenesis, which takes place in the liver and uses lactate, glycerol and amino acids to produce glucose, plays a key role in this process. Furthermore, cells fail to respond to the hormone insulin, a process called *insulin resistance*. This occurs especially in insulin-dependent tissues such as muscle and adipose tissue, which need insulin to regulate glucose intake and therefore glycaemia. Insulin resistance seems to be a consequence of insulin receptor downregulation and reduced transcription of GLUT-4, caused by inflammatory mediators, and is one of the mechanisms responsible for *stress-induced hyperglycaemia* (SIH), and in critical patients it is associated with a worse outcome. In addition, it shows up an imbalance in plasma levels of metabolic hormones. The hormonal response includes augmented levels of catecholamines, cortisol and glucagon and a strengthening of gluconeogenesis and glycolysis in the liver, hence the further higher levels of glycaemia. This condition is particularly emphasised in critical patient as part of an adaptive response whose final aim is survival. When the stress response is maintained without adequate treatment, it leads to energy reserve depletion, with severe consequences. It is therefore crucial to accurately assess the metabolic state of patients in ICU. Some of the causes of stress in critical patients are illustrated in Fig. 12.1, along with the relative resting metabolic rate. Patients undergoing hypermetabolism are frequently inadequately fed, but their clinical condition is different from the underfeeding provoked by short-term or long-term starvation.

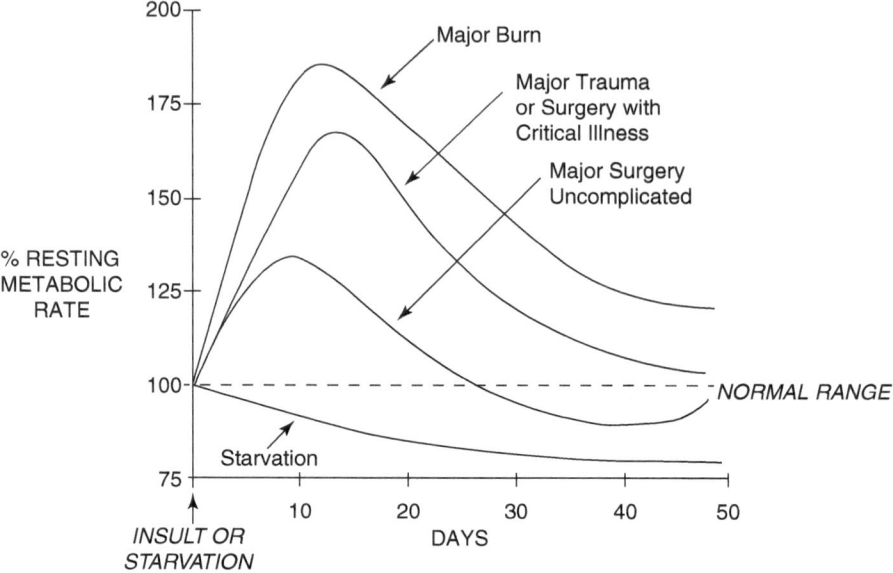

Fig. 12.1 Variation in resting metabolic rate in different types of critical patient. The graph was taken from [9]

Glucose transporters (GLUT) are a group of membrane proteins that facilitate the transfer of glucose across the cell membrane, from interstitial space into cytoplasm. These carriers are usually sequestered in cytoplasmic vesicles. In humans, seven types of glucose transporters have been identified, and each one of them has a different distribution depending on the tissue. In insulin-dependent tissues and in those who directly regulate glycaemia according to variations in the level of glucose, there are three types of glucose transporters:
- GLUT-4 (insulin-dependent glucose transporter)
- GLUT-2 (acts as an insulin-independent glucose sensor)
- GLUT-1 (responsible for the low level of basal glucose required by all cells)

In insulin-dependent tissues such as striated muscle (skeletal and cardiac muscle) and adipose tissue, the main glucose transporter is GLUT-4, which is strictly regulated by insulin concentration. The release of insulin increases both the synthesis of GLUT-4 and its translocation from the intracellular vesicles to the plasma membrane: the vesicles fuse with the membrane, and GLUT-4 transporters are inserted and become available for their function, augmenting glucose uptake from interstitial space into cytoplasm. Once glycaemia is reduced to basal concentration and insulin is cleared from the bloodstream, endocytosis sequesters GLUT-4 in vesicles. GLUT-4 concentration can also be influenced by other factors: hypercortisolaemia reduces it, while stress, physical exercise and any mechanism causing a decrease in the ATP/ADP ratio or an increase in levels of calcium ion

(Ca^{2+}), augmented blood flow and reduced levels of glycogen determine raising in GLUT-4 activity.

In skeletal muscle, GLUT-4 uptake of glucose is more intense in type I fibres (also called red fibres). Striated muscles usually take 60% of the glucose available in the bloodstream, while other tissues take the rest, and only a very small fraction goes to the adipose tissue. It has been shown that at least 80% of glucose consumption, induced by insulin, takes place in the skeletal muscle, while adipose tissue only uses 5–10% of it.

Glycogenolysis

Every day, the human organism needs to regulate a lot of different reactions and functions to preserve its balance. One of the parameters that needs to be controlled is glycaemia. When hypoglycaemia occurs, glucagon is released in the bloodstream, causing a raise in plasmatic glucose levels. Glucagon acts as a signal to the liver, leading to an increased production and release of glucose into plasma. Adrenaline induces an augmentation in glycaemia too, but, unlike glucagon, it influences mostly the muscle tissue. When these hormones bind to their receptors (both in the liver and muscle tissue), protein kinase A is activated: this enzyme starts up phosphorylase kinase. This kinase converts glycogen phosphorylase b in its activated form (glycogen phosphorylase a) by phosphorylation (while glycogen phosphorylase can be inactivated by a protein phosphatase). Glycogen phosphorylase is the first enzyme in glycogenolysis. It removes terminal glucose residue from a glycogen branch, producing glucose-1-phosphate. The latter is converted by phosphoglucomutase into glucose-6-phosphate. This can either be used for glycolysis, in muscle tissue, or be released in the bloodstream, in the liver (in hepatocytes there is a particular enzyme, glucose-6-phosphatase, which can remove the phosphate group from glucose 6-phosphate).

12.3 Starvation vs Stress [17, 20]

Unlike stress-induced metabolic alterations, the *metabolic response to fasting* consists in a reduction of energy expenditure (*metabolic rate* is reduced to 20–25 kcal/kg/day). During the first hours, the glucose stored in the liver as glycogen is depleted; after that, 90% of energy is produced by lipolysis, while proteins are used as a substrate for gluconeogenesis to synthetize glucose. This would result in a decreased protein biosynthesis, if it were not for the *protein-sparing* response which minimises the loss of muscle mass. Starvation induces adaptive responses that, in time, can result in malnutrition.

Fig. 12.2 Haemodynamic changes associated with different types of shock. Systemic vascular resistance (SVR). Pulmonary capillary wedge pressure (PCWP)

Shock	Cardiac output	SVR	PCWP
Cardiogenic	⬇	⬆	⬆
Hypovolemic	⬇	⬆	⬇
Neurogenic	⬇	⬇	⬇
Septic	⬇	⬇	⬇

12.4 Hypermetabolism and Hyperdynamic Circulation

Biochemical and metabolic alterations are not the only changes caused by hypermetabolism. Also *haemodynamics is altered*. The augmented oxygen consumption in peripheral tissues leads to an increased cardiac output (CO) and a reduction in systemic vascular resistance (SVR). Typical clinical conditions presenting with hyperdynamic circulation are sepsis (when vasoplegia causes hypotension or dysoxic septic shock), intense adrenergic stimulation (e.g. due to postoperative pain), hyperthyroidism and hyperthermia. In a patient with hyperdynamic circulation, we should always consider underlying hypermetabolism.

In hyperdynamic circulation, the most common changes in haemodynamic parameters are *increase of cardiac index and systolic volume index*, possibility of hypertension or hypotension (depending on the level of vasoplegia) and reduction of systemic vascular resistance, central venous pressure and wedge pressure (changes in haemodynamic parameters in different types of shock are shown in Fig. 12.2).

12.5 Hypermetabolism and Sepsis [5, 11, 18, 23]

Stress response is particularly emphasised in patients with sepsis: it can be induced by SIRS (systemic inflammatory response syndrome), hypermetabolism (with an increase in resting metabolic rate), hypercatabolism (protein breakdown takes place especially in muscle tissue), shock and *multiple organ failure (MOF)*. In this case the inflammatory response can be triggered by components of the bacterial cell wall (endotoxins or exotoxins) which induce a massive release of inflammatory mediators, increasing the stress action. Augmented energy expenditure can be also explained by fever. It induces a 10–15% increase in energy expenditure for each degree Celsius elevation of temperature, even though the relation between the two parameters in critically ill patients is complicated.

Fig. 12.3 The Cori cycle

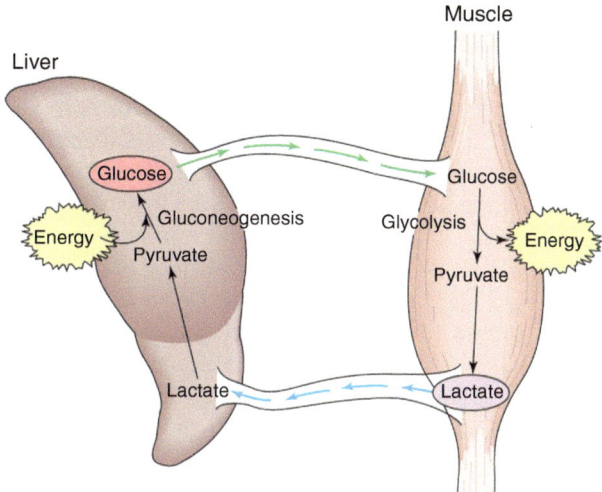

We cannot address hypermetabolism and sepsis without mentioning lactate metabolism. *Hyperlactatemia*, due to hypoxia and hypoperfusion, is present in every low cardiac output condition, such as shock. Understanding lactatemia levels in septic shock has been shown to be a much more complex task though. In the early phase of septic shock, the clinical presentation is similar to that of cardiogenic and haemorrhagic shock. The administration of sympathomimetic drugs (adrenaline, noradrenaline, dopamine and dobutamine) causes an increase in lactatemia per se. A peculiar metabolic condition called "accelerated aerobic glycolysis" occurs in septic patients, and its main features are increased synthesis of glucose transporters across the cell membrane, augmented glycolysis (induced by endogenous and exogenous catecholamines) and inflammation. The rate of glycolysis exceeds the oxidative capacity of mitochondria: this imbalance, together with protein hypercatabolism, causes an increase in pyruvate concentration, especially in muscle cells. Pyruvate is then converted to lactate by fermentation. The increased lactate production acts as an adaptive mechanism in order to keep the carbohydrate metabolism from stopping when oxygen delivery is reduced. Lactate can be used both as an alternative fuel to glucose and a source of glucose itself. Cells keep it for producing energy and this protects from acidosis. Lactate is transported out of the cell by diffusional cotransport with protons (H^+ ions), thus regulating intracellular pH. In septic shock, lactate produced in myocytes is used as a substrate in the Cori cycle (illustrated in Fig. 12.3), an effective but highly energy-consuming pathway. Lactate is transported to the liver, where it is used for gluconeogenesis: it is first converted to pyruvate and then to glucose. In this way, lactate serves to deliver additional glucose that can be used by the organism. It is also important to point out that, when the patient undergoes stress, the heart and the brain are able to use lactate as main fuel: these organs can oxidise lactate instead of glucose during anaerobic conditions, leaving glucose for other cells.

Septic patients are extremely frail, both during the early and the late phase of illness. *SIRS* is a pro-inflammatory syndrome: its aim is to remove the organism responsible for the infection by increasing the activity of the immune system. When this response goes out of control or is overly prolonged, it damages the patient. Studies on septic patients have shown the existence of an anti-inflammatory response, usually occurring after SIRS, called *CARS (compensatory anti-inflammatory response syndrome)*. CARS consists in a suppression of the immune system in order to restore homoeostasis after a severe inflammatory state. SIRS and CARS are the two sides of the same coin: each one is characterised by a particular set of cytokines, and, although they are separate responses, most of the times one follows the other (even though often they take place simultaneously with different relevance). Like SIRS, CARS can be dangerous too if it is not regulated or it fails to restore homoeostasis, making the patient vulnerable to infections. Some of the clinical features of CARS are cutaneous anergy, leucopenia, hypothermia, susceptibility to infections and failure to clear infections.

12.6 Hypermetabolism in Cancer Patients [21]

In neoplastic patients, especially at advanced stages, cachexia is frequently associated with an increased *resting energy expenditure* (REE). The condition is even more complicated due to the presence of symptoms such as anorexia, pain and depression, which can often cause malnutrition, both in quantitative and qualitative terms. Malnutrition affects the metabolic state of the patient, which is already impaired.

12.7 Hypermetabolism in Postoperative Patients [7, 13]

Patients undergoing surgery are an ideal model for the study of hypermetabolism caused by stress response. Surgery is in fact a clear example of a stressful event: even though anaesthesia reduces afferent neural transmission to pain centres, the organism interprets surgery as a threat. The activation of different hormonal axis causes the release of stress hormones such as cortisol, catecholamines, glucagon and growth hormone. These hormones are responsible for the condition of hypermetabolism, whose biochemical aspects have been previously discussed. This mechanism takes place in elective operations, but even more in emergency surgery, major surgery and when postoperative complications occur. The stress response purpose is the survival of the critically ill patient, by using the energy reserves and retaining water. The response becomes a harmful condition when prolonged in time. Regional and local anaesthesia has been shown to be an important factor in both reducing the stress response to surgery and influencing the postoperative outcome by bringing beneficial effects on organ function.

12.8   Hypermetabolism in Trauma Patients [4, 6, 7]

In trauma patients, the systemic inflammatory reaction is similar to the one previously described. The splanchnic region appears to be the main source of hypermetabolic response. The increased energy expenditure is not adequately matched by an implementation in blood flow, especially right after the trauma, when the patient is often hypovolaemic due to loss of blood. Hypovolaemia causes splanchnic vasoconstriction which is an important risk factor for inadequate perfusion of splanchnic region.

12.9   How Can Energy Expenditure Be Accurately Determined [1, 2, 24, 25, 26]?

Once the complex condition of the critical patient in hypermetabolic state has been analysed and understood, it is essential to think about the correct way to manage the administration of nutrients. That is important to satisfy needs and prevent negative consequences of catabolism and malnutrition. First of all, it is crucial to accurately determine energy expenditure (EE).

Historically we know two different ways to solve this problem: the use of predictive equations and the calorimetry procedure (whether direct or indirect).

Predictive equations are really manageable since no measuring instrument is required and the results can be comfortably calculated at a desk; the required data are easily available and at no great expense, either! It should not, however, be forgotten that they represent only a mere approximation of the energetic consumption of the individual being examined. Even in the analysis of healthy subjects, it is well known that predictive equations are not particularly accurate. Each of the available formulas was derived from a cohort of individuals who, potentially, could have had extremely different features from the patient that we want to examine. Let us consider, for example, the Harris-Benedict (which, when the correction factor 1.2 is applied, is the least discordant among the calorimetric measures for the male sex). This formula was worked out, in 1919, from the study of a specific population of 239 *healthy* adults. It is evident that the physical features of the subjects examined were dramatically different from those of people living nowadays. Changes in lifestyle, working conditions, services and facilities available, alimentary regimen and disposition to physical exercise are only some of the differences we can find between these two different groups.

Secondly, even when resorting to these formulas, we have to choose which one, from the large number available, is the most suitable for our patient. There are indeed differences that may reach 20–30% of the estimated value when choosing one rather than another (Table 12.1). It has been proven that the use of these equations can frequently lead to *underfeeding* (in formulas that underestimate the EE) or to *overfeeding* (in equations that overestimate the EE) the patient concerned. This can, obviously, compromise the patient's prognosis. Considering the extreme

Table 12.1 Comparison of REE values obtained by indirect calorimetry and with the different predictive equations in 49 elderly male subjects who were being mechanically ventilated

Predictive equation	REE (kcal/24 h)	ICC	95% CI	P value
Indirect calorimetry	1701.9 ± 387.4	–	–	–
Lührmann	1579.6 ± 267.68	0.574	0.353–0.735	<0.001
Fredrix	1569.4 ± 268.7	0.597	0.384–0.750	<0.001
Ireton-Jones	1590.5 ± 178.4	0.465	0.216–0.658	<0.001
Mifflin St-Jeor	1470.9 ± 265.0	0.446	0.193–0.644	0.001
Harris-Benedict × 1.2	1707.6 ± 339.7	0.668	0.480–0.798	<0.001
ESPEN minimum	1553.3 ± 424.9	0.579	0.360–0.738	<0.001
ESPEN average	1747.5 ± 478.0	0.617	0.410–0.764	<0.001
ESPEN maximum	1941.7 ± 531.1	0.505	0.265–0.686	<0.001

The table was taken and adapted from [24]
REE resting energy expenditure, *ICC* intraclass correlation coefficient, *CI* confidence interval, *ESPEN* European Society for Clinical Nutrition and Metabolism

variations of energy expenditure in the different conditions of stress that can occur in a critical patient, it is obvious how only the correct measurement of how much energy (EE) the patient *actually consumes*, and not the estimate of how much the patient *should theoretically consume*, can represent the baseline for the institution of a correct caloric supply.

This is especially true when treating critical patients and, in particular, hypermetabolic ones. Using predictive equations with these subjects, their real energetic consumption is almost always underestimated. We will determine how much energy they *should theoretically* consume and not what they are *really* wasting, in energetic terms, to support the hypermetabolic state in which they are. The arrangement of artificial nutrition, based on energy expenditure obtained using predictive equations, will lead to a negative energetic balance that will inevitably deteriorate the state of intensive catabolism. Literature supports how "hospital malnutrition" is associated with unfavourable prognostic factors such as an increased risk of contracting nosocomial infections, prolongation of hospitalisation and, not least, increased risk of mortality. An absolutely necessary goal in the management of artificial nutrition must be the strict recording of the patient's daily energy expenditure. This represents best practice with the aim of identifying the correct calorie intake to prevent a negative energy balance in the critical patient.

In the light of all this, we can understand how calorimetry acquires overriding importance. This is the reference tool for the measurement of energy expenditure. Unfortunately, this method is still not widely practised. Considering how cumbersome the early instruments were and how difficult they were to use, it is understandable why such instrumental investigation was rarely resorted to in the past. Nowadays, thanks to the portability of the equipment and its ever-increasing simplicity of use, there is no longer any justification for omitting to measure this sort of data at the patient's bedside. This is actually even easier, as we shall see later, where patients are being ventilated through an endotracheal tube or a tracheostomy cannula.

Calorimetry assessment is, therefore, the real issue of the metabolic and nutritional study of critically ill patients.

In current scientific literature, *the calorimeter* is the "gold standard" reference tool for the measurement of *energy expenditure*. Yet, today, the use of these instruments is limited to only a few artificial nutrition centres and even fewer intensive care units. The rather high cost of the equipment, together with the fact that they are still hardly user-friendly and that certain measurements—especially the more accurate ones—take a long time to calculate, still seems to be a problem.

We are confident, however, that the main obstacle to the use of calorimetry at the critically ill patient's bedside is *a less than perfect understanding* of the importance of these figures which obviously do not only tell us about calorie consumption but also provide an assessment of the metabolic or hypermetabolic state of the critically ill patient.

12.10 Which Calorimetry [8, 12, 16, 19]?

Direct calorimetry measures the heat produced by the metabolic processes to quantify total energy expenditure. For this survey to be carried out, the subject must be transferred into a whole room calorimeter. This is, undoubtedly, the most accurate method to determine the consumption of substrates for energetic aims. The costliness, lack of availability and the complexity of performance have limited the chances of widespread use of this method, so direct calorimetry is out of the question for critical patients.

With *indirect calorimetry*, on the other hand, energy expenditure is defined by the analysis of respiratory gases based on the principle of respiratory thermochemistry: the organism gets energy through the oxidation of energetic sublayers held in food; these are metabolised according to known stoichiometric reactions in which oxygen is consumed and carbon dioxide is produced. Indirect calorimetry can be carried out using two different types of circuit. In closed circuit, the patient inspires and expires from the same chamber the gases, after a certain period, will be analysed. In this case only the consumption of oxygen is measured, and energy expenditure is estimated considering a thermal equivalent per litre of oxygen (i.e. 4.82 Kcal/L).

In open-circuit indirect calorimetry, the inspiratory air is supplied one way, while the expiratory gases are collected by another separate one for examination. So we can observe both O_2 consumption and CO_2 production. In this way we can define energy expenditure and respiratory quotient (which is useful for detecting nutritious substances that the patient is burning). This is the preferred method for clinical and diagnostic use because it is easy to perform either on ventilated patients or on patients that are in spontaneous breath. In this second class of patients, the gases are collected by using helmets, masks or nozzles—applying a nasal clamp to prevent any gas dispersion.

In patients with orotracheal intubation or with tracheotomy, the analytic circuit should simply be inserted between airway and ventilator (the latter can be set on just any ventilation mode). With these subjects, furthermore, there is far less chance of gas leaks leading to any misrepresentation of the results of the analysis.

Accuracy of execution is fundamental. Aspects that could distort the determination are:

- Concomitant use of anaesthetic gases
- Gas leaks along the circuit
- Absence of appropriate calibration and validation of the equipment
- The failed achievement of a patient's steady state characterised by continuous changes in FiO_2 administration, in alimentary regimen and in drug prescription
- Fractions of inspired oxygen above 60%

Oversights in these fields can lead to imprecise metabolic measurements and data that are clinically absolutely useless.

As mentioned above, the determination of energy expenditure is possible through *the analysis of oxygen consumption (VO_2) and carbon dioxide production (VCO_2)*. It is obvious how any factor that continuously alters the dynamic of O_2 consumption and/or CO_2 production falsifies a quick reading (limited in time to 20–30 min) as an estimation of daily energy expenditure.

It is helpful to make sure the patient has reached a steady state before calorimetry is carried out and, then, to check that the same is maintained during measurement. This is important if we are to achieve reliable and clinically useful data using this method.

To verify the stability of the patient's energy consumption, it is enough to check temporary progress of VO_2 values. This parameter, after energy consumption variations, will settle on its new value in a maximum time of 2–3 min—unlike CO_2 that can take up to 30 min. If during calorimetric measurement the excursion of VO_2 values does not exceed 10%, it would be reasonable to assume that the patient is in stable metabolic conditions. Otherwise, it is worth considering a 24-h respiratory gas analysis.

The use of *sedatives and/or neuromuscular blocking agents* has been seen to lead to a reduction of energy expenditure. That being said, it is easy to understand how, whenever we introduce or remove these drugs, it is necessary to carry out the calorimetric determination once more in order to adjust artificial nutrition to the new metabolic attitude.

If we introduce these drugs and go on with caloric administration based on the indirect calorimetry already done, even if carefully, before the administration of sedatives and/or neuromuscular blocking agents, we will risk overfeeding our patient with deleterious consequences. Conversely, the nutritional provision might even prove wholly inadequate for the patient's needs.

Special consideration has to be given to patients undergoing *haemodialysis or continuous renal replacement therapy (CRRT)*. Haemodialysis removes a large share of carbon dioxide from the venous circulation. This leads, inevitably, to a reduction in the proportion of CO_2 released from the lungs with consequent underestimation of VCO_2 and contemporary overestimation of VO_2. To these, one should add the side effects of the change in the acid-base balance, due to dialytic depuration, that could further influence VCO_2. At this point it is to be recommended that patients undergoing intermittent haemodialysis do not have indirect calorimetry until 24 h after their last dialytic session. This will favour an accurate measurement of energy expenditure.

In patients undergoing CRRT, as well as those undergoing continuous venovenous haemodialysis (CVVHD), the gas removal rate depends on the dialysate flow rate.

The loss of CO_2 will lead to an underestimation of energy expenditure. Furthermore, these techniques often cause a reduction in body temperature with consequent decline in metabolic demands. At the present time, it is not yet entirely clear how CRRT affects the accuracy of indirect calorimetry. In the light of this, it is advisable to carry out a "temporary" indirect calorimetry to be repeated 24 h after the end of the dialysis cycle.

Since the 1990s, the biomedical industry has offered a contribution to spread clinical use of indirect calorimetry. The technological prerequisite is the availability of sensors for oxygen and carbon dioxide integrated in ventilators: it is therefore easier to measure the expiratory fraction of O_2 that in addition to the already known inspiratory fraction of CO_2 (equal to zero), expiratory fraction of CO_2 (measured by capnography) and inspiratory fraction of O_2 (imposed by the physician) provides a complete picture of the input and output of these two gases and therefore production and consumption of the same (VO_2 e VCO_2).

Many *respirators* from various companies offer the option to perform calorimetry: of particular interest is the opportunity to measure the change in energy expenditure during weaning from mechanical ventilation. Weaning that requires excessive energy consumption likely represents an attempt that it is better not to pursue.

12.11 Metabolic Calculations

Indirect calorimetry, performed at rest, quantifies the basal metabolic rate (REE) which, as we shall see, constitutes the bulk of daily energy expenditure. Energy expenditure is estimated from oxygen consumption (VO_2), production of carbon dioxide (VCO_2) and urinary excretion of nitrogen (uN_2). VO_2 and VCO_2 can be transformed into energy expenditure, corrected for protein metabolism (through uN_2), by applying the *Weir equation*:

$$M = 3.941VO_2 + 1.106VCO_2 - 2.17uN_2$$

where M represents the metabolic energy expenditure expressed in kcal/min. Weir himself pointed out how, by neglecting the protein metabolism, you make an error of 1% each 12.3% of the proportion of calories provided by the same. If we accept an approximation of this order of magnitude, we can simplify *the Weir equation*:

$$M = 3.941VO_2 + 1.106VCO_2$$

Multiplying M to 1440 min/day, you get the REE expressed in kcal/day. These calculations are performed automatically by open-circuit indirect calorimeters that are used in clinical practice, accurately and in real time during the examination.

The *respiratory quotient*, which is the relationship between the CO_2 produced and the O_2 consumed, is a useful parameter to assess the metabolic mixture used during the investigation. The complete metabolisation of fats, proteins and carbohydrates leads to the production of different amounts of CO for the same values of O_2 consumed (the RQ of carbohydrates is equal to 1, for the lipids the value is 0.7, while for proteins is 0.8). In a fasting subject under physiological conditions, the expected RQ is around 0.82 (assuming as a physiological limit the range 0.707–1.000). Values below the lower physiological limit are associated with gluconeogenesis and ketogenesis, while values above the upper limit are associated with lipogenesis. Among the most frequent causes of *increase of RQ*, let us remember hyperventilation, metabolic acidosis, overnutrition, exercise and hyperthermia. Frequent factors that, conversely, *negatively affect the RQ* are hypoventilation, food deprivation, diabetic ketoacidosis, ethanol metabolism and hypothermia.

The RQ has been used, in the past, to guide the choice of the mixture of macronutrients to be administered as a nutritional support. It has been noted that such use of the RQ is inadequate. In fact, an increase in respiratory quotient may reflect an intolerance to excessive calorie intake which can lead to respiratory distress; that fact is especially common in debilitated patients, subjected to great stress, in hypermetabolic state or suffering from chronic obstructive pulmonary disease with reduced CO_2 elimination capacity.

12.12 How to Use Data Obtained [10, 15, 22]?

The total daily energy expenditure (TDEE) is given by three components: the basal metabolic rate (or *resting energy expenditure REE*) which accounts for 60–80%, the *diet-induced thermogenesis* (*SDA, specific dynamic action* of nutrients) which constitutes about 10% and the *energy consumption due to physical exercise (PAEE, physical activity energy expenditure)* that identifies the remaining 10–30% (Fig. 12.4). This is what happens in the healthy and autonomously mobile subject.

Calorimetry, performed in rest conditions, identifies, therefore, the *MREE* (*measured REE*). At this point it is worth thinking about the use of the data obtained. In particular, one might wonder if the value obtained from the calorimetric measurement needs an additional quota of calories to cover also the PAEE and SDA. With in-patients who are bedridden and immobilised, you can safely assume that the MREE is comparable to TDEE. Recovering from the sickness process, the resumption of mobilisation, deambulation and, then, routine daily activities affect the total daily energy expenditure. It is only at this point that, to define the TDEE, one must also add the PAEE to the MREE. In the past it was common practice to implement caloric administration in patients admitted to the ICU of a further 10% compared with MREE. This actually cannot help but lead to *overfeeding* of patients. It is now established that, if the determination is performed in the patient's steady state (or, alternatively, for 24-h investigation), the MREE closely approximates the total daily

Fig. 12.4 Components of the total daily energy expenditure. The total daily energy expenditure is made up of the resting energy expenditure (REE), which accounts for approximately 70%, plus the share due to the specific dynamic action of nutrients (SDA) and physical activity energy expenditure (PAEE). In young individuals, the REE may be increased by active anabolic processes. The graph was taken and adapted from [15]

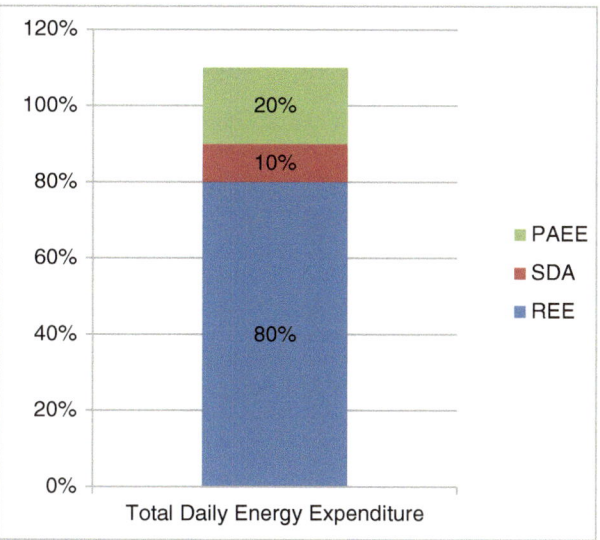

energy expenditure (even in conditions of hypermetabolism—the hypermetabolic processes are not interrupted while measuring takes place and thus contribute to the energy expenditure), and this should be the only reference value in determining the artificial nutrition dose to be administered.

References

1. Harris AJ, Benedict FG. A biometric study of basal metabolism in man. Carnegie Inst. 1919;279(3):48–9.
2. Weir JB. New methods for calculating rate with special reference to protein metabolism. J Physiolol. 1949;109:1–9.
3. Barton R, Cerra FB. The hypermetabolism. Multiple organ failure syndrome. Chest. 1989;96(5):1153–60.
4. Monk DN, Plank LD, Franch-Arcas G, Finn PJ, Streat SJ, Hill GL. Sequential changes in the metabolic response in critically injured patients during the first 25 days after blunt trauma. Ann Surg. 1996;223(4):395–405.
5. Chioléro R, Revelly JP, Tappy L. Energy metabolism in sepsis and injury. Nutrition. 1997;13(9 Suppl):45S–51S.
6. Takala J. Regional contribution to hypermetabolism following trauma. Bailliere Clin Endocrinol Metab. 1997;11(4):617–27.
7. Desborough JP. The stress response to trauma and surgery. Br J Anaesth. 2000;85(1):109–17.
8. Ruzicka J, Novak I, Rokyta R, et al. Effects of ultrafiltration. Dialysis, and temperature on gas exchange during hemodiafiltration: a laboratory experiment. ArtifOrgans. 2001;25:961–6.
9. Demling, RH, De Santi L Posted. Effect of a catabolic state with involuntary weight loss on acute and chronic respiratory disease 2002.www.medscape.org.
10. Griffiths RD. Specialized nutrition support in critically ill patients. Curr Opin Crit Care. 2003;9(4):249–59.
11. Clemmesen O, Ott P, Larsen FS. Splanchnic metabolism in acute liver failure and sepsis. Curr Opin Crit Care. 2004;10(2):152–5.

12. Holdy KE. Monitoring energy metabolism with indirect calorimetry; instruments, interpretation and clinical application. Nutr Clin Pract. 2004;19:447–54.
13. Ljungqvist O, Nygren J, Soop M, Thorell A. Metabolic perioperative management: novel concepts. Curr Opin Crit Care. 2005;11(4):295–9.
14. Vanhorebeek I, Langouche L, Van den Berghe G. Glycemic and nonglycemic effects of insulin: how do they contribute to a better outcome of critical illness? Curr Opin Crit Care. 2005;11(4):304–11.
15. Da Rocha EE, Alves VG, da Fonseca RB. Indirect calorimetry: methodology, instruments and clinical application. Curr Opin Clin Nutr Metab Care. 2006;9(3):247–56.
16. Haugen HA, Chan LN, Li F. Indirect calorimetry: a practical guide for clinicians. Nutr Clin Pract. 2007;22(4):377–88.
17. Ward NS, Casserly B, Ayala A. The compensatory anti-inflammatory response syndrome (CARS) in critically ill patients. Clin Chest Med. 2008;29(4):617. -viii
18. Sobotka L, et al. Basics in clinical nutrition: metabolic response to injury and sepsis. Eur e-J Clin Nutrition Metabol. 2009;4(1):e1–3.
19. Lev S, Cohen J, Singer P. Indirect calorimetry measurements in the ventilated critically ill patient: facts and controversies—the heat is on. Crit Care Clin. 2010;26(4):e1–9.
20. Finnerty CC, et al. The surgically induced stress response. J Parenter Enter Nutr. 2013;37(5): 21S–9S.
21. Dev R, Hui D, Chisholm G, Delgado-Guay M, Dalal S, Del Fabbro E, Bruera E. Hypermetabolism and symptom burden in advanced cancer patients evaluated in a cachexia clinic. J Cachexia Sarcopenia Muscle. 2015;6(1):95–8.
22. Preiser J-C, van Zanten AR, Berger MM, et al. Metabolic and nutritional support of critically ill patients: consensus and controversies. Crit Care. 2015;19(1):35.
23. Wu C, Wang X, Yu W, Tian F, Liu S, Li P, Li J, Li N. Hypermetabolism in the initial phase of intensive care is related to a poor outcome in severe sepsis patients. Ann Nutr Metab. 2015;66(4):188–95.
24. Segadilha NL, Rocha EE, Tanaka LM, Gomes KL, Espinoza RE, Peres WA. Energy expenditure in critically ill elderly patients: indirect calorimetry vs predictive equations. J Parenter Enter Nutr. 2016;41(5):776–84.
25. Rousing ML, Hahn-Pedersen MH, Andreassen S, Pielmeier U, Preiser JC. Energy expenditure in critically ill patients estimated by population-based equations, indirect calorimetry and CO_2-based indirect calorimetry. Ann Intensive Care. 2016;6(1):16.
26. Singer P, Singer J. Clinical guide for the use of metabolic carts: indirect calorimetry—no longer the orphan of energy estimation. Nutr Clin Pract. 2016;31(1):30–8.